LIFE STYLE AND HEALTH
RESEARCH PROGRESS

Life Style and Health Research Progress

Anna B. Turley
and Gertrude C. Hofmann
Editors

Nova Biomedical Books
New York

For permission to use material from this book please contact us:
Telephone 631-231-7269; Fax 631-231-8175
Web Site: http://www.novapublishers.com

NOTICE TO THE READER

The Publisher has taken reasonable care in the preparation of this book, but makes no expressed or implied warranty of any kind and assumes no responsibility for any errors or omissions. No liability is assumed for incidental or consequential damages in connection with or arising out of information contained in this book. The Publisher shall not be liable for any special, consequential, or exemplary damages resulting, in whole or in part, from the readers' use of, or reliance upon, this material.

Independent verification should be sought for any data, advice or recommendations contained in this book. In addition, no responsibility is assumed by the publisher for any injury and/or damage to persons or property arising from any methods, products, instructions, ideas or otherwise contained in this publication.

This publication is designed to provide accurate and authoritative information with regard to the subject matter covered herein. It is sold with the clear understanding that the Publisher is not engaged in rendering legal or any other professional services. If legal or any other expert assistance is required, the services of a competent person should be sought. FROM A DECLARATION OF PARTICIPANTS JOINTLY ADOPTED BY A COMMITTEE OF THE AMERICAN BAR ASSOCIATION AND A COMMITTEE OF PUBLISHERS.

LIBRARY OF CONGRESS CATALOGING-IN-PUBLICATION DATA

Life style and health research progress/[edited by]Anna B. Turley and Gertrude C. Hofmann.
        p.;cm.
Includes bibliographical references and index.
ISBN 978-1-60456-427-3(hardcover)
1. Health behavior.2.Lifestyles—Health aspects.3.Health—Psychological aspects.4.Medicine and psychology.I.Turley,AnnaB.II.Hofmann,Gertrude C.
[DNLM: 1.health Behavior.2.Life Style.3.Health Promotion.4.Risk Reduction Behavior.
W85L72245 2008]
RA776.9.L553 2008
613—dc22   2008005354

Published by Nova Science Publishers, Inc. ✣ *New York*

Contents

Preface

Good health apparently derives from at least these different developments: genetic programming, environmental factors, and lifestyle. This new book is devoted to new and important research on the effects of lifestyle on health. Lifestyle includes a wide range of activities that can be detrimental to a normal lifespan or health status of the organism. These include smoking, diet, addictions, exercise or the lack thereof, stress, socio-economic status, and personal hygiene.

Expert Commentary A - With the rising prevalence of preventable disease caused by our modern lifestyles, population approaches to health promotion are becoming an essential part of healthcare. Nursing is the largest occupational group within the National Health Service and nurses play a significant role in promoting health for chronic disease prevention and management. Nurses spend a significant proportion of their time engaging patients in health promotion activities such as healthy eating and increased physical activity and encouraging others to make healthy lifestyle choices and sustained behaviour changes. But do they practice what they preach? Demands on our limited healthcare resources are increasing and this profession is physically and mentally challenging, leaving individuals susceptible to stress, burnout and poor morale, resulting in chronic disease, reduced efficiency or poor performance and absenteeism. Ironically, the consequence is a significant economic burden which puts more pressure on the healthcare services. Maintaining the health of the nursing workforce is becoming as important as healthcare activities for patients, and the NHS as a 'socially responsible' employer should take actions in a supportive direction. There is a need for a nationwide drive to initiate change through workplace wellness programmes targeted at healthcare staff.

Expert Commentary B - Health psychology – a branch of psychology with a brief three decades of history – appeared in Hungary in the late 1990s and has become an organic part of local psychology studies in recent years.

Health psychology courses are now organic parts of both the BA and the MA programs, and specialised psychologist training courses. Health psychologist training was launched in 2007 in Hungary.

Health psychology courses were introduced at several universities in the country and there are many research groups who undertake studies in health psychology. In order to improve communication and collaboration among the research groups and the training

Anna B. Turley and Gertrude C. Hofmann

institutions, and to promote health psychological awareness in a broader context, a conference titled Egészségpszichológia Magyarországon: Oktatás, kutatás, együttműködés [Health Psychology in Hungary: Education, Research, Collaboration] was organised in Budapest on 23 April, 2004, and was followed by other similar events.

The College of Nyíregyháza's Department of Psychology, within the Faculty of Education, formed its Health Psychology Group in 2005. The College of Nyíregyháza (www.nyf.hu) operates in the Eastern region of Hungary, in Nyíregyáza, a county seat of 120,000 inhabitants. Presently there are five faculties at the college (Arts, Economics and Social Studies, Science, Engineering and Agriculture, Education) which run 24 BA and BSc courses. There are more than 12,000 students pursuing studies at the college.

The major research areas of the Health Psychology Group are the following:

- The background factors of coping with depressive experiences (2005-2006)
- The connections between individual aspirations and religiousness/spirituality, and subjective well-being and emotional intelligence (2007-2008)

It is hoped that the results of this research can contribute to the effectiveness of prevention programmes which deal with the mental health of young people, and, furthermore, provide information for the work of those professionals who specialise in young adults.

Short Communication - Evidence is accumulating to support the importance of association between sleep disorders and depression. The authors reviewed the literature on this subject by conducting a PubMed search entering the keywords "insomnia" and "sleep apnea" crossed by the search term "depression". They restricted articles for inclusion to those published in English in the past ten years featuring human subjects and which were obtained from core clinical journals (n = 24). Briefly stated, while one of the hallmark signs of depression is alteration of sleep, recent research suggests that sleep interruption may foster depressive symptomatology. Moreover, sleep disorders may frequently co-occur, thus complicating the association between depression and impaired sleep and the impact of comorbid chronic disease – often disrupting sleep – must also be considered. Adverse childhood experiences may also yield sleep impairment, thereby attesting to the importance of environmental factors to sleep even decades after their occurrence. These results suggest that assessment of depressive status is a vital aspect of the care of persons with sleep disturbance and that monitoring sleep sufficiency is an important consideration in the management of depression.

Chapter I - To understand what causes peer victimization, some researchers have suggested that certain qualities of victimized children and adolescents (e.g., shyness) may invite or reinforce aggression from bullies. However, a factor that has received relatively little empirical attention is a physical factor that influences the physical appearance of a victimized child or adolescent (i.e., obesity). The present research was designed to address this and examine the relationship between peer victimization, physical activity, and social-psychological adjustment in obese youth. Parents completed a measure of child internalizing and externalizing behavior. Children completed measures of peer victimization, depressive symptoms, general anxiety, loneliness, and physical activity. Findings indicated positive relationships between peer victimization and a range of social-psychological adjustment variables, but no significant relationship with physical activity. Such data may prove valuable for physicians and mental health clinicians working with victimized obese youth.

Over the past decade, research has improved the understanding of the dynamics, nature, and consequences of peer victimization in childhood and adolescence for both victims and perpetrators. From this research, the definition of peer victimization has expanded to include other aspects besides physical assaults. Traditional definitions of peer victimization primarily focused on physical acts of aggression (e.g., kicking, punching, slapping). Research studies have shown that a definition that includes both overt and relational assaults (i.e., spreading rumors, damaging relationships, verbal abuse) more fully captures peer victimization.

Chapter II - Of all developed, wealthy nations, the U.S. has the highest rate of sexually transmitted infections (STI). More than 65 million people in this country are living with an incurable STI, and more than half of Americans will have an STI at one point in their lifetime. Each year, 19 million STI diagnoses are made. Of these, roughly 40,000 are new cases of HIV infection, contributing to the estimated 1 to 1.2 million people living with HIV/AIDS (PLWHA) in the U.S. today. In terms of the vulnerability of the U.S. to increases in HIV infection rates, the high rate of STI in this country is prima facie evidence that levels of condom use and levels of avoidance of unsafe sexual situations are disturbingly low.

The risk of HIV infection, particularly for heterosexuals, has grown since the late 1990s. Yet, the number of Americans who regard HIV as a top health concern for the country has been steadily declining. As recently as the year 2000, HIV was perceived to be the dominant health threat facing the country; today, only around 7% of the population holds this view (Gallup, 2003). This change in perception is attributable to the advent of antiretroviral (ARV) medications, which have been effective in helping PLWHA lead longer, healthier lives. Effective ARV medications were introduced in 1996, and by 1998, HIV plummeted from being the 8th leading cause of death for all Americans to being the 14th.

In part, the phenomenon which Demmer (2003) refers to as "HIV complacency" can be partially attributed to a lack of knowledge among members of the public – specifically, although PLWHA do in fact lead longer, healthier lives as a result of the new medications, these medications are not a cure, they do not work for everyone, they produce severe, sometimes disfiguring side-effects, and the medications themselves can produce life-threatening toxicities. The phenomenon of HIV complacency can only be fully appreciated, however, in the context of the social stratification of the U.S. by race, ethnicity, and socio-economic status. Even though HIV is by no means a leading cause of death in the general population, the most recent available data suggest that HIV remains the 7th leading cause of death among African American men and is the leading cause of death among African American women between the ages of 25 and 34. One goal of this chapter will be to encourage the reader to reflect on the bases and practical implications of the conclusion that HIV/STI-related health disparities are the result of a complex web of contributing factors, many of which may be described as "lifestyle factors."

The phrase "lifestyle factors contributing to HIV transmission" refers to sexual activity involving HIV-infected partners, and the illicit use of intravenous drugs. In this sense, the term "lifestyle" denotes simply "the way a person lives," just as sedentary lifestyle may be said to increase the risk of obesity. HIV prevention researchers refer to individuals as "high risk" when their lifestyles place them at elevated risk of HIV infection. However, it is a mistake to suppose that fixed categories exist, such that some lifestyles are "high risk" and others are "low risk." It has been shown, for example, that many young people will report having had one or two lifetime sex partners and having used condoms on most occasions. This lifestyle is significantly less likely to result in HIV infection for a late adolescent white woman than it is for a late adolescent black woman living in comparable communities. Hence, understanding an individual's sexual lifestyle does not enhance our predictions of health outcomes with quite the same precision that knowledge of an individual's eating habits and level of physical activity enhances our ability to predict obesity risk.

In this chapter, the authors consider the association between lifestyle and HIV transmission from an "ecological" perspective. To this end, their emphasis is on reciprocal person-environment interactions. An ecological perspective asserts that environments exert measurable effects on individual behavior. It also views behavior as a succession of discrete acts manifesting over time and in a variety of *behavior settings*. Here, the term "behavior setting" is understood as the immediate environment, such as a discrete location or social interaction. In the case of a single individual, the same behavior may bring (or may be expected by the actor to bring) desirable consequences in one behavior setting and undesirable consequences in another. Hence, an individual may refuse unsafe sex as a rule, but nonetheless encounter sets of circumstances in which violations of this rule occur. Likewise, two individuals may generally exhibit quite different patterns of behavior, but nonetheless exhibit similar patterns of behavior when they occupy similar behavior settings.

Although behavioral scientists are generally aware of the powerful effect of setting on behavior, this source of variability is conspicuously absent from the most influential and widely-used theories of health behavior change that guide their research and interventions. Instead, definable settings that are associated with increased risk – cruising venues, for example – are viewed as amenable locations for recruiting participants for research and intervention projects, or as suitable locations for distributing condoms or prevention-oriented print materials. The extent to which these settings account for unique variance in the prediction of behavior, how settings affect behavior, and how to address the motivations that bring people into these settings remain understudied questions. This is in large measure the result of the practical difficulties associated with measuring the effects of setting, and transitions between settings, on behavior. To say that research on context-dependent facets of behavior has been neglected implies an over-emphasis on the facets of behavior which may be construed as unvarying. In this chapter, the authors seek to highlight some of the consequences of this over-emphasis on a static conceptualization of behavior. The authors will also highlight novel theoretical and methodological approaches which provide the means of mitigating some of the practical difficulties which have historically stood in the way of context-sensitive observational research. In this discussion of person-environment interactions, they approach the environment as an inherently multilevel construct. Here, a good point of reference is Bronfenbrenner's (1979) model. He described the environment, as it acts upon the person, as a series of concentric circles. At the outermost ring, the *macrosystem* describes broad influences on individual behavior including political decisions at the national level, cultural values, and the media environment. The innermost circle, or the *microsystem,* describes the array of familial, social and physical behavior settings that the individual enters on a day-to-day basis. Between the macrosystem and the microsystem,

Bronfenbrenner identified the *mesosystem* as the level of environmental analysis involving interactions between microsystems as well as the points of contact (e.g., institutions) between the macrosystem and the microsystem.

Chapter III - Background: Assisted reproductive technology (ART) including in vitro fertilization (IVF), intracytoplasmic sperm injection (ICSI), gamete intrafallopian transfer (GIFT), and zygote intrafallopian transfer (ZIFT) are universally available for infertile couples. Currently, 123,200 ART cycles are performed each year in the US, and >99% of these are IVF treatments. It is well documented that live birth success rates decrease significantly with advancing age, from 37% (<35 years), to 29% (35-37 years), to 20% (38-40 years), and finally 11% (41-42 years). Female and male lifestyle habits such as psychological stress could additionally influence IVF success rates, although there is no conclusive experimental evidence that lower stress levels result in better fertility treatment outcomes. Inconsistent and contradictory findings on the effects of psychosocial stress on IVF outcomes could be explained by the lack of distinction made between acute (i.e., procedural) and chronic (i.e., lifetime) emotional stress responses. This discrepancy could also pertain to anxiety, depression, and coping styles. Hence, the purpose of this chapter is to assess the impact of procedural and chronic psychological factors on IVF endpoints.

Methods: An exhaustive computerized search of the published literature was conducted using 8 databases and employing strict eligibility criteria. A total of 372 abstracts were retrieved, and 322 were excluded. Only a smattering of articles (n=50) met the inclusion criteria. Studies that examined the effects of chronic and procedural anxiety, depression, coping styles, marital satisfaction, and stress on IVF outcomes were evaluated. Gender effects were also considered.

Results: Higher levels of anxiety and ineffective coping at the time of the procedure were both associated with decreases in pregnancy, implantation, and fertilization rates in women. In addition, higher procedural stress negatively impacted pregnancy. In contrast, chronic depression and negative mood were associated with lower pregnancy rates. Marital satisfaction and gender related stress differences had no effect on any IVF endpoints. Thus, procedural anxiety, coping, and stress (i.e., hormones) appeared to affect pregnancy success rates, whereas the effects of depression and mood on pregnancy were found at baseline. Consequently, different psychological factors may have diverse effects at various IVF endpoints.

Summary: The field of reproductive endocrinology requires more prospective studies that simultaneously evaluate the relationship among multiple psychological factors, and the time points at which these factors are measured (i.e., baseline vs. procedural), on the array of IVF endpoints (i.e., live births). If the results suggested in this chapter are confirmed in subsequent studies, then reducing stressors at the time of the procedure may diminish the number of treatment cycles and increase pregnancy and live birth delivery success rates after undergoing IVF. Similarly, treatment of existing depression and negative mood prior to beginning the IVF cycle may be beneficial.

Chapter IV - This study assessed the extent and efficacy of three regulatory modalities of the emotions elicited by negative life events: rumination, distraction and social sharing. Despite the wide literature existing on this subject, to the author's knowledge this is the first study comparing these regulatory modalities, from adolescence to old age, in order to estimate their use and their effectiveness in function of the significance of the negative event and of the participants' gender and age.

Eight hundred persons (400 female, 400 male) participated in this study: 200 adolescents (13-19); 200 young people (20-29); 200 adults (30-59); 200 old people (60-89). They were randomly assigned to two research conditions: very significant vs. not very significant negative life events.

Participants were asked to describe a very important negative life event or a not very important one and assess on 7-point scales when the event occurred, its appraisal, perceived importance and impact upon their beliefs, emotional intensity, the extent of rumination, distraction and social sharing, along with their relative frequency and duration, and their effectiveness to re-establish cognitive equilibrium and modulate the negative emotional burden; finally, the recovery from the event was assessed.

Qualitative data were treated through log-linear analyses. Quantitative data were first reduced by performing principal component analyses and then submitted to mediational regression analyses to evaluate the incidence of event significance on the three regulatory modalities through mediator variables (referred to the perceived cognitive and emotional event impact), controlling for gender and age. Finally, multiple regression analysis was performed to assess the effectiveness of rumination, distraction and social sharing in recovering from the event.

In brief, results showed that the significant events produced a higher cognitive and emotional impact than the less significant ones. Such impact, in turn, elicited a greater use of rumination and social sharing, a more consistent sense of pervasiveness of rumination and paradoxical effect of distraction. Instead, a suppression effect emerged on the use and perceived effectiveness of distraction.

The recovery from the event was positively predicted by the temporal distance from the event and the perceived effectiveness of rumination and social sharing, whereas it was negatively predicted by the use and extent of rumination, the cognitive impact of the event and the paradoxical effect of distraction. Females were more affected by the event impact and resorted to rumination and social sharing more than males. With age the use of social sharing and distraction grew. The theoretical implications of these results are discussed.

Chapter V - Measuring the antibody response to medical vaccination is regarded as a useful model for studying the influence of psychological factors on immunity. It allows an assessment of the impact of psychosocial variables on an *in vivo* integrated immune response and within the context of other bodily systems. The response to vaccination is also clinically relevant in that it provides an estimation of protection against infectious disease. Positive psychosocial factors, such as support from close friends and family, are associated with a stronger antibody response. Negative psychosocial factors, on the other hand, have been shown to attenuate the response to vaccination. The chronic stress consequence on caregiving for a spouse with dementia has consistently been related to a poorer antibody response to a range of vaccinations and even more everyday stressful life events have been associated with a poorer antibody response in both young and older adults. In contrast, acute or short-term stress may actually potentiate the antibody response to vaccination. This review will discuss the scientific evidence regarding the impact of both chronic and acute stress and other behavioural and psychosocial variables on the antibody response to vaccination. Implications for interventions to improve immunity and protection against infectious disease will be suggested.

Chapter VI - Women, especially those who enter adulthood with a higher BMI, have a greater risk of age-related weight gain. Weight gain from early adulthood has been associated with an increased risk of heart disease, ischemic stroke, cancer, diabetes, kidney stones, asthma, and even premature death in mid-adulthood. Carrying excess weight poses an additional burden on young women as it increases the risk of infertility, reduces the success of assisted reproductive techniques and increases the risk of complications during pregnancy and delivery. Data from national surveys, population studies and intervention studies suggests a number of reasons for weight gain in young women. The main reason for weight gain is likely to be due to changes in lifestyle that occur in young adulthood, resulting in higher levels of energy intake and lower levels of physical activity. Further investigations reveal that life events such as getting married, having children, or starting work coincides with weight gain and undesirable changes in lifestyles of young women. Social roles acquired at these milestones may affect the priorities and time availability of young women, which in turn influence their ability to maintain a healthy lifestyle. On the other hand, individual psychological characteristics such as the sense of control over one's health mediate the impact of these life events on the lifestyles of young women. The authors have noted the high prevalence of weight loss attempts and costly investments on weight management strategies in this group which indicated their strong desire to lose weight. Current research in weight loss suggest that lifestyle modification involving a combination of energy-restricted diets, exercise and behavioural therapy are effective for short term weight loss and metabolic improvements in young women. However, weight loss interventions consistently report a higher dropout rate among young women, suggesting that current weight loss approaches do not meet the needs of this group. From what the authors have learned about the causes of weight gain in young women, future interventions may need to address the underlying broader issues which shape the lifestyles of young women in order to produce sustainable behavioural change in this group.

Chapter VII - Although diagnostic rates of eating disorders (e.g., anorexia, bulimia) are relatively small in the United States, disordered eating behaviors (including weight control behaviors through excessive exercise and restrictive eating, as well as body dissatisfaction, are much more common (Anorexia Nervosa and Related Eating Disorders, Inc., 2005a, sub clinical eating disorders section). Fifty-one percent of U.S. adults did something to control their weight in 2001-2002. However, it is difficult for many to keep the weight off, in large part because a post-diet binge occurs in nearly half of people who end a diet (successfully or not; Tribole and Resch, 1995). The 'dieting lifestyle' is beginning at younger and younger ages. Half of 3rd to 6th graders want to weigh less and half of 8- to 10-year-olds have done something to try to alter their weight. Although disordered eating behaviors are not considered serious enough to be diagnosed as eating disorders, these behaviors do need attention as they can have damaging mental, social, and physical effects. With over half of children, adolescents, and adults currently engaging in some type of disordered eating or exercise behavior, these cultural trends can no longer be ignored. The purpose of this chapter will be to discuss factors influencing disordered eating and exercise behaviors in children, adolescents, and adults. In addition, possible solutions at the familial and societal levels will be proposed. This chapter should be informative for parents, school officials, and those who are either suffering from disordered eating behaviors or know someone who is.

Chapter VIII - Body image is the picture of one's own body in the mind. Body image contains the body mass estimation and the emotional attitude towards body. For the purpose of the research study, four aspects of body image were separated: declarative (the way of thinking about body), sensory (feeling body), imaginable (imaginary body) and perceptive (a picture of body in a mirror). The research study included 150 overweight women who participated in an outpatient complex obesity treatment. The average age of the examined was 42.97 ± 13.55. The average body mass before the treatment was 97.93 ± 16.47 kg, and the average Body Mass Index (BMI) was 37.17 ± 6.42 kg/m^2. Two research methods were used for body mass estimating: Silhouette Test and the Assessment Scale of a Body Mass. The Scale of Satisfaction with One's Own Body was used to assess an emotional attitude towards body. The following aspects of body were analyzed with respect to the level of satisfaction: attractiveness, charm, agility, shapeliness, proportionality and firmness. All research methods were used separately for each aspect of body image at each stage out of four research stages: at the beginning of the treatment, and after weight reduction by 5%, 10% and 15% of initial body mass. The research results confirmed that at following stages of the research study an objective weight of participants was reducing considerably ($F(3.144)=987.038$; $p<0.001$). As far as a subjective assessment of body mass is concerned, the participants estimated their weight as decreasing in relation to the following aspects: declarative (Assessment Scale: $\chi^2=78.775$; $p<0.001$; Silhouette Test: $\chi^2=87.123$; $p<0,001$), sensory (Assessment Scale: $\chi^2=39.963$; $p<0.001$; Silhouette Test: $\chi^2=60.269$; $p<0.01$), and perceptive (Assessment Scale: $\chi^2=67.728$; $p<0.001$; Silhouette Test: $\chi^2=88.182$; $p<0.001$). A subjective estimation of body mass in an imaginable aspect was not changing, and it was defined as an average weight (The Assessment Scale: $\chi^2=2.727$; $p=0.436$; Silhouette Test: $\chi^2=4.211$; $p=0.240$). The adequacy of a subjective body mass estimation was decreasing at following stages of the research study with respect to a declarative aspect (Assessment Scale: $Q=21.578$; $p<0.001$; Silhouette Test: $Q=43.108$; $p<0.001$), a sensory aspect (Silhouette Test: $Q=25.114$; $p<0.001$), and a perceptive one (Assessment Scale: $Q=18.677$; $p<0.01$; Silhouette Test: $Q=51.283$; $p<0.01$). As far as an imaginable aspect is concerned, the adequacy of the assessment was at a constant level (inadequate assessments outnumbered the adequate ones). At next research stages the increase in satisfaction with one's own body was examined, with respect to all the following aspects: declarative ($Q=31.299$; $p<0.001$), sensory ($Q=22.444$; $p<0.001$), imaginable ($Q=8.250$; $p<0.05$), and perceptive ($Q=40.880$; $p<0.001$). The conducted research shows that from the beginning of the treatment to its end, imaginable aspect of body image differed from declarative, sensory and perceptive aspects. Imagined body was younger ($t(149)=13,234$; $p<0.001$), slimmer ($t(149)=17.774$; $p<0.001$), and more attractive in respect to the appearance than the body that was declared ($Z=9.460$; $p<0.001$), felt ($Z=9.345$; $p<0.001$), and seen in a mirror ($Z=9.455$; $p<0.001$).

Chapter IX - The purpose of the chapter is to present results obtained from the contribution of an innovative research approach about the life style of persons with chronic conditions. The Brazilian population has undergone substantial changes in the number of individuals who are exposed to different illnesses. There has been a reduction of transmitted diseases, but, at the same time, an increase in chronic degenerative diseases. Chronic diseases are considered to be a result of a disorderly lifestyle; however, the lifestyle they live is not only the individuals' fault. Yet, individuals can only take on greater responsibility for their lifestyles if they have access to education and economic support to make healthy decisions. It is up to health professionals to take on part of the responsibility, since those diseases require continued assistance to support people not only with the medicinal, and clinical treatment, but mainly in preparing them to manage their lifestyles. A new qualitative research approach was developed by the authors of this abstract in 1999, and it was named Converging Assistance Research (Pesquisa Convergente Assistencial – PCA). The approach maintains a strict link with daily health practices. This study was conducted by searching 100% of the studies on lifestyle carried out with people with chronic conditions in Southern Brazil and used the PCA as a methodological reference. The results showed that there were changes in two dimensions: 1) direct changes in people's life styles such as a) minimizing feelings of loneliness and seeking occupational and leisure activities; b) increased well-being and improved self-esteem; c) reducing of stress, anxiety and depression; d) access to help support the new reality of the new life relationships; e) replacement of stereotyped movements; f) intensified relationships with peers; g) changing from learning to continuous learning; 2) changes in the approach of health professionals; a) acting modes from the individual to the collective; b) contents originating from themes generated by people in chronic conditions as well as political, social, and technical themes related to the rights assured by the Health Services; c) interpreting news and technological innovations focused on improving the qualification in the lifestyles of people in chronic situations. Conclusion: PCA has been contributing effectively to improving the lifestyles of individuals in chronic conditions and in the way the professional care is given to those individuals.

Chapter X - *Aims:* The authors' research aimed to find out what role the risk mechanisms, as described in Goodman and Gotlib's (1999) model (genetic-biological, interpersonal, social learning related cognitive and stress related factors), play in the development of increased risk for depression in the case of men and women.

Methods: The genetic-biological factors were examined with certain temperament characteristics, the interpersonal factors with parental educational purpose, educational attitudes, educational style and parental treatment. In the case of factors related to social learning the authors looked at the dysfunctional attitudes and the attributional style. As far as the stressors are concerned, they observed the quality of family atmosphere, and the number of the positive and negative life events of the preceding six months and their subjective evaluation. Six hundred and eighty-one students took part in the research (465 female and 216 male).

Results: The research results show that all of the increased risk mechanisms, namely the genetic-biological, interpersonal, social learning related cognitive, and stress related factors are connected with the development of vulnerability to depression, explaining 41.4% of the depression symptoms' variance in the case of women, and 36.5% in the case of men. Harm avoidance, a genetic-biological factor, proved to be the most significant risk mechanism, irrespective of the sexes. From among the environmental factors – irrespective of the sexes – one stress-related factor, the subjective evaluation of negative life experiences, which implies an increased sensitivity to stress, proved to be the strongest risk mechanism. While the above factors played an important role in the development of vulnerability to depression in both sexes, the social learning-related cognitive and interpersonal risk mechanisms differed in their degree in women and men. In the case of women, the social learning-related mechanisms proved to be stronger and higher impact risk factors than in the case of men. The effect of interpersonal factors seemed to be relatively the weakest in the development of increased risk for depression.

Limitations: The results of the authors' research cannot be generalised to represent present-day 18- to 23-year-old Hungarian youth due to the limitations of their sample.

Conclusion: The mental hygienic interpretation of their research findings is that in the future there should be more emphasis put on the personality development of college and university students, especially on the development of such competencies which aid them in effectively coping in their struggle with the depressive mood.

Chapter XI - Adherence to treatment may be considered the coincidence degree observed between the patient's behavior and healthcare professional's therapeutic recommendations. Several cognitive-behavioral mechanisms are likely to interfere with this process. Low-level treatment compliance shows to be related to situations requiring long-term treatments or those of preventive nature, or else, when patients´ lifestyles are affected by alterations. From either the behavioral and economic points of view, long-term perceived rewards show lower reinforcement strength. Objective: The present study was intended to examine predictive factors related either to pharmacological with selective serotonin reuptake inhibitor and cognitive-behavioral treatments in patients with Social Phobia. Method: Evaluation of the following items as possible predictive factors in treatment adherence included personality traits, personality disorders, social abilities and comorbidity depression in 144 patients with patronized scales. Results: Social abilities were not included into the proposed adherence treatments. A correlation between depression, dependent personality trait, and anti-social and borderline personality disorders were observed when based on the proposed adherence treatments findings. Conclusion: Study findings suggest that significant factors in those patients´ treatment adherences, were their personality characteristics and symptoms of depression.

In: Life Style and Health Research Progress
Editors: A. B. Turley, G. C. Hofmann

ISBN: 978-1-60456-427-3
© 2008 Nova Science Publishers, Inc.

Expert Commentary A

Practising What We Preach: Worksite Wellness Intervention for Healthcare Employees

[1]*Holly Blake*[*] *and* [2]*Sandra Lee*

[1]Faculty of Medicine and Health Sciences, University of Nottingham
[2]Nottingham University Hospitals NHS Trust

ABSTRACT

With the rising prevalence of preventable disease caused by our modern lifestyles, population approaches to health promotion are becoming an essential part of healthcare. Nursing is the largest occupational group within the National Health Service and nurses play a significant role in promoting health for chronic disease prevention and management. Nurses spend a significant proportion of their time engaging patients in health promotion activities such as healthy eating and increased physical activity and encouraging others to make healthy lifestyle choices and sustained behaviour changes. But do they practice what they preach? Demands on our limited healthcare resources are increasing and this profession is physically and mentally challenging, leaving individuals susceptible to stress, burnout and poor morale, resulting in chronic disease, reduced efficiency or poor performance and absenteeism. Ironically, the consequence is a significant economic burden which puts more pressure on the healthcare services. Maintaining the health of the nursing workforce is becoming as important as healthcare activities for patients, and the NHS as a 'socially responsible' employer should take actions in a supportive direction. There is a need for a nationwide drive to initiate change through workplace wellness programmes targeted at healthcare staff.

[*] Corresponding Author: Dr. Holly Blake; Faculty of Medicine and Health Sciences; School of Nursing; University of Nottingham; Queen's Medical Centre; Nottingham; NG7 2UH; Tel: +44 115 8231049; Fax: +44 115 8230999; Email: Holly.Blake@nottingham.ac.uk

With the rising prevalence of preventable disease, caused by our modern lifestyles, population approaches to health promotion are becoming an essential part of healthcare. Nursing is the largest occupational group within the National Health Service and as specified by professional bodies (RCN, 2002; DH, 2002), nurses play a significant role in promoting health for chronic disease prevention and management. Nurses spend a significant proportion of their time engaging patients in health promotion activities such as healthy eating and increased physical activity and encouraging others to make healthy lifestyle choices and sustained behaviour changes. But do they practice what they preach? Demands on our limited healthcare resources are increasing and this profession is physically and mentally challenging leaving individuals susceptible to stress, burnout and poor morale, resulting in chronic disease, reduced efficiency or poor performance and absenteeism. Ironically, the consequence is significant economic burden which puts more pressure on the healthcare services. Maintaining the health of the nursing workforce is becoming as important as healthcare activities for patients, and the NHS as a 'socially responsible' employer should take actions in a supportive direction.

Patients are regularly advised by nurses to modify health behaviours. To consume a healthy balanced diet, to reduce their alcohol consumption, to stop smoking, to increase physical activity levels, to reduce or manage stress and so on. However, there is an intuitive argument which suggests that if healthcare staff are not healthy themselves, or have access to resources to engage in healthful behaviours, how can they be reasonably expected to promote health to their patients? Recent surveys conducted with pre and post-registration nurses at a large teaching hospital in the UK showed that the concepts of health promotion with patients do not necessarily translate to their own behaviour as nurses do not always seem to act on their own health recommendations. Health was poor in the nursing students, with a large proportion not meeting current recommendations for physical activity or nutrition, a many smoking or binge drinking and reporting low levels of sleep and low mood. Health promotion education is included within taught courses although knowledge of recommended levels of physical activity was poor in this group and many nursing students were unclear as to what constitutes 'moderate' physical activity. Furthermore, only a small percentage of students reported engaging in incidental activities throughout the working day including active travel, stair-use and walking. There is also a lack of knowledge that daily activity can be broken down into 'chunks' of time rather than being continuous or structured activity. There is still a clear need to increase awareness about health issues such as nutrition, smoking and alcohol consumption and a need to increase awareness about *why* students need to increase their activity levels and *how* they might achieve this, in order to educate our health care providers of the future and encourage them to look after their own health which is high on the government agenda. A significant proportion of their professional counterparts also reported poor health behaviours and low mood which reflects a 'do as I say, not as I do' ethos, and this could have a negative effect on health promotion efforts and impact on patient compliance with health messages.

Current government policy advocates health promotion within a 'settings' approach and workplace wellness programmes have been developed across the UK in diverse environments including schools, hospitals, prisons and corporate groups. Employers who actively promote health and wellbeing amongst their staff present a positive image both to employees and to the wider community, and can impact on attraction, retention and productivity of staff. Through organisational changes and health-related policy, employers can create access to services and facilities which allow their staff to make healthy lifestyle choices, thus protecting their health and welfare. Changes to 'health culture' of organisations means that healthcare staff can be targeted with services that are accessible during the working day, to help them to cope with the pressures of their role and promote healthy, active lifestyles and employee wellbeing. From a cost-effectiveness angle, research has shown that employers who promote physical activity and health in the workplace benefit from substantial reductions in sickness absence.

Nurses are involved in the delivery of targeted actions resulting from the recent government White Paper Choosing Health (DH, 2004). It is essential that nurses benefit themselves from the implementation of this policy in order to protect their own health and as a result, protect the quality of care that is provided to others. This philosophy extends also to pre-registered nurses undergoing training as they are the healthcare providers of our future. Despite our longstanding knowledge of the benefits of workplace intervention coupled with the need to invest in population health, it remains a frustrating fact that action to implement workplace programmes is not universal. Nevertheless, an innovative evidence and theory-based workplace wellness scheme at a NHS Trust was developed according to staff need and serves approximately 11,000 employees, offering activity and wellbeing classes offered at a range of times to accommodate diverse work patterns. The award-winning 'Q-active' programme includes physical activity sessions (e.g. nordic walking, pilates, yoga, dancing), a range of holistic therapies, educational sessions (e.g. nutrition advice, weight management, stress management), free health screening and opportunities for staff to become a 'health champion'. Loyalty schemes and health promotion campaigns, together with health-promoting environmental initiatives (e.g. motivating signage to encourage stair use and increased facilities to encourage active travel) have ensured that many aspects of the programme will be self-sustaining in the long-term. The service has been rolled out to over 5,000 nursing, medical and allied healthcare students in a bid to change the health culture of both present and future professionals. eHealth is emerging as a promising vehicle to promote health behaviour change and so integral to the student service will be the use of interactive web-based health technologies in educating the next generation of health professionals about the benefits of physical activity and workplace health. Electronic communication media are becoming increasingly popular for health promotion and such methods have shown to be inexpensive and often effective in initiating behaviour change in key public health areas including physical activity. Web-based learning packages will be developed as part of this workplace health programme for healthcare staff and students.

Previous reviews of workplace health schemes have commented on the lack of UK evidence and an economic argument for workplace wellness programmes. However, the need to tackle health in this population is incontrovertible. From experience we know these schemes are feasible, well-received and well-utilised in an NHS setting. Further, the government support for health promotion and corporate responsibility in this arena is without question. The main obstacle is therefore accessibility of funds for implementation and scientific evaluation and whilst the research evidence in this area is on the increase, there is still a need for a nationwide drive to initiate change in practice.

REFERENCES

Department of Health (2002) *Liberating the Talents: Helping Primary Care Trusts and Nurses to Deliver the NHS Plan.* Department of Health, London.

Department of Health 'Choosing Health' White Paper, 2004.

RCN (2002) *The Community Approach to Improving Public Health: Community Nurses and Community Development.* Royal College of Nursing, London.

In: Life Style and Health Research Progress
Editors: A. B. Turley, G. C. Hofmann

ISBN: 978-1-60456-427-3
© 2008 Nova Science Publishers, Inc.

Expert Commentary B

Health Psychological Research at the College of Nyíregyháza, Hungary

Ferenc Margitics and Zsuzsa Pauwlik
Department of Psychology at College of Nyíregyháza, Hungary

Health psychology – a branch of psychology with a brief three decades of history – appeared in Hungary in the late 1990s and has become an organic part of local psychology studies in recent years.

Health psychology courses are now organic parts of both the BA and the MA programs, and specialised psychologist training courses. Health psychologist training was launched in 2007 in Hungary.

Health psychology courses were introduced at several universities in the country and there are many research groups who undertake studies in health psychology. In order to improve communication and collaboration among the research groups and the training institutions, and to promote health psychological awareness in a broader context, a conference titled Egészségpszichológia Magyarországon: Oktatás, kutatás, együttműködés [Health Psychology in Hungary: Education, Research, Collaboration] was organised in Budapest on 23 April, 2004, and was followed by other similar events.

The College of Nyíregyháza's Department of Psychology, within the Faculty of Education, formed its Health Psychology Group in 2005. The College of Nyíregyháza (www.nyf.hu) operates in the Eastern region of Hungary, in Nyíregyáza, a county seat of 120,000 inhabitants. Presently there are five faculties at the college (Arts, Economics and Social Studies, Science, Engineering and Agriculture, Education) which run 24 BA and BSc courses. There are more than 12,000 students pursuing studies at the college.

The major research areas of the Health Psychology Group are the following:

- The background factors of coping with depressive experiences (2005-2006)
- The connections between individual aspirations and religiousness/spirituality, and subjective well-being and emotional intelligence (2007-2008)

It is hoped that the results of this research can contribute to the effectiveness of prevention programmes which deal with the mental health of young people, and, furthermore, provide information for the work of those professionals who specialise in young adults.

The Health Psychology group launched a research project in 2005 which focused on the study of the subclinical depression syndrome. The subclinical depression syndrome refers to an emotionally negative state which significantly influences level of achievement and quality of life, but which cannot be yet classified as an illness. Based on the seriousness of the symptoms, it could be measured on different scales of depression as mild or moderate.

One of the aims of the research was to find out what characterises the state of mind of college students, whether the hopelessness, despondency and subclinical depressive mood, nationally found among Hungarian citizens, are also typical of them.

The other aim of the research was to examine and discover in their complexity those factors which have a role in the development of subclinical syndrome.

The results of the study show that more than half of college students suffered from feelings of remorse, tiredness, and dissatisfaction. Besides these, inability to work, hopelessness, and indecision were typical of every second subject.

In our research we tried to approach the factors responsible for the development of the subclinical syndrome in their complexity, taking into account the biological, psychic, and social relations, as well.

The results show that certain factors which are also found to be predispositional in the development of depression may have an important role in the development of subclinical syndrome. It was found that one of the most important of these was the hereditary nature of depression, while the other was the feeling of loss (death of parents, divorce, long separation) in the early years of personality development. The findings also show that – besides pre-dispositional factors – one of the most important background factors in the development of subclinical syndrome is the lack of effective coping strategies. Those people who can be characterised by subclinical syndrome have not learned to effectively face problems, or cope in stressful situations in the course of their socialization process. They are unable to perform constructive problem solving, cognitive restructuring. They develop faulty coping strategies, and are liable to unprincipled conformity, or emotionally driven coping, primarily for emotional acts or introvertedness. They are afraid of danger and risk, and are careful, inhibited, and worried, while their character is undeveloped.

Another important background factor of college students' subclinical depression syndrome was the development of certain dysfunctional attitudes and a passive attributional style. Out of the dysfunctional attitudes, they were mostly characterised by external control. Drifting, a lack of control, and a passive inability state may undermine their self-evaluation, making them dissatisfied, hopeless, and indecisive, which have the direct consequence of the development of the pessimistic attributional style. Besides the lower need for achievement, their remorse may stem from their perfectionism because they believe they are unable to meet the expectations of their context.

When family socialising effects were examined, it was discovered that certain endangering family socialising factors may predispose the development of subclinical depression syndrome. It was found that the most endangering family socialising factor, as far as the development of the subclinical depression syndrome is concerned, was the family conflict, which was accompanied by the indifference of parents toward their children, and the lack of parental care, love, and support. A child who grows up in a bad family environment may react to these – as one of the responses – by producing subclinical depression symptoms. Furthermore, maternal overprotection, which makes the individual dependent and passive, can also lead to the development of subclinical depression syndrome, just like the inconsistent parental attitude, the heterogeneity of the parental effects of the mother and the father.

These family socialising effects do not appear in isolation in the life of the individual; rather, they are embedded in the overall effects of society. In the development of subclinical depression syndrome one should pay attention to the social components: the individualistic value system of the modern consumer, civic society; self-actualization becoming a value category; prosperity and fame replacing the values of personal contacts, identity problems, alienation and anomy, the increased social stress, psychic problems caused by a widening socio-economic cleavage, disintegrating communities, and the ineffectiveness of community and contact networks to protect the individual.

Our research, starting in 2007, investigates the connections between subjective values, individual and spirituality), and subjective well-being and emotional intelligence (the data is being analysed at present).

The results of the research indicate that in the future there should be more emphasis put on the personality development of college and university students, with special attention on raising their self-awareness levels, and the development of adequate coping strategies. The mental hygienic interpretation of our research findings indicate that professionals during the support and therapy work with families should make their clients aware of the discovered risk factors, and reinforce protective factors in order to prevent the development of a more serious form of depression which requires clinical treatment.

The findings of our research – due to the limitations of the sample – cannot be generalised to and called valid for the present day Hungarian 18-23 year old youth. However, the results may also be useful in the wider area of prevention, promotion of adequate parental childcare views and the development of prevention forms which promote the healthy development of families.

In: Life Style and Health Research Progress
Editors: A. B. Turley, G. C. Hofmann

ISBN: 978-1-60456-427-3
© 2008 Nova Science Publishers, Inc.

Short Communication

The Relationship between Depression and Sleep Apnea and Insomnia: A Brief Review

Daniel P. Chapman, Lela McKnight-Eily,
Geraldine S. Perry and Robert F. Anda
Centers for Disease Control and Prevention
National Center for Chronic Disease Prevention and Health Promotion
Divisions of Adult and Community Health

ABSTRACT

Evidence is accumulating to support the importance of the association between sleep disorders and depression. We reviewed the literature on this subject by conducting a PubMed search entering the keywords "insomnia" and "sleep apnea" crossed by the search term "depression". We restricted articles for inclusion to those published in English in the past ten years featuring human subjects and which were obtained from core clinical journals (n = 24). Briefly stated, while one of the hallmark signs of depression is alteration of sleep, recent research suggests that sleep interruption may foster depressive symptomatology. Moreover, sleep disorders may frequently co-occur, thus complicating the association between depression and impaired sleep and the impact of comorbid chronic disease – often disrupting sleep – must also be considered. Adverse childhood experiences may also yield sleep impairment, thereby attesting to the importance of environmental factors to sleep even decades after their occurrence. These results suggest that assessment of depressive status is a vital aspect of the care of persons with sleep disturbance and that monitoring sleep sufficiency is an important consideration in the management of depression.

Keywords: Depression, Sleep apnea, Insomnia.

While depression, insomnia, and sleep apnea represent distinct entities in diagnostic nomenclature, they also may be characterized by an interrelated presentation. In this Brief Review, we examine the literature addressing these areas, as well as research suggesting common underlying pathways in the presentation of these disorders. We also identify areas where further research is needed in order to better understand the complex relationships between depression and both insomnia and sleep apnea.

METHODS

Articles were identified for review by PubMed, using the search terms "sleep apnea," or "insomnia," "depression," and "epidemiology". Studies included in this review were restricted to publications written in English and featuring human subjects. To assure the timeliness and relevance of selected articles, this review was restricted to studies published in the previous ten years and in core clinical journals. Use of this search strategy resulted in 9 articles pertaining specifically to sleep apnea and 17 relevant to insomnia. Removal of two duplicates and four articles which did not provide adequate definitional criteria or a specified time course yielded an N=20 articles for review. Other articles were added by expert input.

RESULTS

Sleep Apnea

In a study pertaining to the growing obesity epidemic, Bell et al. [1] studied normal weight (n=73) and overweight (n=53) children between the ages of 6 and 13 years. These investigators reported that each increase of 1.0 in BMI z-score was associated with odds ratios of 1.89 (95% CI=1.54, 2.83) and 3.38 (95% CI=1.13-10.11) for subjects reporting obstructive sleep apnea (OSA) and depressive symptoms, respectively. Thus, in this study, increased BMI emerged as a common risk factor for both sleep apnea and depression, corroborating previous research suggesting the urgency of overweight and obesity as marked health risk factors [2].

In addition to sharing common risk factors, specific sleep disorders may also be significantly associated with other sleep disorders. Examining data from the 2005 National Sleep Foundation *Sleep in America* poll, a random sample of U.S. households (N=1,506, with a mean age of 49 years), Phillips et al. [3] found that persons reporting symptoms consistent with restless legs syndrome (RLS) appeared to be at increased risk for sleep apnea and insomnia. Moreover, respondents with depression were more likely to report suffering from RLS. Thus, these investigators sagely conclude that adequate assessment of medical and psychiatric issues is vital to identifying the underlying precipitants of the presenting sleep disorder.

Excessive daytime sleepiness (EDS) is considered a cardinal sign of sleep apnea, as individuals with sleep apnea characteristically experience nonrestorative sleep [4]. Bixler et al. [4] examined the association between complaints of EDS and sleep apnea, as well as BMI, diabetes, and depression in a random sample of 16,583 community-dwellers from central Pennsylvania (n=16,583). A random sample of these subjects (n=1,741) were further evaluated in a sleep laboratory for one night. Notably, logistic regression indicated that EDS was significantly more strongly associated with depression and metabolic characteristics than with sleep-disordered breathing (SDB), a hallmark sign of sleep apnea, or sleep disruption. The results of this study suggest that patients presenting with a complaint of EDS be carefully evaluated for depression, obesity, and diabetes, regardless of whether SDB is evident [4]. This recommendation stands in stark contrast to the results of elicitation of sleep-related complaints among patients, who were much more likely to attribute impaired quality of life to somatic factors than to emotional ones [5].

Notably, specific psychosocial factors appear to be associated with an increased prevalence of SDB which may be symptomatic of sleep apnea. Specifically, out of 187 women who survived sexual assault with sustained posttraumatic symptoms, 168 were judged to be confirmed or suspected SDB cases. Compared to the 19 remaining women who had been sexually assaulted but whom did not show signs of SDB, those manifesting SDB reported significantly worse nightmares, sleep quality, depression, and posttraumic stress symptoms [6].

Moreover, the potential gravity physiological consequences of sleep apnea- hypopnea should not be minimized. Relative to controls, patients with sleep apnea display a higher frequency of cardiac rhythm disturbances, most notably ST-segment changes. Specifically, apnea-related ST-segment alterations are related to sleep fragmentation and impairment in sympathetic tone [7], which suggests sleep abnormalities pose serious threats to optimal cardiac and neuromuscular functioning.

It is thus not surprising that sleep apnea patients used 23-50% more healthcare resources relative to control patients in the 5 years prior to their diagnosis with sleep apnea. Notably, prior to their diagnosis with sleep apnea, examination of odds ratios revealed that sleep apnea patients were at significantly increased risk for being diagnosed with hypertension, OR=2.5 (2.0-3.3), congestive heart failure, OR=3.9 (1.7-8.9), cardiac arrhythmias, OR=2.2 (1.2-4.0), cardiovascular disease, OR=2.6 (2.0-3.3), chronic obstructive airways disease, OR=1.6 (1.2-2.0), and depression, OR=1.4 (1/0-1.9) [8]. Having received a wide array of potentially relevant diagnoses undoubtedly fostered delays in receiving the warranted diagnosis of sleep apnea, which, in turn, likely fostered the suboptimal use of healthcare resources and, potentially, impaired patient care.

INSOMNIA

Notably, insomnia or hypersomnia are among the diagnostic criteria for both major depressive disorder and dysthymic disorder [9]. As a syndrome, insomnia may be fostered by a variety of precipitants. Most notably, antidepressant medications, such as serotonin-specific reuptake inhibitors, commonly disturb sleep [10] and may increase rapid eye movement (REM) sleep latency and reduce the total amount of REM sleep [11]. Generally, however, the sleep-disturbing properties of antidepressants are short-lived, with objective measures of sleep among patients receiving antidepressant medications indicating improvement in sleep after 3-4 weeks of treatment [11].

Complementary and alternative medicine (CAM) appears to be assuming an increasingly popular role in the management of insomnia. Using data from the 2002 National Health Interview Survey, Pearson et al. [12] reported that 17.4% of respondents indicated a 12-month prevalence of insomnia or difficulty sleeping. Notably, insomnia or trouble sleeping was positively associated with obesity, adjusted odds ratio (AOR) = 1.15 (1.01-1.31), hypertension AOR = 1.32 (1.16-1.51), congestive heart failure AOR= 2.24 (1.60-3.14), and anxiety or depression AOR = 5.64 (5.07-6.29). Of those respondents reporting insomnia or difficulty sleeping, 4.5% indicated that they had used some form of CAM to attempt to improve their sleep [12]. These findings suggest it is important for clinicians to assess the use of CAM among patients with insomnia as, potentially, some forms of CAM may adversely interact with pharmacotherapies for insomnia and depression. Inquiry about the use of CAM appears particularly warranted as 50% of 3,445 patients in clinical settings with chronic medical or psychiatric conditions reported to experience insomnia some or all of the time [13].

Notably, adverse childhood experiences (ACEs) – including physical, sexual, and emotional abuse, and emotional and physical neglect – appear to be associated with primary insomnia, decades after their occurrence [14]. In an investigation conducted by Bader et al. [14], thirty-nine adults suffering from primary insomnia completed questionnaires concerning ACEs, present stress levels, predelicition towards heightened arousability, and depression.

By use of wrist actigraphy, participants were monitored for sleep-related activity for seven consecutive nights in their homes. Strikingly, ACEs emerged as significant predictors of actigraphically monitored sleep onset latency, number of body movements and moving time, and sleep efficiency. As the mean age of participants in this study was 43.0 years of age, these results suggest the importance of ACE to sleep – even decades after their onset, and further suggest the relevance of inquiry about ACEs among patients reporting insomnia [14]. These results are of further interest as ACEs or childhood physical or sexual abuse have been found to also be associated with depression [15,16].

The relationships between insomnia and depression in older adults has also emerged as an area of considerable investigation. In a review by Buysse [17], it was noted that age-related changes in sleep make the epidemiologic association between depression and insomnia particularly strong. While epidemiologic research has indicated that depression is one of the most robust predictors of current insomnia, recent evidence has suggested that this relationship is bidirectional. Specifically, current insomnia is a risk factor for the emergence of subsequent depression [17,18]. This finding suggests that clinicians should routinely inquire among their older patients about both sleep difficulties and depression [17].

In an investigation of a consecutive series of 670 patients with probable Alzheimer's disease (AD) assessed with the Structured Clnical Interview for DSM-IV, 52% were judged to manifest clinically significant depression. Notably, among depressed patients with AD, insomnia was significantly associated with sad mood, thus rendering its presentation multi-faceted [19]. As not all depressed individuals manifest sad mood, the presence of the latter may be an important marker of the potential presence of insomnia, which may further complicate clinical presentation and treatment.

Given the prevalence of depression-related insomnia among older adults, it is not surprising that the relationship between depression and insomnia has emerged as clinically relevant among populations with chronic disease. Noting that while depression was an important contributor to sleep problems among persons with arthritis, Power et al. [20] found that the relationship between arthritis and insomnia is largely mediated by pain. Concluding that insomnia and unfreshing sleep are approximately twice as prevalent among persons with arthritis as among those without this condition, Power et al., conclude that improved pain management could appreciably improve sleep in persons with arthritis [20]. Likewise, pain management – as well as the evaluation and treatment of psychological symptoms (depression, anxiety, and/or depression) – have emerged as important aspects of the care of lung cancer patients nearing the terminal stage of their disease [21].

In an investigation of 120 outpatients with systemic lupus erythematosus (SLE), the results of questionnaires administered to these individuals revealed that abnomal fatigue was reported by 81% of patients and 60% reported poor sleep quality. Notably, fatigue was significantly correlated with depression and anxiety and negatively associated with all measures of functioning, leading Tench et al [22] to conclude that treatment of depression and insomnia appear to be important components in the care of SLE patients.

CONCLUSION

The relationship between sleep apnea, insomnia, and depression is complex. While sleep disturbance has commonly been recognized as a sign of depression, recent investigation suggests that depression may be precipitated or exacerbated by sleep impairment. Some antidepressant medications may foster insomnia, although this adverse effect typically diminishes over time. Older adults may, in particular, experience difficulty sleeping with sleep impairment associated with sad mood among persons with AD and depression contributing significantly to sleep disturbance among persons with arthritis. These data suggest the advisability of assessment of sleep among clinicians treating persons with depression, as well as gauging the presence of depression among persons suffering from sleep impairment. Heightened awareness of the importance of sleep as a vital facet of physical and mental health among both clinicians and the public may promote prompt treatment of both sleep impairment and depression and thus appears to be an important aspect of public health research and intervention.

ACKNOWLEDGMENTS

The opinions expressed by the authors do not necessarily reflect the opinions of the U.S. Department of Health and Human Services, the Public Health Service, the Centers for Disease Control and Prevention, or the authors' affiliated institutions. Use of trade names is for identification only and does not imply endorsement by any of the groups named above.

REFERENCES

[1]   Bell LM, Byrne S, Thompson A, Ratnam N, Blair E, Bulsara M, Jones TJ, Davis EA. Increasing body mass index z-score is continuously associated with complications of overweight in children, even in the health weight range. *J. Clin. Endocrinol. Metab.* 2007;92:517-522.

[2]   O'Brien PE, Dixon JB. The extent of the problem of obesity. *Am. J. Surg.* 2002;184:4S-8S.

[3]   Phillips B, Hening W, Britz P, Mannino D. Prevalence and correlates of restless legs syndrome: Results from the 2005 National Sleep Foundation Poll. *Chest.* 2006;129:76-80.

[4]   Bixler EO, Vgontzas AN, Lin HM, Calhoun SL, Vela-Bueno A, Kales A. Excessive daytime sleepiness in a general population sample: The role of sleep apnea, age, obesity, diabetes, and depression. *J. Clin. Endocrinol. Metab.* 2005;90:4510-4515.

[5]   Goncalves MA, Paiva T, Ramos E, Guilleminault C. Obstructive sleep apnea syndrome, sleepiness, and quality of life *Chest.* 2004;125:2091-2096.

[6]   Krakow B, Melendrez D, Johnston L, Warner TD, Clark JO, Pacheco M, Pedersen B, Koss M, Hollifield M, Schrader R. Sleep-disordered breathing, psychiatric distress, and quality of life impairment in sexual assault survivors. *J. Nerv. Ment. Dis.* 2002; 190:442-452.

[7]   Alonso-Fernandez, Garcia-Rio G, Racionero MA, Pino JM, Ortuno F, Marinez I, Villamor J. Cardiac rhythm disturbances and ST-segment depression episodes in patients with obstructive sleep apnea-hypopnea syndrome and its mechanisms. *Chest.* 2005;157:15-22.

[8]   Smith R, Ronald J, Delaive K, Walld R, Manfreda J, Kryger MH. What are obstructive sleep apnea patients being treated for prior to this diagnosis? *Chest* 2002;121:164-172.

[9]   American Psychiatric Association. *Diagnostic and statistical manual of mental disorders: DSM-IV* -- 4th ed. Washington, DC: American Psychiatric Association, 2004.

[10]   Mayers AG, Baldwin DS. Antidepressants and their effect on sleep. *Hum. Psychopharmacol.* 2005;20:533-559.

[11]   Wilson S, Argyropoulos S. Antidepressants and sleep: A qualitative review of the literature. *Drugs.* 2005;65:927-947.

[12]   Pearson NJ, Johnson LL, Nahin RL. Insomnia, trouble sleeping, and complementary and alternative medicine: Analysis of the 2002 National Health Interview Survey data. *Arch. Intern. Med* .2006;166:1775-1782.

[13]   Katz DA, McHorney CA. The relationship between insomnia and health-related quality of life in patients with chronic illness. *J. Fam. Prac.* 2002;51:229-235.

[14]   Bader K, Schafer V, Schenkel M, Nissen L, Kuhl H-C, Schwander J. Increased nocturnal activity associated with adverse childhood experiences in patients with primary insomnia. *J. Nerv. Ment. Dis.* 2007;195:588-595.

[15] Chapman DP, Whitfield CL, Felitti VJ, Dube SR, Edwards VJ, Anda RF. Adverse childhood experiences and the risk of depressive disorders in adulthood. *J. Affect Disord.* 2004;82:217-225.

[16] Levitan RD, Parikh SV, Lesage AD, Hegadoren KM, Adams M, Kennedy SH. Major depression in individuals with a history of childhood physical or sexual abuse: Relationship to neurovegetative features, mania, and gender. *Am. J. Psychiatry.* 1998;155:1746-1752.

[17] Buysse DJ. Insomnia, depression and aging. Assessing sleep and mood intereactions in older adults. *Geriatrics.* 2004;59:47-52.

[18] Roberts RE, Shema SJ, Kaplan GA, Strawbridge WJ. Sleep complaints and depression in an aging cohort: A prospective perspective. *Am. J. Psychiatry.* 2000;157:81-88.

[19] Starkstein SE, Jorge R, Mizrahi R, Robinson RG. The construct of minor and major depression in Alzheimer's Disease. *Am. J. Psychiatry.* 2005;162:2086-2093.

[20] Power JD, Perruccio AV, Badley EM. Pain as a mediator of sleep problems in arthritis and other chronic conditions. *Arthritis Rheum.* 2005;53:911-919.

[21] Skaug K, Eide GE, Gulsvik A. Prevalence and predictors of symptoms in the terminal stage of lung cancer: A community study. *Chest.* 2007;131:389-394.

[22] Tench CM, McCurdie I, White PD, D'Cruz DP. The prevalence and associations of fatigue in systemic lupus erythematosus. *Rheumatology. (Oxford)* 2000;39:1249-1254.

In: Life Style and Health Research Progress
Editors: A. B. Turley, G. C. Hofmann
ISBN: 978-1-60456-427-3
© 2008 Nova Science Publishers, Inc.

Chapter I

A Further Examination of the Relationships among Peer Victimization, Physical Activity, and Social Psychological Adjustment in Obese Youth

Charisse Williams*, Eric A. Storch
and Marilynn Paradora
University of Florida

ABSTRACT

To understand what causes peer victimization, some researchers have suggested that certain qualities of victimized children and adolescents (e.g., shyness) may invite or reinforce aggression from bullies. However, a factor that has received relatively little empirical attention is a physical factor that influences the physical appearance of a victimized child or adolescent (i.e., obesity). The present research was designed to address this and examine the relationship between peer victimization, physical activity, and social-psychological adjustment in obese youth. Parents completed a measure of child internalizing and externalizing behavior. Children completed measures of peer victimization, depressive symptoms, general anxiety, loneliness, and physical activity. Findings indicated positive relationships between peer victimization and a range of social-psychological adjustment variables, but no significant relationship with physical activity. Such data may prove valuable for physicians and mental health clinicians working with victimized obese youth.

Over the past decade, research has improved the understanding of the dynamics, nature, and consequences of peer victimization in childhood and adolescence for both victims and perpetrators. From this research, the definition of peer victimization has expanded to include other aspects besides physical assaults. Traditional definitions of peer victimization primarily focused on physical acts of aggression (e.g., kicking, punching, slapping). Research studies have shown that a definition that includes both overt and relational assaults (i.e., spreading rumors, damaging relationships, verbal abuse) more fully captures peer victimization (Crick and Grotpeter, 1996).

CONSEQUENCES OF PEER VICTIMIZATION

Research has also linked peer victimization to negative social-psychological adjustment in children and adolescents. More specifically, studies have found positive correlations between peer victimization and depression, social and general anxiety, and loneliness in child and adolescent samples (Bond, Carlin, Thomas, Rubin, and Patton, 2001; Crick and Bigbee, 1998; Crick and Grotpeter, 1996; Nansel et al., 2001; Storch, Nock, Masia, and Barlas, 2003; Storch, Zelman, Sweeny, Danner, and Dove, 2002; Storch et al., 2004a, b; Storch et al., 2006a; Storch et al., 2007).

PEER VICTIMIZATION RISK FACTORS

In effort to understand the causes of peer victimization and to determine why certain children are bullied, several researchers have suggested that victimized children may possess certain qualities that invite or reinforce aggression from bullies. For example, victims tend to be socially passive and compliant (Perry, Kussel, and Perry, 1988; Schwartz, Dodge, and Coie, 1993), physically weak (if boys), low in self-esteem (Olweus, 1992), average or poor students, and less popular in school (Pellegrini, 1998). Bullies are often reinforced when victims offer little to no resistance, display signs of distress, and/or do not retaliate (Schwartz et al., 1993). Additionally, socially ostracized children, like those with special needs, are particularly vulnerable to peer victimization. For example, learning-disabled children report higher levels of peer victimization and aggression, and have fewer friends than children who do not have learning disabilities (Martlew and Hodson, 1991; Nabuzoka and Smith, 1993). Little (2001) completed a study that showed children with Asperger's disorder and nonverbal learning disorders reported higher rates of peer victimization than those without Asperger's or nonverbal learning disabilities.

Furthermore, some children with overt physical differences are often targets for peer victimization (Storch et al., 2004a). For example, children with endocrine disorders, specifically gynecomastia, precocious puberty, delayed puberty, and short stature have overt physical differences associated with their disorder, which may cause them to be targets for peer aggressors; additionally, children with chronic medical conditions may display anxiety symptoms and poor social skills which increases their vulnerability to being victimized (Storch et al., 2004a). A study on children with obsessive-compulsive disorder (OCD) showed that not only was peer victimization a common experience (with more than one quarter being regularly victimized), relative to children with diabetes or healthy children (Storch et al., 2006b).

PEER VICTIMIZATION AND OBESITY

Whereas research efforts have improved the understanding of non-physical characteristics of sufferers of peer victimization, little empirical attention has been given to physical characteristics of victims. One physical characteristic that may invite peer victimization is obesity. There are several reasons why peer victimization may be a frequent experience in the life of obese youth. First, obese youth may be labeled as "unattractive" or different, providing bullies with a rationale to victimize. Second, obese youth may be hesitant or unable to participate in school activities or interact with peers due to a fear of rejection or physical limitations, which, subsequently, may lead to a smaller social network of friends. Finally, physical limitations, medical issues, and fewer friends may contribute to the development of social anxiety and low self-esteem. These factors make obese youth prime candidates for peer victimization (Storch et al., 2007).

Besides obesity being a risk factor for peer victimization, it may also impact obese youth's desire to participate in physical activities. For example, obese, victimized youth may avoid physical activity that is not closely monitored (i.e., physical education classes or after-school sports) due to the frequency of peer victimization occurring during these events (Frey et al., 2005). Additionally, peer victimization of obese youth may reduce intrinsic motivation for physical activity due to fear of peer victimization during activities (Faith, Leone, Moonseong, and Pietrobelli, 2002) Whereas there is evidence that weight-based peer victimization may lead to negative attitudes about sports and reduced amounts of physical activity (Faith et al., 2002), overall, there is little research on how peer victimization affects physical activity for obese youth.

Storch et al. (2007) examined the relationships between physical activity, peer victimization, and child, adolescent, and parental reports of psychosocial adjustment in at-risk-for overweight and overweight youth. Participants (child and parent) completed measures on peer victimization, depression, anxiety, social physique anxiety, loneliness and physical activity and both internalizing and externalizing behaviors (Storch et al., 2007). Results showed peer victimization was positively correlated to youth's reported depression, anxiety, social physique anxiety, loneliness and parental reports of internalizing and externalizing symptoms; additionally, peer victimization was negatively related to physical activity and depressive symptoms and loneliness mediated the relationship between peer victimization and physical activity (Storch et al., 2007).

The primary purpose of this study is to examine the relationships among peer victimization, social-psychological adjustment, and physical activity in obese youth. We had the following four goals:

1. To examine the relationship between peer victimization and physical activity.
2. To examine the relationship between peer victimization and social-psychological adjustment indices. We expected to find positive relationships between these variables.
3. To determine if the relationship between peer victimization and physical activity is moderated by age. Younger children (aged 8-12 years) may not be able to avoid physical activity as much as an older adolescent (aged 13-17 years). It is

hypothesized that older adolescents have more experience addressing bullying behaviors and subsequently, have developed more coping strategies than a younger child. Furthermore, an older adolescent may have more autonomy in deciding to participate in physical activity than a younger child. In regards to directionality, it is hypothesized that older age (adolescents between the ages of 13-17 years) will positively moderate the relationship between peer victimization and physical activity.

4. To determine if the relationship between peer victimization and physical activity is mediated by social-psychological adjustment.

METHOD

Participants

Participants in the current study were 64 children and adolescents ages 8-18 years and their parent/guardian. Participants attended a scheduled appointment at the University of Florida Pediatric Lipid Clinic. This clinic is a multidisciplinary clinic that serves children and adolescents with lipid problems. It is staffed by a clinical psychologist, a nutritionist, and a medical doctor. Children and adolescents diagnosed by the attending clinical psychologist with mental retardation, a psychotic disorder, or who were unable to read the questionnaire packets, were excluded from participation. The sample of 64 children and adolescents consisted of 38 females and 24 males (missing data from 2 subjects) with a mean age of 13.4 years (SD = 2.6). Approximately half of the children and adolescents self-identified as Caucasian (45.3%), followed by African-American (39.1%), Hispanic (4.7%), and "other ethnicity" (4.7%).

Procedure

The University of Florida Institutional Review Board has approved this study. After it was determined the child or adolescent met the criteria for the study, the first or third author asked the family if they would like to participate. If the family refused to participate, they still received the standard of care provided by the Pediatric Lipid Clinic. This standard of care includes obesity information, diet and exercise information, medical treatment, and psychological consultation during their scheduled appointment. If the family was interested in participating, the parent or guardian was asked to read and sign a consent form and the child or adolescent was asked to provide written assent. After consent and assent were received, the parent or guardian was asked to complete the demographic form and the Child Behavior Checklist. The child or adolescent was asked to complete the Child Depression Inventory—Short Form, the Multidimensional Anxiety Scale for Children, the Asher Loneliness Scale, the SPARK Physical Activity Measure, and the Schwartz Peer Victimization Scale. Both the parent and child or adolescent received instructions on how to complete the questionnaires, and the principal investigator (PI) or trained research assistant remained available to answer any questions. The parent or guardian was informed their participation would take approximately 20 minutes and the child or adolescent was informed their participation would take approximately 35 minutes. Parents and their children or adolescents were notified that they were still receiving their regular standard of care. After the completion of the questionnaires, participants were thanked for their time.

Measures

Schwartz Peer Victimization and Aggression Scale (Schwartz, Farver, Change, and Lee-Shin, 2002)

This 5-item scale assesses overt and relational forms of peer victimization and aggression among children and adolescents that occurred over the past two weeks. Items are consistent with contemporary definitions of peer victimization which include both overt and relational forms of bullying behaviors (Crick and Gropeter, 1996). For example, one item reads, "How often do other kids make fun of you?" The items are rated on a 4-point scale ranging from ("never") to ("almost every day"). This measure has a good internal consistency (Cronbach's alpha of .75), a stable one-factor structure, and correlated modestly and positively with teacher and peer reports of peer victimization (Schwartz, Farver, Change, and Lee-Shin, 2002). Cronbach's alpha for this study was .89.

Children's Depression Inventory—Short Form (Kovacs, 1992)

This commonly used 10-item version of the CDI assesses depressive symptomlogy over the past two weeks for school-aged children and adolescents (Kovacs and Beck, 1977). There are 10 items that ask a child or adolescent to assess statements that best describe cognitive, affective, or behavioral symptoms of depression. The CDI has a 3-point scale indicating the absence or presence of mild or definite symptoms, with the child or adolescent choosing the one that is the best fit. The literature supports good reliability with various samples, with a Cronbach's alpha ranging from .71 - .89, and test-retest coefficients ranging from .74-.83. Additionally, there has been strong support for the construct validity of the CDI (Craighead, Smucker, Craighead, and Illardi, 1998; Kovacs, 1992). Cronbach's alpha for this study was .83.

The Multidimensional Anxiety Scale for Children (March, Parker, Sullivan, Stallings, and Conners, 1997)

The MASC is a 39-item self-report questionnaire that assesses symptoms of general, social, and separation anxiety in children and adolescents. The items are rated on a 4-point Likert scale ranging from 0 ("never") to 3 ("always"). An example of an item is, "I feel tense or uptight." Higher scores reflect higher levels of anxiety, with the total score being computed by summing all items. The MASC has excellent internal consistency with a Cronbach's alpha of .90 (March et al., 1997). Three week and three month test-retest reliability has been shown to be .88 and .87, respectively (March et al., 1997; March, Sullivan, and Parker, 1999). Cronbach's alpha for this study was .88.

Asher Loneliness Scale (Asher and Wheeler, 1985)

The ALS is a 24-item scale that assesses self-reported loneliness in children and adolescents over the past two weeks (Asher, Hymel, and Renshaw, 1984). The ALS was modified to only include those items that focus on feelings of loneliness, social and subjective adequacy, and subjective estimations of peer status. The items are rated on a 5-point scale ranging from 1 ("not true about me at all") to 5 ("always true about me"). The ALS has good psychometric properties including, good internal consistency (alpha = .91), a stable factor structure, and high convergent validity (Asher and Wheeler, 1995; Bagner, Storch, and Roberti, 2004). Cronbach's alpha for this study was .89.

SPARK Physical Activity Measure (Sallis et al., 1993)

This is a 21-item self-report measure that examines physical activity in youth. The child or adolescent reflects on a list of physical activities and then writes how often they were done in the last week, for at least 15 minutes, between a) Monday-Friday and b) the weekend. A metabolic equivalent score is used to group the list of activities by their levels of intensity (Sallis et al., 1993). Light activities (e.g., walking, four square, gymnastics) were scored 3 METS; medium activities (e.g., dancing, hiking/climbing, basketball) were scored 5 METS; and hard activities (e.g., jumping ropes, jumping jacks, running/jogging) were scored 9 METS (Sallis et al., 1993). Multiplying the frequencies of each activity by the appropriate MET value and summing the products will total the final score.

The SPARK was chosen over existing measures because it provides more comprehensive data on when the physical activity occurred (weekday, weekend) and the type of physical activity completed. Furthermore, it is important to note only activities completed before or after school count; engaging in physical activity outside of school displays more volition by the child or adolescent (Sallis et al., 1993). Cronbach's alpha for this study was. 92.

Child Behavior Checklist (Achenbach, 1991)

The CBCL is a widely used 113-item parent-rated scale that assesses the chores, hobbies, activities, and internalizing and externalizing symptoms of children and adolescents over the past 6 months. The CBCL is rated on a 3-point scale ranging from 0 ("never") to 2 ("often or always"). Eight subscales are derived, including Withdrawal/Depression (Cronback's alpha for this study was .83), Somatic Symptoms (.79), Anxiety/Depression (.87), Social Problems (.72), Attention Problems (.86), Rule Breaking Behavior (.74), Aggression (.89). Cronbach's α for the Internalizing and Externalizing Scales were .92 and .94. Cronbach's alpha was .90 for the Externalizing scale and .92 for the Internalizing scale.

Data Analysis

First, to examine correlations among peer victimization, social-psychological adjustment, and physical activity, Pearson product moment correlations will be computed. Pearson-product moment correlations were calculated to assess the relationships between peer victimization, depression, general anxiety, and loneliness. Considering that the current sample was modest in size, correlations between .1-2.9 were considered to be of small effect sizes, correlations between .3-.49 were considered to be of medium effect sizes and correlations above 0.5 were considered to be of a large effect size (Cohen, 1977). Given the modest sample size and preliminary nature of this study, corrections for Type I error were not made for these or subsequent analyses.

Second, one mediational and one moderator model will be tested to ascertain if the relationship between peer victimization and physical activity is moderated by age or mediated by social-psychological adjustment indices. Baron and Kenny's (1986) guidelines for mediation will be followed to test the model for the influence of peer victimization on physical activity via social-psychological adjustment. The following criteria are necessary for mediation: (I) the predictor (peer victimization) is significantly associated with the outcome (physical activity); (II) the predictor is significantly associated with the mediator (social-psychological adjustment variables); (III) the mediator is associated with the outcome variable (with the predictor accounted for); and (IV) the addition of the mediator to the full model reduces the relation between the predictor and criterion variable.

The moderator variable of age will be tested by using hierarchical regression analyses. For step one, age will be added to the regression. For step two, the predictor variable will be added (peer victimization). In step three, age by the physical activity will determine the interaction between the two variables (age and physical activity). Age was defined as children 8-12 years of age and adolescent 13-17 years of age. The split was created to ascertain if there would be differences between younger children and older adolescents in regards to how peer victimization is addressed. For example, are older adolescents better apt to manage peer victimization due to more experience in developing coping strategies?

RESULTS

Descriptive Statistics

An independent samples t-test revealed a significant gender difference in children and adolescents' self-report of peer victimization, t (1, 56) = 2.03, p = 0.048. Females scored significantly higher (M = 8.49, SD = 3.30) in self-reports of peer victimization (than males (M = 6.91, SD = 2.11). There was no significant difference found between age (child, aged 8-12 vs. adolescent, aged 13-17) among youth's self-report of peer victimization, t (1, 54) = -.63, ns. In regards to the other variables, 22.1% of children and adolescents scored 1 SD above the mean or higher on peer victimization, 18.9% on loneliness, 19.3% on depressive symptoms, and 15% on anxiety.

Correlational Analyses

Pearson product moment correlation revealed no significant relationship between peer victimization and physical activity (r = -.034, p > .05) (see table 1).

Table 1. Pearson correlation coefficients among study variables

	(1)	(2)	(3)	(4)	(5)	(6)	(7)	(8)	(9)	(10)	(11)	(12)	(13)	(14)
(1) Peer Victimization	1.0													
(2) CDI	.45**	1.0												
(3) MASC	.37**	.39**	1.0											
(4) ALS	.55**	.50**	.38*	1.0										
(5) CBCL WD Scale	.33*	.34*	.39**	.46**	1.0									
(6) CBCL SPRB Scale	.44**	.25	.45**	.34*	.63**	1.0								
(7) CBCL SOM Scale	.14	.09	.27	.029	.37**	.27*	1.0							
(8) CBCL ANXD Scale	.14	-.00	.39*	.23	.66**	.63**	.638	1.0						
(9) CBCL TPRB Scale	.10	.10	.12	.29	.44**	.39**	.32*	.58**	1.0					
(10) CBCL ATT Scale	.22	.16	.23	.30*	.63**	.73**	.24	.67**	.74**	1.0				
(11) CBCL DEL Scale	.22	.09	.21	.34*	.46**	.58**	.21	.57**	.42**	.73**	1.0			
(12) CBCL AGGR	.21	.23	.39**	.29	.44**	.71**	.43**	.69**	.59**	.84**	.66**	1.0		
(13) CBCL INT	.29	.19	.41*	.59**	.88**	.64**	.71**	.90**	.56**	.69**	.59**	.62**	1.0	
(14) SPARK	-.03	.13	.00	-.10	.00	-.12	-.23	-.16	.15	-.03	-.25	-.09	-.16	1.0
Mean (Standard deviation)	7.9 (2.9)	13.1 (3.4)	35.0 (14.4)	29.7 (12.1)	3.6 (3.5)	4.2 (3.4)	3.3 (2.7)	3.5 (3.5)	.888 (1.1)	4.1 (4.2)	1.9 (2.1)	7.5 (6.3)	10.7 (8.8)	104.8 (89.3)

Note: PVS=Peer Victimization Scale; *CDI* = Children's Depression Inventory; *MASC* = Manifest Anxiety Scale for Children; *ALS* = Asher Loneliness Scale; *CBCL* = Child Behavior Checklist; *SPARK*=Weekly Physical Activity Measure; * $p < .05$, ** $p < .01$.

Pearson product moment correlations were conducted between reports of peer victimization and both child and parent reports of social-psychological adjustment, which are presented in table 4. Pearson product moment correlations revealed significant and positive correlations between child-rated indices of peer victimization and depressive symptoms [$r = 0.45$, $p = 0.001$], general anxiety symptoms [$r = 0.37$, $p = 0.007$], and loneliness [$r = 0.55$, $p < 0.001$]. Additionally, child-rated peer victimization was positively correlated with parent-rated indexes of withdrawal behavior/depression $r = 0.33$ [$p = 0.012$] and social problems [$r = 0.44$, $p = 0.001$], but not with physical activity and parent-rated indexes of child internalizing behaviors (i.e., somatic symptoms, anxiety/depression, thought problems, attention problems) and externalizing behaviors (aggressive behavior, rule-breaking behavior).

A hierarchical linear regression was conducted to investigate whether or not child age would be a moderator variable between peer victimization and physical activity (see table 2). The child peer victimization scores and child age were the predictor variables and physical activity was the criterion variable. Per guidelines by Baron and Kenny (1986), the child age and peer victimization scores were entered together in step one, and then the interaction age and peer victimization were entered in step two.

Results revealed a main effect for age as a predictor of child-rated physical activity ($\beta = -.36$, $p = .021$), however, there was no significant main effect for peer victimization as a predictor physical activity ($\beta = -.12$, ns). There was no significant effect for the interaction of age by peer victimization [R^2 change = 0.008; $F(1, 38) = .56$, ns].

Per Baron and Kenny (1986), the following criteria were necessary for mediation: (I) the predictor (peer victimization) is significantly associated with the outcome (physical activity); (II) the predictor is significantly associated with the mediator (social-psychological adjustment variables); (III) the mediator is associated with the outcome variable (with the predictor accounted for); and (IV) the addition of the mediator to the full model reduces the relation between the predictor and criterion variable. These guidelines for mediation were not met to test the influence of peer victimization on physical activity via social-psychological adjustment due to the lack of a significant relationship between peer victimization and physical activity ($r = -.034$, ns).

Table 2. Fixed effects for the model testing the peer victimization as a predictor of child physical activity with age as a moderator

Predictor Variable	B	SE	t
Age as Moderator			
Peer Victimization	10.20	24.42	.42
Age	-3.33	16.94	-.20
Age * Peer Victimization	-1.15	1.95	-.59

B = Unstandardized Regression Coefficient, SE = Standard Error, t = t-statistic.

DISCUSSION

The current study investigated the relationships between peer victimization, physical activity, and social-psychological adjustment in obese youth. Although the study was correlational and does not provide causal information regarding the relationships between the variables, it does provide supporting evidence to the existent literature reflecting the damage peer victimization has on with obese youth. Overall, peer victimization was significantly and positively correlated with child and adolescent reports of depressive symptoms, general anxiety symptoms, and loneliness. Additionally, peer victimization was also significantly and positively correlated with parental reports of withdrawal/depressive symptoms and social problems.

Females scored significantly higher in self-report of peer victimization than males. There was no significant difference found between age (child vs. adolescent) in self-reports of peer victimization. In regards to the other variables, less than 20% of the sample reported being peer victimized and experiencing symptoms of depression, anxiety, and loneliness. Further discussion and examination of results, clinical implications, and limitations are to follow.

The first research aim of the study was to examine the relationship between peer victimization and physical activity. It was predicted that peer victimization would negatively correlate with physical activity. The current study did not reveal a significant relationship between peer victimization and physical activity, which has been shown in a prior study (Storch et al., 2007). This surprising finding raises the question of what differences existed between this study and that of Storch et al. (2007). One contributing factor to the difference in results may be attributed to the use of a different physical activity measure. In Storch et al. (2007), the two-item PACE measure was utilized. The PACE asks youth to report how many days they have been physical active for at least 60 minutes in the prior week (Prochaska, Sallis, and Long, 2001). The SPARK physical activity measure used in the current study is a relatively new measure and has not demonstrated strong stability and convergent validity with other physical activity measures as with the PACE. For example, the PACE+ has demonstrated stability (intraclass correlation coefficient =.77) and convergent validity with other measures of physical activity (Prochaska, Sallis, and Long, 2001). The SPARK had low validity (.47) with an objective measure of physical activity, the Caltrac accelerometer, which is an electronic assessment tool that measures both the quantity and intensity of movement. (Sallis et al., 1993). Furthermore, Sallis et al. (1993) reported that caution should be used when interpreting SPARK data due to the low validity and the self-report nature of the SPARK which calls for subjects to have the ability to recall variable physical activities which may be a difficult cognitive task for youth..

The SPARK's utilization in the current study was based upon its ability to provide more detailed accounts of when physical activity occurred (weekdays and weekends) and provided more details on the type of physical activity completed (i.e., running, jumping rope, playing basketball). Whereas the SPARK does provide more comprehensive information on physical activity than the PACE, it may have been too overwhelming or complex for participants to complete, particularly in the time constraints of their appointment. Considering the differential results regarding the relationship between peer victimization and physical activity, future research should focus on pilot testing physical activity measures in order to assess which one would be most appropriate for the sample.

There is also a possibility that peer victimization does not impact physical activity in the same manner (or at all) for obese youth. For example, obese youth may elect to participate in physical activities despite the possibility of being peer victimized. Parents may be able to override children or adolescents fears of being victimized by offering incentives, assisting them with the development of anti-bullying strategies, or offering to speak with school officials. Additionally, with an increase in technology, children and adolescent television programming, and computer and video games, obese youth may prefer sedentary activities over physical ones.

The second research aim of the study was to examine the relationships between peer victimization and social-psychological adjustment reports by children, adolescents, and parents. It was predicted that peer victimization would positively correlate with child-rated indices of depressive symptoms, generally anxiety, and loneliness, and parent-rated indices of internalizing and externalizing behavior. As previous studies have shown (see Hawker and Boulton, 2000 for a review), peer victimization was positively associated with depressive symptoms, anxiety, and loneliness, which provides further support of the distressing and problematic aspects of peer victimization. These findings may reflect not only the damaging effects of peer victimization, but also that frequently peer victimized children and adolescents may internalize the content of peer attacks, thus impacting important social-psychological development (Storch et al., 2007). For example, a child who is victimized and frequently belittled may believe attackers' comments, which could potentially reduce their confidence and compromise their ability to approach or befriend others. Obese and victimized youth often lack opportunities to develop positive peer relationships in childhood and adolescence, which is crucial task in successful social-psychological development (Stern et al., 2007).

Obese youth who are victimized may be at particular risk for poorer psychosocial outcomes due to childhood and adolescence being an important time period for physical changes and self-awareness of physical changes (Janssen et al., 2004). Furthermore, the association of peer victimization and low self-esteem of obese children and adolescents is persistent in the literature due to bullying negatively affecting quality of life issues (Stern et al., 2007; Storch et al., 2006). Additionally, significant implications exist for children and adolescents who have medical conditions (i.e., obesity, endocrine disorders) including suicidal ideation, suicide attempts, and non-adherence to important self-management of potentially life threatening diseases (Eisenberg et al., 2003; Storch et al., 2006).

The third aim was to examine age as a moderator of the relationship between peer victimization and physical activity. Age was chosen as a moderator variable to investigate potential differences between children (aged 8-12-years) and adolescents (aged 13-17-years) in levels of peer victimization and physical activity.

However, the current study did not find significant results for peer victimization and physical activity being moderated by age. This could be mean that regardless of age, peer victimization is difficult to address and has negative consequences for all ages. The final research aim was to examine the relationship between peer victimization, physical activity, and social-psychological adjustment. It was predicted that the relationship between peer victimization and physical activity would be mediated by social-psychological adjustment.

Inconsistent with expectations, results did not support social-psychological adjustment as a mediator of peer victimization and physical activity. Although the current study did not find the relationship between peer victimization and physical activity being mediated by social-psychological adjustment, one other study has demonstrated supporting evidence for mediation (Storch et al., 2007). Non-significant findings may also be attributed to familial relationships providing additional protective factors. For example, parents may be able to provide support and unconditional positive regard that assists children and adolescents in addressing peer victimization, participate in physical activities and navigate social-psychological adjustment positively than their counterparts who lack strong family bonds.

Clinical Implications

Considering the strong evidence that supports peer victimization as being significantly associated with poorer social-psychological outcomes (Hawker and Boulton, 2000; Storch et al., 2007), these findings have several clinical implications. First, it may be beneficial for healthcare providers treating obese youth to discuss peer victimization and problem-solve ways to develop counter-bullying strategies. For example, healthcare providers can consult with school officials and parents in order to raise the level of awareness of the problem of peer victimization. Motivational strategies, like empowerment workshops, unconditional positive regard, incentives, anti-bullying information, and continuous support, may also help victims confront challenging situations (Faith et al., 2002).

Children and adolescents who express depressive symptoms, anxiety, loneliness, withdrawal behaviors, and social problems at clinic appointments need to be assessed and subsequently, may need psychotherapeutic or psychotropic interventions. Cognitive-behavioral treatment and psychotropic medications (i.e., Lexapro, Paxil, Zoloft) for depression and anxiety have been empirically-supported as appropriate and successful measures (Messer, 2004). Therefore, treatment of symptoms associated with peer victimization via psychological and/or psychiatric intervention is important. It would also prove beneficial to teach social skills to children and adolescent (i.e., assertiveness, conflict management).

An example of such a bullying intervention was completed with 40 girls that were identified as peer victimizers; they were randomly recruited to participate in brief strategic family therapy (BSFT) for three months with a follow-up occurring 12 months after treatment (Nickel et al., 2006). It was revealed that girls who participated in BSFT (in comparison to the control group) not only showed reduction in bullying behaviors there were also statistically significant reductions in all risk-taking behaviors including aggression, anger, interpersonal conflict, and health-related problems (i.e., smoking cigarettes; Nickel et al., 2006). Findings suggested that those exhibiting bullying behaviors also suffer from psychological and social problems that may be remedied or reduced with therapeutic intervention (Nickel et al., 2006).

Due to the negative outcomes associated with peer victimization, it is important for schools to establish and maintain programs that effectively address the problem of peer victimization including, but not limited to, development of stricter penalties for aggressors, reduction of opportunities for bullying, and meetings with parents (Eisenberg and Aalsma, 2004). Furthermore, it would be beneficial to have school staff trained in being able to identify bullying behaviors. For example, school officials and staff should be trained to identify perpetrators and peer victimization (both overt and relational forms). Also, more supportive programming and policies that celebrated size diversity, consulted with healthcare professionals and providers, provided equality of opportunity in school events and activities, educated parents on the consequences of peer victimization, and developed a no-tolerance policy on bullying that was closely monitored and enforced would be helpful in creating a better climate for all students.

For example, peer victimized children and adolescents are often fearful that reporting bullying behaviors will have even more disastrous outcomes, like not resolving the problem, retribution, or an exacerbation of the situation (Newman and Murray, 2005). Furthermore, anti-bullying programs have not only been shown efficacious, but also distribute more of the responsibility to end peer victimization on all involved parties, not just the victim (Frey et al., 2005). In a previous study (Frey et al., 2005), six schools were randomly assigned to an anti-bullying program called "Steps to Respect;" results revealed that students in the intervention group reported increases in agreeable interactions, an increase in bystander responsibility, greater perceived adult responsiveness, and less aggression or bullying than the control group.

Future research should focus on identifying moderators and mediators between the relationships of peer victimization, physical activity, and social-psychological adjustment to continually provide data for the existence or non-existence of these relationships, to evaluate if these relationships are constant over time (longitudinal studies), and how peer victimization may influence adulthood adjustment and psychological functioning . Several potential variables that should be explored include family variables, socio-economic status, treatment seeking vs. non-treatment seeking populations, and access to healthcare.

Limitations

Limitations of the current study should be considered. First, the correlational nature of the study does not provide causal data or directionality of the relationships. Therefore, it is difficult to ascertain how these relationships are established and maintained. Second, this study depends on accurate self-report by youth and their parents, which may not capture the relationships between peer victimization, physically activity, and social-psychological adjustment in its entirety. For example, self-report measures are vulnerable to potential confounds of response bias (Storch et al., 2007). Additionally, considering the variable nature of physical activity (e.g., changes daily) and the need to recall physical activity, objective measures of physical activity may be beneficial in future research. Additionally, children, adolescents, and parents may provide socially desirable responses or underreport symptomology for fear of negative consequences or being negatively judged by others.

Third, all of the children and adolescents who participated in the study were seeking medical treatment at a lipid clinic, which in and of itself may play a factor in the relationships between these variables. For example, results may not generalize to non-seeking treatment obese youth due to additional variables and difference between those who seek and do not seek treatment (that may be related to socio-economical status, the ability to pay for healthcare). For example, a prior study showed smaller quality of life issues among non-seeking treatment youth (Williams, Wake, Hesketh, Maher, Watrs, E, 2005). Therefore, future research should focus on studying both clinical and non-clinical obese youth to ascertain if differences exist between the two populations.

Fourth, the SPARK's less strong validity properties could have negatively impacted results. Therefore, not including the PACE+ as one of the measures is an additional limitation. Fifth, the study does not take into account obese youth that have physical limitations that may prevent or limit their ability to exercise and be physically active. Sixth, the timing of the study, could have impacted the results. The majority of data collection was completed during the summer in a tropical climate which could have impacted youth's ability or desire to participate in physical activity (especially physical activity that would occur outside). Seventh, body mass index was not collected, which could have potentially provided information regarding differences between youth of varying weight. However, Storch et al. (2007) did not find significant differences between youth's weight which may reveal that regardless of the exact weight, youth that obese share similar experiences.

AUTHOR NOTE

This research was conducted as part of Charisse Williams' dissertation. The contributions of Marni Jacob, Janet Silverstein, Milagros Huerta, and Valerie Crawford are gratefully acknowledged.

REFERENCES

Achenbach, T.M. (1991). *Manual for the Child Behavior Checklist/4-18 and 1991 Profile.* Burlington, VT: University of Vermont, Department of Psychiatry.

Asher, S. R., Hymel, S., and Renshaw, P.D. (1984). Loneliness in children. *Child Development, 55*, 1457-1464.

Asher, S. R., and Wheeler, V. A. (1985). Children's loneliness: A comparison of rejected and neglected peer status. *Journal of Consulting and Clinical Psychology, 53,* 500-505.

Bagner, D. M., Storch, E. A., and Roberti, J. W. (2004). A factor analytic study of the Loneliness and Social Dissatisfaction Scale in a sample of African American and Hispanic American children. *Child Psychiatry and Human Development, 34,* 237-250.

Baron, R. M., and Kenny, D. A. (1986). The moderator-mediator variable distinction in social psychological research: Conceptual, strategic, and statistical considerations. *Journal of Personality and Social Psychology, 52*, 1173-1182.

Bond, L., Carlin, J. B., Thomas, L., Rubin, K. and Patton G. (2001). Does bullying cause emotional problems? A prospective study of young teenagers. *British Medical Journal, 323,* 480-484.

Broder, H. L., Smith, F. B., and Strauss, R. P. (2001). Developing a behavior rating scale for comparing teachers' rating of children with and without craniofacial anomalies. *The Cleft Palate-Craniofacial Journal, 38,* 560-565.

Bronfenbrenner, U. (1979). *The ecology of human development: Experiments by nature and design.* Boston: Harvard University Press.

Craighead, W. E., Smucker, M. R., Craighead, L. W., and Ilardi, S. S. (1998). Factor analysis of the Children's Depression Inventory in a community sample. *Psychological Assessment, 10,* 156-165.

Crick, N.R. (1996). The role of overt aggression, relational aggression, and prosocial behavior in the prediction of children's future social adjustment. *Child Development, 67,* 2317-2327.

Crick, N. R., and Bigbee, M. A. (1998). Relational and overt forms of peer victimization: A multi-informant approach. *Journal of Consulting and Clinical Psychology, 66,* 337-347.

Crick, N. R., Casas, J. F., and Ku, H. (1999). Relational and physical forms of peer victimization in preschool. *Developmental Psychology, 35, 376-385.*

Crick, N. R., Casas, J. F., and Mosher, M. (1997). Relational and overt aggression in preschool. *Developmental Psychology, 33,* 579-588.

Crick, N. R., and Grotpeter, J. K. (1996). Children's treatment by peers: Victims of relational and overt aggression. *Development and Psychopathology, 8,* 367-380.

Eisenberg, M. E., and Aalsma, M. C. (2004). Bullying and peer victimization: Position paper of the Society for Adolescent Medicine. *Journal of Adolescent Health, 36,* 88-91.

Eisenberg, M. E., Neumark-Sztainer, D., and Story, M. (2003). Associations of weight-based teasing and emotional well-being among adolescents. *Archives of Pediatrics and Adolescent Medicine, 157,* 733-738.

Espelage, D. L. and Swearer, S. M. (2003). Research on school bullying and victimization: What have we learned and where do we go from here? *School Psychology Review, 32,* 365-383.

Faith, M. S., Leone, M. A., Ayers, T. S., Moonseong, H., and Pietrobelli, A. (2002). Weight criticism during physical activity, coping skills, and reported physical activity in children. *Pediatrics, 110,* e23.

Fekkes, M., Pijpers, F. I. M., Fredriks, A. M., Vogels, T., and Verloove-Vanhorick, S. P. (2006). Do bullied children get ill, or do ill children get bullied?: A prospective cohort study on the relationship between bullying and health-related symptoms. *Pediatrics, 117,* 1568-1574.

Frey, K. S., Hirschstein, M. K., Snell, J. L., Edstrom, L. V., MacKenzie, E. P., and Broderick, C. J. (2005). Reducing playground bullying and supporting beliefs: an experimental trial of the steps to respect program. *Developmental Psychology, 41,* 479-490.

Gladstone, G. L., Parker, G. B., and Malhi, G. S. (2006).Do bullied children become anxious and depressed adults?: A cross-sectional investigation of the correlates of bullying and anxious depression. *Journal of Nervous and Mental Disease, 194,* 201-208.

Grills, A.E., and Ollendick, T.H. (2002). Issues in parent-child agreement: the case of structured diagnostic interviews. *Clinical Child and Family Psychology Review, 5,* 57-83.

Grills, A.E., and Ollendick, T.H. (2003). Multiple informant agreement and the anxiety disorders interview schedule for parents and children. *Journal of the American Academy of Child and Adolescent Psychiatry, 42,* 30-40.

Hawker, D. S. J. D. and Boulton, M. J. (2000). Twenty years' research on peer victimization and psychosocial maladjustment: A meta-analytic review of cross-sectional studies. *Journal of Child Psychology and Psychiatry, 41,* 441-455.

Hugh-Jones, S., and Smith, P. K. (1999). Self-reports of short- and long-term effects of bullying on children who stammer. *British Journal of Educational Psychology, 69,* 141-158.

Jackson, T. D., Grilo, C. M., and Masheb, R. M. (2002). Teasing history and eating disorder features: An age and body mass index-matched comparison of bulimia nervosa and binge-eating disorder. *Comprehensive Psychiatry, 43,* 108-113.

Jacobsen, A. M., Hauser, S. T., Wertlieb, D., Wolfsdorf, J. I., Orleans, J., and Vieyra. (1986). Psychological adjustment of children with recently diagnosed diabetes mellitus. *Diabetes Care, 9,* 323-329.

Janssen, I., Craig, W. M., Boyce, W. F., and Pickett, W. (2004). Associations between overweight and obesity with bullying behaviors in school-aged children. *Pediatrics, 113,* 1187-1194.

Khatri, P., Kupersmidt, J. B., and Patterson, C. (2000). Aggression and peer victimization as predictors of self-reported behavioral and emotional adjustment. *Aggressive Behavior, 26,* 345-358.

Kim, Y. S., Leventhal, B. L., Koh, Y., Hubbard, A., and Boyce, W. T. (2006). School bullying and youth violence. *Arch of General Psychiatry, 63,* 1035-1041.

Kochenderfer, B. J., and Ladd, G. W. (1996). Peer victimization: Cause or consequence of school adjustment? *Child Development, 67,* 1305-1317.

Kovacs, M. (1992). *The Children's Depression Inventory.* Manual. Toronto, Ontario, Canada: Multi-Health Systems, Inc.

Kovacs, M. A., and Beck, A. T. (1977). An empirical-clinical approach toward a definition of childhood depression. In J. G. Schulterbrandt and A. Raskin (Eds.), *Depression in childhood: diagnosis, treatment, and conceptual model* (pp. 1-25). New York: Raven Press.

Little, L. (2001). Peer victimization of children with Asperger spectrum disorders. *Journal of the American Academy of Child and Adolescent Psychiatry, 40,* 995-996.

March, J. S., Sullivan, K., and Parker, J. D. (1999). Test-retest reliability of the Multidimensional Anxiety Scale for Children. *Journal of Anxiety Disorders, 13,* 349-358.

March, J. S., Parker, J. D., Sullivan, K., Stallings, P., and Conners, C. K. (1997). The Multidimensional Anxiety Scale for Children (MASC): Factor structure, reliability, and validity. *Journal of the American Academy of Child and Adolescent Psychiatry, 36,* 554-565.

Masten, A. S. (2005). Peer relationships and psychopathology in developmental perspective: Reflections on progress and promise. *Journal of Clinical Child and Adolescent Psychology, 34,* 87-92.

Martlew, M., and Hodson, J. (1991). Children with mild learning difficulties and in a special school: Comparisons of behavior, teasing, and teachers' attitudes. *British Journal of Educational Psychology, 61,* 355-372.

Messer, S. B. (2004). Evidence-based practice: Beyond empirically supported treatments. *Professional Psychology: Research and Practice, 35,* 580-588.

Montes, G. and Halterman, J. S. (2007). Bullying among children with autism and the influence of comorbidity with ADHD: A population-based study. *Ambulatory Pediatrics, 7,* 253-257.

Nabuzoka, D., and Smith, P. K. (1993). Sociometric status and social behaviour of children with and without learning difficulties. *Journal of Child Psychology and Psychiatry, 34,* 1435-1448.

Nansel, T. R., Craig, W., Overpeck, M. D., Saluja, G., Ruan, W. J., and the Health Behaviour in School-aged Children Bullying Analyses Working Group. (2004). Cross-national consistency in the relationship between bullying behaviors and psychosocial adjustment. *Archives of Pediatric and Adolescent Medicine, 158,* 730-736.

Nansel, T. R., Overpeck, M., Pilla, R. S., Ruan, W. J., Simons-Morton, B., and Scheidt, P. (2001). Bullying behaviors among US youth: Prevalence and association with psychosocial adjustment. *Journal of the American Medical Association, 285,* 2094-2100.

Neumark-Sztainer, D., Falkner, N., and Story, M. (2002). Weight-teasing among adolescents: correlations with weight status and disordered eating behaviors. *International Journal of Obesity and Related Metabolic Disorders, 26,* 123-131.

Neumark-Sztainer, D., Story, M., and Faibisch, L. (1998). Perceived stigmatization among overweight African-American and Caucasian adolescent girls. *Journal of Adolescent Health, 23,* 264-270.

Nickel, M., Luley, J., Krawczyk, J., Nickel, C., Widermann, C., Lahmann, C., Muehlbacher, M., Forthuber, P., Kettler, C., Leiberich, P., Tritt, K., Mitterlenner, F., Kaplan, P., Gil, F. P., Rother, W., and Loew, T. (2006). Bullying girls-changes after brief strategic family therapy: A randomized, prospective, controlled trial with one-year follow-up. *Psychotherapy and Psychosomatics, 75,* 47-55.

Olweus, D. (1992). Victimization by peers: Antecedents and long-term outcomes. In K. H. Rubin and J. B. Asendorpf (Eds.), *Social withdrawal, inhibition, and shyness in childhood* (pp.315-341). Hillside, NJ: Erlbaum.

Pearce, M. J., Boergers, J., and Prinstein, M. J. (2002). Adolescent obesity, overt and relational peer victimization, and romantic relationships. *Obesity Research, 10,* 386-393.

Pellegrini, A. D. (1998). Bullies and victims in school: A review and call for research. *Journal of Applied Developmental Psychology, 19,* 165-176.

Perry, D. G., Kusel, S. J., and Perry, L. C. (1988). Victims of peer aggression. *Developmental Psychology, 24,* 807-814.

Perry, D. G., Williard, J. C. and Perry, L. C. Peers' perceptions of the consequences that victimized children provide aggressors. *Child Development, 6,* 1310-1325.

Prinstein, M. J., Boergers, J., and Vernberg, E. M. (2001) Overt and relational aggression in adolescents: Social-psychological adjustment of aggressors and victims. *Journal of Clinical Child Psychology, 30,* 479-491.

Prochaska, J. J., Sallis, J. F., and Long, B. (2001). A physical activity screening measure for use with adolescents in primary care. *Archives of Pediatric and Adolescent Medicine, 155,* 554-559.

Sallis, J.F., Condon, S.A., Goggin, K.J., Roby, J.J., Kolody, B., and Alcaraz, J.E. (1993). The development of self-administered physical activity surveys for 4th grade students. *Research Quarterly for Exercise and Sport, 64,* 25-31.

Sandberg, D. E. (1999). Experiences of being short: Should we expect problems of psychosocial adjustment. In: Eiholzer, U., Haverkamp, F., Voss, L. (Eds). *Growth, stature, and psychosocial well-being.* Seattle: Hogrefe and Huber Publishers.

Schwartz, D., Dodge, K. A., and Coie, J. D. (1993). The emergence of chronic peer victimization in boys' play groups. *Child Development, 64,* 1755-1772.

Schwartz, D., Farver, J., Change, L., and Lee-Shin, Y. (2002). Victimization in South Korean children's peer groups. *Journal of Abnormal Child Psychology, 30,* 113-125.

Stern, M., Mazzeo, S. E., Gerke, C. K., Porter, J. S., Bean, M. K., and Laver, J. H. (2007). Gender, ethnicity, psychosocial factors, and quality of life among severely overweight, treatment-seeking adolescents. *Journal of Pediatric Psychology, 32,* 90-94.

Storch, E. A., Heidgerken, A. D., Geffken, G. R., Lewin, A. B., Ohleyer, V., Freddo, M., Silverstein, J. H. (2006a) Bullying, regimen self-management, and metabolic control in youth with Type 1 diabetes. *Journal of Pediatrics, 148,* 784-787.

Storch, E. A., Krain, A. L., Kovacs, A. H., and Barlas, M. E. (2003). The relationship of communication attitudes and abilities to peer victimization in elementary school children. *Child Study Journal, 32,* 231-240.

Storch, E. A. and Ledley, D. (2005). Peer victimization and psychosocial adjustment in children: current knowledge and future directions. *Clinical Pediatrics, 44,* 29-38.

Storch, E. A., Ledley, D. R., Lewin, A. B., Murphy, T. K., Johns, N. B., Goodman, W.K., and Geffken, G.R. (2006b). Peer victimization in children with Obsessive-Compulsive Disorder: Relations with symptoms of psychopathology. *Journal of Clinical Child and Adolescent Psychology, 35,* 446-455.

Storch, E. A., Lewin, A., Silverstein, J. H., Heidgerken, A. D., Strawser, M. S., Baumeister, A., and Geffken, G. R. (2004a). Social-psychological correlates of peer victimization in children with endocrine disorders. *Journal of Pediatrics, 145,* 784-789.

Storch, E. A., Lewin, A., Silverstein, J. H., Heidgerken, A. D., Strawser, M. S., Baumeister, A., and Geffken, G. R. (2004b). Peer victimization and psychosocial adjustment in children with type I diabetes. *Clinical Pediatrics, 43,* 467-472.

Storch, E. A., and Masia, C. L. (2001). *Peer victimization and social anxiety and distress in adolescence.* In M. Prinstein (Chair), Peer relationships, social anxiety, and developmental psychopathology. Symposium presented at the annual meeting of the Association for the Advancement of Behavioral Therapy, Philadelphia, PA.

Storch, E. A., and Masia-Warner, C. (2004). The relationship of peer victimization to social anxiety and loneliness in adolescent females. *Journal of Adolescence, 27,* 351-362.

Storch, E. A., Milsom, V. A., DeBraganza, N., Lewin, A. B., Geffken, G. R., and Silverstein, J. H. (2007). Peer victimization, psychosocial adjustment, and physical activity in overweight and at-risk-for-overweight youth. *Journal of Pediatric Psychology, 32,* 80-89.

Storch, E. A., Zelman, E., Sweeney, M., Danner, G., and Dove, S. (2002). Overt and relational victimization, and psychosocial adjustment in minority preadolescents. *Child Study Journal, 32,* 73-80.

Sullivan, H.S. (1953). *The interpersonal theory of psychiatry.* New York: Norton Press.

Sweeting, H., Wright, C., and Minnis, H. (2005). Psychosocial correlates of adolescent obesity, "slimming down" and becoming obese. *Journal of Adolescent Health, 37,* 409-417.

Wilde, M., and Haslan, C. (1996). Living with epilepsy: a qualitative study investigating the experiences of young people attending outpatient clinics in Leicester. *Seizure, 5,* 63-72.

Williams, J., Wake, M., Hesketh, K., Maher, E., and Watrs, E. (2005). Health-related quality of life of overweight and obese children. *Journal of the American Medical Association, 293,* 1525-1529.

Wolke, D., Woods, S., Bloomfield, L., and Karstadt, L. (2000). The association between direct and relational bullying and behaviour problems among primary school children. *Journal of Child Psychology and Psychiatry, 41,* 989-1002.

Young-Hyman, D., Schlundt, D. G., Herman-Wenderoth, L., and Bozylinski, K. (2003). Obesity, appearance, and psychosocial adaptation in young African-American children. *Journal of Pediatric Psychology, 28,* 463-472.

Zeller, M. H., Saelens, B. E., Roehrig, H., Kirk, S., and Daniels, S. R. (2004). Psychological adjustment of obese youth presenting for weight management treatment. *Obesity Research, 12,* 1576-1586.

In: Life Style and Health Research Progress
Editors: A. B. Turley, G. C. Hofmann

ISBN: 978-1-60456-427-3
© 2008 Nova Science Publishers, Inc.

Chapter II

Lifestyle Factors in HIV Transmission: A Functional Contextualist Perspective

William D. Barta and Howard Tennen
University of Connecticut

Of all developed, wealthy nations, the U.S. has the highest rate of sexually transmitted infections (STI). More than 65 million people in this country are living with an incurable STI, and more than half of Americans will have an STI at one point in their lifetime. Each year, 19 million STI diagnoses are made. Of these, roughly 40,000 are new cases of HIV infection, contributing to the estimated 1 to 1.2 million people living with HIV/AIDS (PLWHA) in the U.S. today (Guttmacher Institute, 2006). In terms of the vulnerability of the U.S. to increases in HIV infection rates, the high rate of STI in this country is prima facie evidence that levels of condom use and levels of avoidance of unsafe sexual situations are disturbingly low.

The risk of HIV infection, particularly for heterosexuals, has grown since the late 1990s. Yet, the number of Americans who regard HIV as a top health concern for the country has been steadily declining. As recently as the year 2000, HIV was perceived to be the dominant health threat facing the country; today, only around 7% of the population holds this view (Gallup, 2003). This change in perception is attributable to the advent of antiretroviral (ARV) medications, which have been effective in helping PLWHA lead longer, healthier lives (Kates et al., 2002). Effective ARV medications were introduced in 1996, and by 1998, HIV plummeted from being the 8th leading cause of death for all Americans to being the 14th (Hoyert et al. 1999).

In part, the phenomenon which Demmer (2003) refers to as "HIV complacency" can be partially attributed to a lack of knowledge among members of the public – specifically, although PLWHA do in fact lead longer, healthier lives as a result of the new medications, these medications are not a cure, they do not work for everyone, they produce severe, sometimes disfiguring side-effects, and the medications themselves can produce life-threatening toxicities (Cengiz et al., 2005). The phenomenon of HIV complacency can only be fully appreciated, however, in the context of the social stratification of the U.S. by race, ethnicity, and socio-economic status. Even though HIV is by no means a leading cause of death in the general population, the most recent available data suggest that HIV remains the 7th leading cause of death among African American men (Miniño et al., 2007) and is the leading cause of death among African American women between the ages of 25 and 34 (Fergusson et al., 2006). One goal of this chapter will be to encourage the reader to reflect on the bases and practical implications of the conclusion that HIV/STI-related health disparities are the result of a complex web of contributing factors, many of which may be described as "lifestyle factors."

The phrase "lifestyle factors contributing to HIV transmission" refers to sexual activity involving HIV-infected partners, and the illicit use of intravenous drugs. In this sense, the term "lifestyle" denotes simply "the way a person lives," just as sedentary lifestyle may be said to increase the risk of obesity. HIV prevention researchers refer to individuals as "high risk" when their lifestyles place them at elevated risk of HIV infection. However, it is a mistake to suppose that fixed categories exist, such that some lifestyles are "high risk" and others are "low risk." It has been shown, for example, that many young people will report having had one or two lifetime sex partners and having used condoms on most occasions. This lifestyle is significantly less likely to result in HIV infection for a late adolescent white woman than it is for a late adolescent black woman living in comparable communities (Halpern et al., 2004). Hence, understanding an individual's sexual lifestyle does not enhance our predictions of health outcomes with quite the same precision that knowledge of an individual's eating habits and level of physical activity enhances our ability to predict obesity risk.

In this chapter, we consider the association between lifestyle and HIV transmission from an "ecological" perspective. To this end, our emphasis is on reciprocal person-environment interactions. An ecological perspective asserts that environments exert measurable effects on individual behavior. It also views behavior as a succession of discrete acts manifesting over time and in a variety of *behavior settings*. Here, the term "behavior setting" is understood as the immediate environment, such as a discrete location or social interaction. In the case of a single individual, the same behavior may bring (or may be expected by the actor to bring) desirable consequences in one behavior setting and undesirable consequences in another. Hence, an individual may refuse unsafe sex as a rule, but nonetheless encounter sets of circumstances in which violations of this rule occur. Likewise, two individuals may generally exhibit quite different patterns of behavior, but nonetheless exhibit similar patterns of behavior when they occupy similar behavior settings.

Although behavioral scientists are generally aware of the powerful effect of setting on behavior, this source of variability is conspicuously absent from the most influential and widely-used theories of health behavior change that guide their research and interventions. Instead, definable settings that are associated with increased risk – cruising venues, for example – are viewed as amenable locations for recruiting participants for research and intervention projects, or as suitable locations for distributing condoms or prevention-oriented print materials. The extent to which these settings account for unique variance in the prediction of behavior, how settings affect behavior, and how to address the motivations that bring people into these settings remain understudied questions. This is in large measure the result of the practical difficulties associated with measuring the effects of setting, and transitions between settings, on behavior. To say that research on context-dependent facets of behavior has been neglected implies an over-emphasis on the facets of behavior which may be construed as unvarying. In this chapter, we seek to highlight some of the consequences of this over-emphasis on a static conceptualization of behavior. We will also highlight novel theoretical and methodological approaches which provide the means of mitigating some of the practical difficulties which have historically stood in the way of context-sensitive observational research. In this discussion of person-environment interactions, we approach the environment as an inherently multilevel construct. Here, a good point of reference is Bronfenbrenner's (1979) model. He described the environment, as it acts upon the person, as a series of concentric circles. At the outermost ring, the *macrosystem* describes broad influences on individual behavior including political decisions at the national level, cultural values, and the media environment. The innermost circle, or the *microsystem,* describes the array of familial, social and physical behavior settings that the individual enters on a day-to-day basis. Between the macrosystem and the microsystem, Bronfenbrenner identified the *mesosystem* as the level of environmental analysis involving interactions between microsystems as well as the points of contact (e.g., institutions) between the macrosystem and the microsystem.

THE ECOLOGICAL PERSPECTIVE

To better appreciate what a so-called "ecological" perspective has to offer to the discussion of HIV transmission and the role of lifestyle, we will contrast it with the prevailing conceptual framework that has guided prevention research since the beginning of the HIV epidemic. From the time behavioral scientists first began to formulate a concerted response to the emerging HIV epidemic in the 1980s until now, research has been strongly influenced by social-cognitive models such as the *Theory of Reasoned Action* (Fishbein and Ajzen, 1975), the *Theory of Planned Behavior* (Ajzen, 1991), and the *Health Belief Model* (Becker, 1974). Investigators using these models collect data on constructs such as attitudes toward condom use, perception of the personal risk of HIV infection, and perceived social norms relating to condom use, and relate them to the frequency of condom use behavior.

We offer an (admittedly simplified) example of how these theories are applied: An investigator may find that, in a given sample of individuals, attitudes toward condom use are negative and the rate of condom use is low. This investigator conducts an intervention designed to improve attitudes toward condom use. Weeks or months later, the participants are contacted again and it is found that, among individuals reporting more favorable attitudes, self-reported frequency of condom use has increased. This is taken as evidence in favor of interventions that target attitudes toward condom use. The strength of this evidence depends on the validity of the assumption that attitudes are stable.

Some researchers have, however, suggested that evidence of the stability of attitudes is subject to more than one interpretation. From the perspective of *Self-Perception Theory* (Bem, 1965, Weinstein, 2007), individuals who do not decide to use condoms infer from their own behavior that they possess negative attitudes toward condom use, and individuals who decide to use condoms infer that they have favorable attitudes toward condom use. As Spinoza wrote in his *Ethics,* "in no case do we strive for, wish for, long for, or desire anything, because we deem it to be good, but on the other hand we deem a thing to be good, because we strive for it, wish for it, long for it, or desire it." If we suppose that behavior is influenced by situational factors, the day-to-day consistency of the behavior settings that an individual occupies, rather than the effects of holding certain attitudes, may account for attitude-consistent behavior.

If there is a change that is attributable to an intervention targeting HIV/STI preventive attitudes, it may be a change in the individual's willingness to consider using condoms the next time he or she has sex. That is, whatever it is that is being assessed by an attitude measurement is only an imperfect approximation of a latent factor that is a key ingredient in behavior change. If this is the case, something other than attitudes might approximate the latent factor more closely and produce behavior change in a more efficient manner. If we rely on conventional measurement methods, we can only resolve the question by making comparisons between the attitude measure and other, similar constructs such as "behavioral intention" or "readiness to change." However, even if one takes this step, it begs the question of whether the differences between "attitude" and "intention" reflect a genuine, behaviorally-relevant distinction or merely the capacity of the measurement instruments to elicit distinctive and consistent patterns of responses and distinctive patterns of correlations to other constructs.

Suppose that what has changed as a result of the intervention is the individual's willingness to consider using condoms rather than his or her attitudes toward condom use *per se*. If this increased willingness persists until the next opportunity to engage in sex, and the resulting experience is positive, e.g., the partner reacts favorably, the individual finds the reduction of HIV-related worry rewarding, and does not experience an extreme reduction in the enjoyment of the physical sensation of sex, this behavior is likely to be repeated. If the experience is negative, e.g., sex is less enjoyable, the condom fails, or the partner is uncooperative, it is unlikely to be repeated. The outcomes of the behavior, as suggested above, are likely to impact the individual's attitudes, but this does not mean that the change in attitudes is at all relevant to whether the individual uses condoms on subsequent occasions. In this hypothetical scenario, the contingencies of the behavior may be the sole determinant of HIV preventive behavior and the most reliable predictor of whether the behavior will be repeated on subsequent occasions. At question, though, is how to adequately represent the behavior setting and person x situation interactions in a generalizable model of behavior. Bearing closely on this is the related question of what we mean by "reasons," or more specifically, causal factors.

Features of the Setting and Partner

According to Staats (1996), a situational cue performs at least three functions. Consider a situation in which an individual wishes to use a condom during sex but is also tempted to avoid this sensitive topic. The first function of a situational cue, Staats notes, is to elicit an affective state, e.g., the individual worries about how the partner might react to a condom use request. Secondly, the affective valence of this cue reinforces the behavior, e.g., this worry becomes linked to the thought of requesting condoms. The third function of a situational cue

– which may be described as an "additive" function – is to inform the individual's event-specific decision-making process. That is, a given situational cue is weighed against other situational cues that may also be present, e.g., whether condoms are available, or whether the partner denies having HIV/STI (which in turn forces a confrontation with potentially sensitive "trust issues").

The task of treating the behavior setting as a variable in a model of behavior -- as opposed to the more typical approach of treating the effects of the setting as "error variance" -- depends on the researcher's ability to accurately and reliably identify relevant settings. One of the most important elements of a sexual situation in predicting HIV preventive outcomes is the sex partner. For example, the individual's perception of the partner as someone likely to have an STI, the relative importance placed on prophylaxis versus contraception, and the extent to which one's decision-making is influenced by concern over upsetting the partner as opposed to protecting oneself, are all influenced by how the partner is perceived. Researchers have long recognized that the distinction between "first time" or "casual" partners on one hand, and "steady" or "committed" partners on the other, has a reliable effect on the likelihood of condom use (c.f., Lescano et al., 2007).

Although many HIV/STI prevention counselors promote the message "use condoms every time you have sex" (or "always practice sexual abstinence"), inevitably, recipients of this message find themselves in situations in which they abandon an across the board policy and instead make *ad hoc* assessments of the risks and benefits of unsafe sex. Our experience suggests that, in the urban communities in which we conduct research, awareness of HIV/STI is strong and condom use during first-time sex with a new partner has become a socially normative practice. However, the use of condoms in "established" relationships is more problematic. As noted by other researchers, in as few as 3 weeks, 18-29 year old couples decide that there is sufficient trust and stability in the relationship that the female partner will initiate hormonal birth control and condom use will be discontinued. Given the high rate of relationship dissolution, partner turnover, and partner concurrence (i.e., maintaining two or more simultaneous sexual relationships) observed in the community, discontinuation of condom use in established relationships is concerning.

The point to be made here is that a substantive distinction exists between what may be termed "behavior in general" and "situation-specific behavior." Social cognitive theories of health behavior change (as discussed earlier) focus on the former. Social cognitive theories guide investigators to measure the aggregate effects on condom use of changes in attitudes toward condom use, perception of the personal risk of HIV infection, and perceived social norms relating to condom use.

Situation-specific behavior is addressed, if it is addressed at all, within the curriculum of a given HIV/STI prevention intervention. These interventions are designed, in many cases, by following principles adopted from counseling and educational psychology. The interventionist operating in a small group setting relies on activities such as role-plays to aid participants gain insight into previously unrecognized situational cues which trigger risky behavior. In individual treatment settings, a counselor may ask his/her client to detail the circumstances of past sexual encounters, and as is the case with role-plays, the goal is to identify situational triggers of risk behavior (c.f. Kelly, 1995).

Once these context-dependent cues are recognized, this creates an opportunity to consider personal strategies that might be employed to reduce the individual's exposure to risk. If unsafe sex occurs because condoms are not available during sexual situations, the interventionist may advocate the practice of always carrying condoms or keeping them handy. The interventionist may also recommend *verbal strategies*; for example, in situations in which a sex partner resists using condoms because he or she does not perceive HIV/STI to be a risk, an effective verbal strategy is to highlight the benefits of condoms as an added protection against pregnancy. In simple terms, the interventionist seeks to encourage "if-then" thinking to prepare the client to behave adaptively in challenging situations.

The interventionist is confronting *causes* of unsafe behavior. That is, the failure to anticipate a sexual encounter by carrying condoms creates a situation in which the only choice that is salient to the individual may be between refusing to have sex when the opportunity arises, and engaging in unsafe sex. Hence, the strategy of always keeping condoms handy. If a person fails to use condoms because he or she cannot convince a partner to use condoms, providing that individual with communication and assertiveness skills will, in principle, alleviate this problem.

To underscore the point being developed here, behavior change theory focuses on factors such as "positive attitudes toward HIV preventive behavior" with the understanding that, at the aggregate level, more positive attitudes are associated with more frequent preventive behavior. The interventionist, in contrast, may focus entirely on a case-by-case examination of sexual situations in which a condom was not used or in which the individual felt that using a condom was especially challenging. Whereas the theorist is concerned with constructs which "in general" are correlated with preventive behavior, the practitioner is concerned with situational variables which, *at a specific point in time and for a specific individual*, prevent or complicate preventive behavior.

Consider several of the factors that may determine whether condoms are used on a given occasion:

1. whether condoms were used with the same partner in the past,
2. whether the partner refuses to use condoms or is known to have an aversion to condoms,
3. whether condom use is perceived as a personal responsibility or a decision that is left to one's partner,
4. whether condom use was attempted and failed due to incorrect use,
5. whether the female partner, in a heterosexual encounter, is using hormonal contraception at the time,
6. whether both partners are in a stable monogamous relationship with each other and have been tested for HIV.

Each time one of these factors is identified as a barrier to HIV preventive behavior, the trained interventionist may offer targeted advice or facilitate the development of an appropriate skill. It is sometimes unclear, however, whether the intervention effect is attributable to a change in, for example, attitudes toward the behavior, or whether it is instead attributable to the skill of the interventionist or the effect of the intervention on something other than attitudes toward the behavior, such as willingness to try condoms the next time one has sex. It is also unclear whether it is only one or two components of a multi-component intervention that are driving the outcome or whether several of these components are equally important, whether shifting the emphasis onto certain components will improve intervention outcomes in the future, and whether there are identifiable reasons why some individuals are not benefiting from the intervention.

Functional Contextualism

The perspective presented in this chapter is most widely known as "ecological." However, the term "ecological" has been used to describe such a wide range of fields and topics, so for the sake of precision, the term *functional contextualist* (c.f. Wulfert and Biglan, 1994) will be used instead. The term "functional" refers a focus on the interplay between traits (physical characteristics, personality, habits, learned associations) and states (salient goals, affective states, level of alertness and/or intoxication) in predicting and explaining behavior (Cattell and Johnson, 1986; c.f., Haynes and O'Brien, 2000). In this chapter, "traits" and "states" are recognized as *nomothetic* and *idiographic* variables respectively. The former refers to variables that are treated as though they are temporally stable. Hence, the term "nomothetic" encompasses variables that are clearly invariant (e.g., gender, race) and variables such as coping style, that are typically viewed as "trait-like," although they are not in fact invariant characteristics. The term "idiographic" refers to variables that are recognized as exhibiting meaningful (i.e. systematically related to behavior) within-person fluctuations over time and in diverse behavior settings.

The terms "nomothetic" and "idiographic" also describe epistemological orientations and denote, respectively, a programmatic focus on identifying variables that are reliably associated with an outcome net of the situation, or a focus on identifying variables which, when present, affect the likelihood of behavior on a discrete occasion (c.f., Tennen et al., 2000). This may be summarized as the distinction between a universalist and particularist orientation to the project of developing an empirical, theory-driven, systematic understanding of behavior.

The term "contextual" follows Stokols' (1987) understanding of context as an "everyday environmental setting"; to further clarify the concept, Stokols made a comparison between contextual and non-contextual research:

> "Whereas non-contextual research deals with target predictor[s] and outcome variables, contextual research includes supplementary predictor and outcome variables (e.g., the immediate situations and the person's life situations that impact the relationships between target variables). Moreover, whereas non-contextual analysis does not address relations among target variables, contextual analysis is directed toward assessing relations between situational and target variables" (cited in Wapner and Demick, 2002, p. 4).

From a non-contextual standpoint, randomized controlled trials are sufficient to demonstrate causality. To use this approach, one manipulates the independent variable, i.e., assignment to a treatment or control condition, and assesses changes in the dependent variable. To the extent possible, efforts are made to ensure that members of the treatment and control conditions do not systematically differ from each other at baseline. A randomized controlled trial (RCT) offers strong evidence that the manipulation, rather than some other factor, produces change in an outcome. Evidence of how the change occurred is not as strong – here, the researcher must rely on a mediational analysis. For example, evidence of mediation is shown if the magnitude of association between predictor X and outcome Y can be statistically shown to be influenced by the third variable M. This evidence is not as strong as the evidence of whether a change occurred because, typically, the researcher is unable to establish (a) whether changes in the mediating variable in fact preceded changes in the outcome and (b) whether the mediating variable is in fact related to the predictor (Cole and Maxwell, 2003). This has led some researchers to stress the value of a longitudinal (i.e. repeated measures) approach for addressing mediational hypotheses (Flora et al., 2007).

Randomizing individuals to treatment obscures the interaction between individual and treatment; hence, if a subset of the sample is assigned to Treatment A and a second subset to Treatment B, an RCT may be able to show which treatment performs best overall, but does not establish whether Treatment A or B might have been more effective for a given participant (Aldridge and Pietoni, 1987). This constitutes a limitation in terms of the ability of an RCT to test moderation.

Situational variables may modify the association between person and treatment. In a study that illustrates this problem, Steffensmeier et al (2006) conducted a literature review of studies assessing the association between beta-blockers and symptoms of depression. The authors compared studies that relied on RCTs and studies that relied on structured case reports. The RCTs found no association whereas the case reports did. Of note here is that the case reports relied on Naranjo scores; that is, two independent raters ranked the likelihood that, for a single participant, changes in level of depressive symptoms were consistent with the hypothesized effects of the drug or whether the changes in level of depressive symptoms might be attributable to other factors. The authors note that it is often the case that RCTs incorrectly include what may be termed "non-conforming instances" – such as occasions in which individuals take the drug and experience increased depression but the drug is not the cause of the depression.

Based on the logic of the RCT, when it is inappropriate or impossible to manipulate the independent variable, it is not possible to draw causal inferences. In other words, an observational approach, such as cross-sectional or conventional longitudinal design, cannot demonstrate that the predictor preceded the outcome and cannot rule out alternative explanations for any observed change in the outcome of interest. These alternative explanations revolve around characteristics of the person, and characteristics of the situations in which the outcome manifests. The contextual researcher, in contrast, models person-level and situation-level variables. The issue that we address next is whether the contextual researcher can legitimately claim to draw causal inferences from observational data, particularly with respect to mediating and moderating variables.

Context as Confound and as Explanation

Leigh and Stall (1994), in a discussion of the limitations of conventional observational research methods, point out that HIV prevention research has not depended on causal arguments. They note, for example, that when specific racial minority groups are shown to be at high risk of HIV, this does not imply that race or ethnicity are *causes* of elevated risk. Instead, minority status is a marker for a "complex set of social and psychological variables" (p. 133). By extension, they argue, it is not necessary to assume that the often-observed association between global levels of alcohol consumption and frequency of unsafe sex is causal in nature. Rather, alcohol use is simply a marker variable in the same way as race.

In the past several years, researchers have been considering the association between alcohol use and unsafe sex. In published investigations, one typically finds that a global association reported between frequency of alcohol use and frequency of unsafe sex is reported. The researchers reporting the finding remind the reader that a cross-sectional study does not permit causal inferences. Yet, in the discussion section, they suggest that one implication of finding a global alcohol use / unsafe sex association is that HIV prevention programs may benefit from including warnings that alcohol use is a "risk factor" for unsafe sex. Researchers have gone a step further to suggest that HIV risk-reduction interventions may achieve enhanced results by adding components aimed at alcohol use reduction (c.f., Kongnyey et al 2007; Weiser et al., 2006).

As most researchers recognize, there is a distinct possibility that some unmeasured "third variable" exists, such as sensation seeking or peer influence that may account for both willingness to engage in unsafe sex and excessive alcohol consumption. It is also clear that a global measure of alcohol use does not indicate whether the individual consumes alcohol prior to engaging in sex. For that matter, a correlation between global alcohol use and frequency of unsafe sex is mute with regard to whether the individual engages in protected or unprotected sex when he or she is *not* drinking.

If the "third variable" explanation applies, if the individual does not routinely drink prior to engaging in sex, or if the individual is just as likely to engage in unsafe sex when completely sober as he or she is when intoxicated, it is unlikely that alcohol use reduction will have any bearing on the rate of unsafe sex. Indeed, the most compelling justification for combining alcohol reduction components in an HIV risk reduction intervention would be evidence that acute alcohol impairment affects decision-making during sexual situations. Although supportive data have been found in laboratory studies relying on hypothetical risk scenarios, attempts to establish this association in naturalistic settings are complicated by (a) the existence of multiple motives for using alcohol in sexual situations, and (b) the embeddedness of both alcohol use and the opportunity for sexual risk-taking in multifaceted behavior settings.

If an intervention effective at reducing alcohol consumption produces a corresponding reduction in unsafe sex, the reduction may mean that alcohol use is indeed a proximate determinant of unsafe sex for at least some of the individuals completing the intervention. In some cases, it may mean that feelings of increased self-efficacy or increased emotional self-regulatory competence resulting from a successful reduction in alcohol use may generalize to a second health behavior domain, and thereby enhance the individual's ability to resist situational temptations to engage in unsafe sex. In some cases, it may mean that the individual has ceased visiting social venues where alcohol is served and sexual opportunities exist. The specification of whether, to what extent, or for whom these various explanations apply, could serve as a guide for empirically targeted individualized interventions (see Haynes and O'Brien, 2000).

Ecological Transitions

We have asserted that situations shape behavior, and that constructs such as attitudes toward the behavior, while providing a fairly good means of differentiating individuals who are in general more or less likely to practice the behavior, may be of limited prognostic value on any given occasion of sexual activity. The researcher who obtains a measure of participant attitudes is calling on the respondent to make global self-generalizations. At question is whether (1) an individual is able to accurately identify his or her own stable evaluative judgments in light of situational cues that systematically influence these judgments; (2) an individual is able to accurately weight each of the attitude-relevant situations he or she has experienced in the past in arriving at a global characterization and (3) whether the researcher is in fact calling upon the respondent to endorse an artificial construct that may not resonate with his or her lived experience.

Bronfenbrenner (1979) described *ecological transitions* as the movement from one behavior setting to another. He believed that continuities and discontinuities observed in behavior as the individual passes from one behavior setting to another are important foci for research, as these transitions help define the extent of situational influence. From the standpoint of behavior change, clinically-oriented researchers recognize the central importance of facilitating an individual's ability to recognize the situational triggers that may act as contributing causes to "lapse events" in which the individual deviates from his or her own personal behavior change agenda. That clinical intervention is often necessary before an individual will recognize these situational triggers supports our suspicion that the individual is an unreliable observer with respect to the effects of behavior settings on his or her own behavior.

The context-sensitivity of behavior and the unreliability of the individual as observer are challenges to achieving the goals of understanding, predicting, and changing behavior. One investigational practice that will lessen the magnitude of these challenges is to attempt to quantify the extent to which behavior settings affect the likelihood of a behavior. This will allow the researcher to supplement participant self-reports with additional insights obtained from a knowledge of the effects of the behavior settings through which the participant passes. A second practice is to limit, among participants under observation, the amount of time that passes between the behavior of interest and the participant's report of the behavior. With these concerns in mind we turn to the limits of recalled experience.

The Functional Contextualist Agenda
and the Limits of Recalled Experience

The functional contextualist position asserts that to understand people's behavior, including their sexual risk behavior, we must consider their situational goals, emotional states, and immediate situations. Although most social science research attempts to capture people's goals, emotional states and situations by asking them to recollect particular situations or to describe through recall their typical behavior and emotional reactions across situations, there is now converging evidence that autobiographical memory is not only inaccurate, but also systematically biased.

An impressive body of evidence indicates that people do not typically recall past or recent experience, especially emotional experience. Rather, they *reconstruct* their past experiences based on implicit theories and a variety of cognitive heuristics (Kahneman, 1999; Ross and Wilson, 2003). Because episodic memory fades fairly rapidly, people often draw upon their *beliefs* about past experiences, using identity-related beliefs or their beliefs about how they typically respond to the kind of situation they are being asked to reflect upon. In the domain of emotional experience, Robinson and Clore (2002) have demonstrated that people provide very different answers depending upon whether they report their mood in real-time or retrospectively. Since retrospective reports are heavily belief-based and influenced by narrative coherence, they can easily become dissociated from actual experience. Such dissociation has been demonstrated across several experiential and behavioral domains. For example, Stone, Shiffman, and DeVries (1999) found that a recalled interaction with another person, a critical aspect of retrospective reports of sexual risk behavior, can be affected by events that occurred since the interactions in question. And Carney et al. (1998) showed that the accuracy of recalled experience and behavior can vary dramatically across individuals.

A related corpus of evidence demonstrates how judgments of covariation or contingent relationships are biased through illusory correlation (Chapman, 1967), whereby the individual who expects a relationship between the two variables tends to overestimate the magnitude of any relation that might exist, or even infer a relation when none exists. In other words, people have great difficulty detecting, let alone recalling, covariation (Todd et al. 2005). Such biased judgments should be particularly troubling to investigators in the area of sexual risk behavior, where the accurate recollection of the contingencies among safe sex communication, alcohol, condom use and sexual intercourse is critical.

In sum, the literature on autobiographical memory has identified a myriad of processes that conspire to distort the recollection of personally relevant experiences and behavior, including how accurately people remember their sexual risk behavior. An occasion of unsafe sexual behavior is a discrete historical event. It may be indicative of a general pattern of behavior, or it may be a "non-conforming instance." As we have already noted, a behavior may be attributable to a given predictor on some occasions but not on others, in which case counting the behavior as evidence of the pattern is a misleading, even if common, practice. Investigators who are sympathetic to the functional conextextualist framework presented in this chapter and as such concerned with the connections between experiences and behaviors as they unfold in specific behavior settings, are urged to turn away from popular recall methods, and instead measure behavior, including sexual risk behavior, close to its real-time occurrence.

Probabilistic Causality

For many researchers, a cause is that which is both *necessary* and *sufficient* to produce a result. In terms of experimentation, this involves both the manipulation of an independent variable and the discounting of alternative explanations for the observed result. Yet there is another conceptualization of causality which arose from John Stuart Mill's doctrine of the plurality of causes. Mackie (1974) developed this line of thinking in his presentation of "insufficient and non-redundant parts of unnecessary but sufficient causes" or INUS causes. For example, a discarded cigarette is an insufficient part of a cause of a forest fire, because the outcome is dependent on additional factors such as dry brush and oxygen. It is non-redundant because, if it were not for the cigarette, the fire would not happen. It is unnecessary in that a set of variables that does not include a discarded cigarette – substituting, for example, a lightning strike or arson – could produce the same outcome.

To continue the example of alcohol-involved sexual activity, consider an individual who attends a bar that is frequented by sex workers, and is both more likely to drink as a consequence of entering this social venue and more likely to employ a sex worker. The same individual may drink at home with his wife or at a family gathering, and in these contexts alcohol use does not lead to unsafe sex. He may happen upon a sex worker outside the bar and have unsafe sex even if he is not drinking. Therefore, if alcohol exerts a causal influence on the likelihood of unsafe sex, it is clearly not in the traditional sense of the word "causal." One may fall back to the position of calling alcohol a "risk factor" or a "proximate determinant" of unsafe sex, but this is merely an evasion of the complex relationship between alcohol and unsafe sex.

Although researchers agree that there are situations during which alcohol use is unlikely to lead to unsafe sex, this is only rarely taken into account when attempting to empirically link alcohol use to unsafe sex. In determining the impact of alcohol use on unsafe sex, then, the researcher may opt to collect repeated measures of the individual's behavior over time and attempt to establish a baseline frequency of condom use during sex acts such as those involving sex workers, and determine whether alcohol use immediately prior to the sex act results in a significant change in the likelihood of unsafe sex.

An example of this approach is a diary study conducted by Barta et al. (2008) in which participants, consisting of PLWHA, were asked to record each occasion of sexual activity for five weeks. A total of over 1400 event-level records of discrete occasions of sexual activity were collected from 116 persons. Using a hierarchical linear regression model, event records were nested within participant to facilitate the simultaneous analysis of between-person and within-person effects. The substantial sample size achieved by treating event-records as units of analysis aided us in uncovering a complex interaction consisting of partner type (new versus ongoing) x partner serostatus (HIV-positive versus HIV-negative) x partner drinking (yes or no) x number of drinks consumed. It appears that the estimated likelihood of unsafe sex on a given occasion is influenced by each of these factors. Of particular relevance to the current discussion is the finding that, for men and women, a dose-response association was observed between alcohol consumption and likelihood of unsafe sex, but only in the case of new, HIV-positive partners who were also drinking.

Haynes and O'Brien (2000) propose that, in order to demonstrate a causal relationship, four conditions must be met: (1) the two variables must covary; (2) temporal priority is established; (3) there must be a logical mechanism for the hypothesized causal relation; and (4) alternative explanations for the observed covariance must be reasonably excluded (p. 164). To this list, we propose adding Nock's (2007) proposal that (5) a *gradient* or dose-dependent relationship is observed between the predictor and outcome.[1]

By these five criteria, Barta et al.'s findings, even though they consist of observational data, may be said to support a causal inference. Specifically, in a social context involving a new, seroconcordant partner, alcohol use increases the likelihood of unsafe sex. The statistical model indicates that, for a given individual, the likelihood of unprotected sex on a given occasion of sex is lower if the sex partner is neither new nor seroconcordant and if the individual and his or her partner are not drinking, as compared to the same individual's likely behavior given different configurations of social contextual cues. It is assumed, although impossible to verify, that each of these variables in isolation is an insufficient cause, but when considered collectively, these variables are both sufficient and unnecessary (in Mackie's sense of the word). The term "causal inference" is appropriate because this remains a *theory of a cause*, in acknowledgement that it is not possible to prove that a cause exists, as would be the case even in the most stringent experimental design.

Mechanism of Change

Although Haynes and O'Brien do not offer a formal definition of "mechanism," it is critical to the understanding of a functional-contextual approach. Nock (2007) differentiates between "cause" and "mechanism" by analogy to internal versus construct validity: The former identifies *what* produces a change in the dependent variable, whereas the latter identifies *how* the change occurred. Nock asserts that, in order to establish a causal relationship, an experimental design is necessary; this is based on the reasonable assumption that before one can begin to speak of X as a cause of Y, one must establish that it is X and not some other extraneous variable that is driving the observed effect. This line of reasoning is also based on the assumption that there exists a single cause operating in isolation of other contributing causes. We hold a somewhat different view.

Bechtel (2007) defines the term "mechanism" as "an organized system of component parts and component operations. The mechanism's components and their organization produce its behavior, thereby instantiating a phenomenon (p. 314)." Identifying a mechanism of change and conducting empirical tests to substantiate the functional interrelationships of

---

[1] Nock asserts the principle of *specificity* as a criterion for causal inference. In the case of the alcohol – unsafe sex association, the principle of specificity would require that alcohol be shown to increase the risk of unsafe sex without producing a broader change in the individual's pattern of behavior. Nock also asserts that an experimental design is required to test causal hypotheses. We disagree, provided that the five conditions listed here are met.

the component parts of the mechanism enables the functional-contextualist researcher to satisfy one criterion for establishing a causal association, in that these empirical tests permit the researcher to isolate redundant or spurious predictors.

The notion that one may identify causes by establishing both *which* predictor out of many potential predictors is valid and *how* the predictor effects a change in the outcome is the logic employed by advocates of a causal modeling approach. Causal modeling approaches rely on tests of statistical mediation and moderation to substantiate the "how" question. However, Nock asserts that one establishes a causal association only by means of repeated measurements. According to Nock,

> Demonstration of a mechanism of change requires evidence that change in the independent variable precedes change in the proposed mechanism, and that change in the mechanism precedes change in the outcome of interest …. The common procedure of measuring proposed mechanisms and outcomes of interest at pretreatment and post-treatment is insufficient. Showing a temporal relationship requires simultaneous and repeated assessment of the proposed mechanism and outcome over the course of treatment (p. 6).

We concur with Nock that the demonstration of temporal precedence and *incremental* change over time are critical if one's goal is to isolate and better understand mechanisms of change. Moreover, augmenting randomized controlled designs with a systematic effort to identify mechanisms of action would significantly advance both confidence in the findings and the ability to isolate features of an intervention that are most strongly associated with the observed outcome.

LEVELS OF ENVIRONMENTAL INFLUENCE ON BEHAVIOR

The Macrosystem

The incidence of 40,000 new cases of HIV per year has remained roughly flat for the last ten years, even as the composition of the affected groups has shifted. Some of the risk communities that were hardest hit during the early years of the epidemic, such as men who have sex with men (MSM), have shown steady improvements in terms of adopting HIV/STI preventive behavior and reducing the rate of infection. However, other groups have shown increasing rates of infection; whereas only 5% of HIV infections occurred through heterosexual transmission in 1983, the rate had risen to 28% by 2001. HIV is increasingly prevalent among women, Hispanics, and African Americans (Osmond, 2003). Today, over half of all STIs diagnosed are among individuals aged 15-24, and about once every hour, another young adult is infected by HIV (Futterman, 2005).

In attempting to understand the factors that give rise to the high rate of STI in this country, particularly revealing findings emerged from an empirical comparison of data collected from 15-19 year old women in four countries. When asked to identify what method of contraception was used the first time they had sexual intercourse, American women were the most likely to report "none." Indeed, this was reported by 25% of women, and only 33%

reported using condoms as opposed to the pill or other forms of contraception that do not provide protection against HIV/STI (Darroch et al., 2001).

The most likely explanation for this cross-country disparity in the rate of contraceptive use is that each of the countries included in the comparison, other than the U.S., provides mandated, comprehensive, medically accurate sex education to 15-19 year old youth. Although the mandate to provide some form of sex education exists in three quarters of all states in the U.S., very little guidance is offered on content or duration. In most cases, sex education consists of only a "few" class periods (typically as part of a general health class) and sometimes only a single class period (Kaiser Family Foundation, 2004).

This is, of course, only a partial answer. The politicization of sex education is unlikely to have come about were it not for pre-existing cultural attitudes toward sexuality. Health educators have observed a reticence among Americans to speak frankly about sexual issues, and a particular unwillingness to acknowledge that children below the age of 18 are sexually active (c.f., Donovan and Ross, 2000; Reiss, 1990; Weinberg et al., 2000). It is nonetheless clear that many individuals in this age range are sexually active and lack necessary medical information. Liau et al. (2002) recruited over 500 African American women aged 14-18 from disadvantaged communities. Based on biological data collected from participants, the authors found that a startling 28% tested positive, and had evidently failed to detect or failed to seek treatment for, one of three STIs, including *Neisseria gonorrhoeae*, *Chlamydia trachomatis*, and *Trichomonas vaginalis*.

As evidence of resistance to acknowledging STI as a problem in this age group, a national survey of high school principals conducted by the Kaiser Family Foundation survey revealed that 52% described the risk of STI among their students as "minor" and 12% as "no problem at all." Nearly half felt that STI was less of a problem for their own students as compared to the students of other schools. Further evidence can be found in the recent controversy occasioned by the development of a safe and effective vaccine for human papillomavirus (HPV). From a public health standpoint, the risk-to-benefit ratio supports adding this vaccine to routine childhood immunization schedules. Over half of all women will be exposed to HPV at some point in their lives (Koutsky, 1997), and roughly 70% of all cases of cervical cancer can be directly attributed to HPV infection (Charo, 2007). Yet, state legislators who are comfortable requiring parents to vaccinate their children for measles, mumps, and rubella have balked at mandating vaccination for HPV.

Shortcomings in sex education are also a likely contributor to the high abortion rate observed in the U.S. Even though fewer adolescent pregnancies are resolved through abortion in the U.S. as compared to other developed countries, the high number of adolescents who become pregnant has resulted in the U.S. having one of the highest abortion rates among developed, wealthy nations (Darroch et al., 2001).

Despite these sharp differences in the frequency of adverse sexual health outcomes, in many respects, the behavior of American adolescents is not very different from that of adolescents in other countries. As Darroch et al. note, U.S. adolescents are no more or less likely to report being sexually experienced, as compared to adolescents of the same age range in Canada, France, Great Britain, or Sweden. Nor are American adolescents more likely to report having had intercourse in the last 3 months.

U.S. adolescents do differ in one important respect: they are more likely to report having had a higher lifetime number of sex partners, which is attributable to cross-country differences in the typical duration of intimate relationships. This finding suggests that interventions aimed at improving the quality of adolescent relationships, and thereby reducing the rate of partner turn-over associated with serial monogamy, may have HIV/STI preventive utility. Yet, in light of the macrosystem variables described above, such an approach is unlikely to find traction in the U.S., in that it might be viewed as legitimizing sexual relationships among unmarried adolescents. It may nonetheless be useful to consider what factors might contribute to the instability of adolescent intimate relationships, as will be discussed below.

Sexualized Entertainment Media: A Spurious Predictor?

Longitudinal findings gathered in the U.S. suggest that 12-14 year old youth who report a relatively high exposure to sexually-themed television programs and magazines are more likely to report being sexually experienced two years later (Brown et al., 2006). These findings were marshaled in support of what may be termed a "kindling hypothesis," specifically, that level of exposure to sexually-themed material is a risk factor for precocious sexual activity. Early sexual debut, in turn, is widely regarded as a risk factor for unsafe sexual behavior. The reasonableness of this hypothesis, at face value, is greater if one accepts the premise that this association may be understood without regard for contextual factors.

Indeed, at odds with the kindling hypothesis is the fact that, among the five developed, wealthy nations studied by Darroch et al. (2001), the U.S. is both the most restrictive in terms of the regulation of sexually-themed programming and advertising in mass media outlets, and the most severely affected by STI and unintended pregnancy. In France, although genital organs are not shown, partial nudity and erotic content are accepted in television programming as well as billboard and magazine advertising (Bajos and Durand, 2001). In Sweden, a similar but perhaps even more liberal attitude is evident, and there is a lack of concern regarding potential adverse consequences of children seeing images of human genitalia (Danielsson et al., 2001). The tenor of the sexually-themed material available on the streets and in the living rooms in these countries varies widely, ranging from content that might be considered artistic or inoffensive to content that is likely to be considered degrading even by the most permissive standards.

Of course, it would be reckless to draw any firm conclusions from this cross-country comparison without undertaking a more thorough consideration of the variables that distinguish the U.S. from these other countries. For example, in addition to a greater acceptance of erotic content in public spaces, parents residing in the European nations mentioned here are, in general, more likely than parents in the U.S. to conduct candid conversations about sex with their children (c.f. Bajos and Durand, 2001; Danielsson et al., 2001). These data do, however, suggest that exposure to sexual themes is insufficient in itself to generate an increase in sexual risk behavior.

The theory proposed by Brown et al. that early exposure to sexually themed material may promote early sexual behavior is a reasonable one. However, it is also reasonable to suppose just the opposite -- that the practice of censoring sexual themes may communicate and perpetuate the cultural equation of sexuality with harm, embarrassment, and disgust. This in turn, according to Reiss (1990), may have a chilling effect on conversations about sexual health and STIs among adolescents. To substantiate Reiss' hypothesis, Weinberg et al. (2000) conducted a comparison of attitudes among U.S. and Swedish youth. They found Swedish youth to be more accepting of a "naturalistic" view of sexuality as a normal and healthy part of life, more accepting of gender egalitarianism, less likely to view masturbation, nudity, pornography, and desire for sex with a variety of partners as abnormal, shameful or repugnant, and more likely to oppose restrictions on homosexual behavior and abortion, which is free on demand in Sweden (Edgardh, 2002). Yet, as noted earlier, Swedish youth are far less likely than American youth to report multiple lifetime sexual partners, to engage in unsafe sex, seek abortion, or engage in teenage childbearing. As Edgardh notes, recent upticks in STI among Swedish youth have been reported, but are directly attributable to economic stagnation in Sweden and resulting cutbacks in the level of comprehensive sex education provided in schools.

At question is whether the cross-sectional association between level of association of exposure to sexual themes and early sexual debut supports the first theory or casts doubt on the second. Stated differently, does a correlational finding provide a warrant for intervention? In this instance, the finding that exposure to sexual media is associated with early sexual debut prompts Brown et al. to advise educating parents on the "negative effects of media on youth" (p. 1026). This exhortation may resonate with parents who are already uncomfortable discussing sexual issues with their children, and result in an increase in parental efforts to shelter their children from sexual material of any kind. If Reiss's hypothesis is valid, this would bring about an unwanted outcome.

Earlier, we made the distinction between "contextual" and "non-contextual" research. From a non-contextual standpoint, which focuses on the relationship between the predictor and outcome, one may be inclined to accept the premise that unmeasured extraneous variables are unlikely to be as consistently linked to the outcome as the predictor variable. In contrast, a contextual approach incorporates additional predictor and outcome variables to reflect the effects of situational and life history variables and interactions among these variables. In Brown et al.'s study, exposure to sexually-themed media manifested as consumption of magazines such as *Playboy* and *Maxim* which contain sexual content, and consumption of music produced by artists known for their sexually-themed lyrics. This is not "exposure" in the same sense as exposure to second hand cigarette smoke or indoor mold. Instead, it is exposure resulting from the motivated behavior of seeking sexual material. Therefore, examining the functions of seeking sexual material is an indispensibly important step when considering the effects of context and history on behavior. From this perspective, the influence of so-called "third variables" is not a quirk of a particular study design or sample, but an inevitable occurrence. In this instance, it is reasonable to conjecture that a high pre-existing interest in sex might lead to both increased consumption of sexually-themed material and early sexual debut.

In pursuing the goal of substantiating a single hypothesized relationship, one overlooks the possibility that many exist. For some adolescents, consumption of sexually-themed material may provide a sexual outlet and contribute to the postponement of sexual activity.

For others, consumption of sexually-themed material and early sexual debut may each reap desired social rewards – such as defiance of parents or fitting in with peers. For others still, consumption of sexually-themed material may be a means of compensating for a lack of access to other sources of information about human sexuality. By ascertaining whether these distinct patterns exist in subsets of the sample, the researcher is equipped to develop targeted strategies for intervention or determine whether intervention is likely to have a bearing on sexual risk behavior. Just as the same outward behavior may have a multiplicity of causes, the same behavior may have a multiplicity of functions.

Early Sexual Debut

Early sexual debut is a predictor of STI and early pregnancy. As Nock (2007) and others remind us, a predictor need not be a cause or a contributing factor to the outcome. Early sexual debut is a risk factor in the sense that, once an individual becomes sexually active, he or she is likely to continue having sex with the same partner or with various partners, and each time an opportunity for sex arises, the individual may succumb to the situational temptation to have unsafe sex or have sex with a partner who has an STI. As such, early sexual debut is a marker variable, and individuals who report an early sexual debut are expected to be at higher than average risk of reporting higher numbers of sex partners, to report past experience with STI, or to test positive for STI. For this reason, when reporting the association between early sexual debut and adverse sexual health outcomes, researchers most often do not control for the number of years the individual has been sexually active, number of partners, or frequency of sex.

Nonetheless, there are findings that invite the conclusion that the factors giving rise to early sexual debut are also linked to unsafe sex and unintended pregnancy. Some have linked early age at first intercourse to low parental monitoring of adolescent behavior (Wight et al., 2006). Others have placed early sexual debut within a broader pattern of delinquent behavior, which is in turn linked to either deviant peer affiliations or externalizing behavior (c.f., Alexander et al 1990). Researchers suggest that interventions that successfully delay sexual debut may reap benefits in terms of preventing adverse sexual health outcomes (Kinsman et al., 1998).

To address the basic question of whether the factors that give rise to early sexual debut are in fact the same factors that give rise to sexual risk-taking, Tremblay et al (2004) conducted an empirical investigation and found that self-reported delinquent behavior and adverse peer influences are not associated with early debut, but are associated with sexual risk-taking. Kaestle et al. (2005) carried out an ambitious national probability sample of nearly 10,000 18-26 year old youth which included the collection of biological data to assess current STI; they found that, whereas an early age at sexual debut was associated with a greater likelihood of STI for an 18 year old, this association was no longer evident at age 23. Although efforts to delay sexual debut may confer a short term health benefit, they conclude, this benefit may not sustain itself over the long term. Kaestle et al caution that drawing erroneous conclusions from the seeming association between early age at sexual debut and sexual risk outcomes have the potential to magnify the already worrisome health disparities which exist in the U.S. Adolescents who go on to attend college will be exposed to additional HIV / STI prevention messages and in many cases develop greater health literacy, more accurate risk perceptions, and improved social problem-solving skills as a result of their education. Therefore, the delay of sexual activity may reduce lifetime risk of STI for college-bound children while failing to reduce the lifetime risk of STI for individuals who receive no further education after high school.

Early Sexual Debut (and Age Disparity) in Context

With Kaestle and colleagues' interpretive cautions in mind, it remains possible that early sexual debut will increase the risk of unsafe sex *during* sexual debut. Manlove et al (2006) considered differences based on gender and focused not on global associations but on the event-specific association between young age and contraceptive use at the first sexual encounter. For girls, young age was associated with a markedly lower likelihood of contraceptive use; however, the association between young age and lower contraceptive use was attenuated after taking into account the age difference between sex partners. Girls who reported both young age at sexual debut and having debuted with a partner who was at least five years older were half as likely to have used contraceptives. They were also twice as likely to report having given birth during their teenage years. Among those reporting both early age at sexual debut and partner age disparity, a relatively high percentage also reported that the first-time sexual experience was unwanted or involuntary. An additional likely contributor to unsafe sex at first intercourse, Manlove et al. note, is the power imbalance that may manifest when there is an age disparity between intimate partners.

The age disparities mentioned here are also of concern because older partners are also more likely to have an STI than same-age partners (Hallett et al., 2007). It is not merely a matter of older men seeking younger partners. In resource-deprived settings in which sexual partnerships provide tangible economic benefits, women are more likely to prize older men because they are more likely to have realized their earning potential. When a young woman is 14 years old and her partner is 20, age disparity is the most conspicuous feature of this situation. However, structural, gender-based inequalities continue to exist for women as they progress into young adulthood, even if the age disparity narrows.

In the African American community, young men are at an advantage in the mating market owing to an unbalanced sex ratio. This unbalanced sex ratio is attributable to multiple factors, such as the higher mortality rate of African American men as compared to women, the substantial numbers of young African American men who are incarcerated (Khan et al., 2007; Lane et al., 2004), and the fact that African American men are more likely than women to obtain partners who are not African American, thereby removing themselves from the pool of available partners (Gullickson et al., 2006). The fact that men are more likely than women to seek both younger and same age partners also results in fewer men being available to older adolescent and young adult women. Both because there are substantially fewer available men than women and because of the economic pressure to form heterosexual partnerships, women are more likely to form partnerships with men that they might otherwise reject (Lane et al., 2004). Fergusson et al. (2006) found this to be the case even among African American college women. The perceived scarcity of African American male partners was found to be associated with women being more tolerant of their partner conducting outside sexual relationships (i.e. concurrence) and lower assertiveness during condom use negotiation. Women are also more likely to seek concurrent sex partners as insurance against the economic and emotional costs of losing a partner (Adimora et al., 2002). These converging social patterns are particularly concerning in light of the fact that partner concurrence greatly accelerates the rate at which STI spreads throughout a community (Adimora et al., 2002) and because formerly incarcerated men are between three and five times more likely than other men to have HIV (Khan et al., 2007).

The structural and economic factors that influence women's selection of partners and their ability to assert themselves in sexual relationships illustrate the importance of a contextual approach. Researchers who have not adopted a contextualist orientation have examined effective HIV prevention interventions of the past – such as those that target women and provide communication and assertiveness skills – and attempted to bring these interventions into communities in which women are highly disadvantaged in terms of their decision-making power, with limited success (Donovan and Ross, 2000). Researchers who are more aware of these issues have focused on the development of topical microbicides as an HIV preventive measure, in that microbicides, unlike male condoms, are "woman-controlled" (Woodsong, 2004). This prophylactic method is still under development. However, researchers may eventually be forced to confront the question of whether, or under what circumstances, microbicides should be more strongly promoted than condoms even if (as may be the case) they are less effective than condoms in terms of protection against HIV. A careful consideration of contextual determinants is necessary if one is to arrive at an answer to this question that is both broadly generalizable and highly reliable with respect to a specific community.

The Microsystem

Early age at sexual debut and alcohol use during sexual situations have each been discussed as correlates of sexual risk behavior. A combinatorial effect may also exist, such that alcohol use is more strongly associated with unsafe sex during sexual debut among individuals who are relatively young at sexual debut (Dye and Upchurch, 2006). It is plausible that age disparity will predict a greater likelihood that alcohol will be used during the sexual debut of a minor. It is also plausible that age disparity will predict a greater likelihood of unsafe sex in situations in which alcohol is involved. Consistent with the notion of INUS causation mentioned earlier, all three of these predictors (young age, a prospective sex partner who is at least five years older, and alcohol use) may result in unsafe sex, but only if all three are present at a given point in time. From the standpoint of intervention research, the goal becomes one of empirically testing which of these component causes are the most reliably associated with the outcome and which of them is most readily modifiable through intervention.

In ecological research, Bronfenbrenner (1979) noted, "the principal main effects are likely to be interactions." He used these terms, taken from experimental design, loosely.

Nonetheless, he makes an important point. If one's goal is to predict whether condoms will be used during a discrete occasion of sexual activity, in all likelihood there are multiple factors acting in concert that will affect the outcome. It may be that no two sexual situations, like no two snowflakes, are entirely alike. Yet, it is reasonable to suppose that sexual situations are socially scripted events, and as such, there are properties of sexual situations that exist independently of the actors who happen to be involved in a particular sexual situation.

The two lifestyle factors that place the greatest number of young adults at risk for HIV/STI are the failure to use latex condoms consistently, and the practice of *serial monogamy with concurrence*. Concurrence, defined earlier, refers to the practice of maintaining two or more sexual relationships, and so technically, we are referring to ostensible monogamy. Within the context of serial monogamy, as enacted by adolescents and young adults, relationships often follow a certain progression. During the early phase, the likelihood that condoms will be used is variable and likely dependent on a range of situational factors such as the availability of condoms (Bryan et al., 2002), partner attractiveness (Agocha and Cooper, 1999), level of sexual arousal (Parsons et al., 2000), the age difference between partners (noted above), and other factors. During the middle phase, marked by increasing emotional intimacy and trust, the couple may discuss condom use and other contraceptive choices, or if condoms were used during the early phase, that may become a behavioral norm which carries into the middle phase. During the late phase, couples often make the transition from condom use to hormonal birth control.

Obstacles to Preventive Behavior During the Early Phase of a Relationship

Manlove et al (2003) found that adolescents who waited a longer time between the start of the relationship and the initiation of sex with that partner were more likely to discuss contraception before having sex and were more likely to use dual contraceptive methods (e.g., using both condoms and hormonal birth control to achieve maximum protection against both pregnancy and STI). Bryan et al (2002) found that mentioning condoms prior to having sex was a reliable predictor of whether condoms were ultimately used. Halpern-Felsher et al (2002) found that individuals who felt comfortable talking about condoms also tended to have more positive attitudes toward condoms. Some researchers have found that individuals who do not assume that a partner will react negatively if they bring up the subject of condoms, and are comfortable talking about condoms, are more likely to use condoms; moreover, this absence of negative outcome expectancies is a more reliable predictor of condom use than measures of attitudes, self-efficacy to negotiate condom use, or knowledge of various facets of STI-related health information and prevention strategies (Crosby et al., 2003).

A multiplicity of factors may increase the perceived costs of raising the subject of condom use. In a classic and influential study, Fisher, Fisher and Byrne (1977) demonstrated that individuals who stammered or blushed when requesting to buy condoms at a pharmacy were less likely to use condoms during sex; the idea that individuals may find sexual topics sufficiently anxiety-provoking that it obstructs sexual communication, but not so anxiety-provoking that it prevents them from having sex, has been borne out by subsequent research (Halpern et al., 2002). As noted above, macrosystem factors that are evident in the U.S. may deter individuals from talking openly about sexual issues. Power imbalances, as noted in connection with age disparity during sexual debut and in connection with communities where an unbalanced sex ratio exists, can also magnify the perceived barriers to safer sex communication. And personal experience with eliciting a negative partner reaction to a condom use request or the expectation that a negative reaction is likely will present a barrier to enacting the behavior.

Obstacles to Preventive Behavior During the Later Phases of a Relationship

Another social script manifests in established relationships, in which the transition from condoms to hormonal contraceptives is regarded as a symbolic gesture of both partners' intention to remain in the relationship indefinitely and to trust one another to remain faithful or at least HIV/STI free. Some of the pressures militating against condom use by established couples include the worry that the desire to continue using condoms implies distrust of the partner's fidelity, his/her claims to be free of HIV/STI, or his/her intention to remain committed to the relationship indefinitely. Moreover, the individual wishing to continue using condoms may fear the partner's inferences, worrying that the desire to continue using condoms may be construed as a sign that he/she has an STI or does not trust the partner (East et al., 2007). The factors that are germane to condom use by members of established dyads are both similar to and different than the factors guiding condom use decisions in first-time sexual encounters. Among the relevant factors are the competence of individuals to communicate and assert themselves effectively within the context of sexual relationships, and the degree to which a mature and rational approach is adopted over a highly romanticized social script.

Summary

By remaining cognizant of the multiple levels of environmental influence on individual behavior, the researcher is better able to evaluate competing hypotheses and better prepared to appreciate that behaviors are determined by multiple causal influences. We identified serial monogamy as a risk factor for HIV infection. However, this is a far more serious risk factor in the U.S. as compared to other developed countries. To appreciate why this may be the case, one may consider cross-country comparisons and comparisons between demographic groups within the U.S. in order to gain a better understanding of what role macrosystem variables play. These data indicate that: (1) many U.S. adolescents lack the socio-emotional competence to hold frank conversations with their sexual partners about safer sex; (2) there exists institutional resistance in the U.S. to recognizing and confronting sexual activity among minors; and (3) structurally-imposed gender-based power imbalances in the African-

American community lead to increased sexual risk behavior and disproportionately high rates of HIV infection.

Whereas early, global findings suggested that a global association exists between frequency and volume of alcohol use and likelihood of unsafe sex, newer research has incorporated contextual variables, and suggests that sexually inexperienced adolescents who attend social events where alcohol is served and who encounter an opportunity to have sex are less likely to use condoms during first-time sex with that partner (c.f., Weinhardt and Carey, 2000). A functional-contextual research may probe even further and inquire whether feelings of shame and discomfort associated with sexuality – for a given individual or a given subset of prospective intervention recipients -- affect: (a) the amount of alcohol consumed in sexual situations; (b) susceptibility to situational cues promoting sexually disinhibited behavior; (c) whether or not safer sex is discussed; (d) level of trepidation at the thought of using condoms with a sex partner; and (e) the likelihood of unsafe sex. By recognizing these multiple determinants and the potential for multiple, reciprocal interactions among them, the researcher may then consider which of these is most readily modifiable through behavioral intervention, which of these has the strongest impact on behavior, and which of these are most likely to generalize across behavior settings (c.f. Haynes and O'Brien, 2000).

Striking a feasible balance between the richness of idiographic data and the generalizability of nomothetic data has been a perennial challenge for behavior change specialists. Krueger and Piasecki (2002), for example, note that "the idiographic functional analyst is likely to develop a tailored, multivariate causal model that describes the patient's functioning in rich detail. While this is extremely useful for treating the patient, its tailored nature limits its applicability beyond the patient in question (p. 496)." Technological advances in electronic data capture and statistical advances in analyzing intensive repeated measures data demand that we take a fresh look at the existing idiographic-nomothetic divide.

CONCLUSION

In this chapter we have described the intersections between lifestyle and HIV transmission. In the course of doing so, we outlined a functional-contextualist theoretical framework in the hope of encouraging future research that is more attentive both to the mechanisms by which theorized associations between predictors and outcomes occur, and the context-sensitivity of behavior. We have discussed nomothetic variables such as race and gender, which are understood to be unchanging and which distinguish between persons. We have also identified, as equally important, idiographic variables such as the situation-specific and partner-specific cues that either instigate or inhibit HIV preventive behavior on a specific occasion of sexual activity, and that may help us to better understand sources of within-person behavioral consistency and inconsistency across situations.

Our focus on factors that influence within-person consistency or situational variability in HIV preventive behavior is intended to stimulate the search for the kind of evidence that is of greatest interest to adolescents and young adults at risk for STI, their parents, and interventionists who seek to reduce HIV risk. As Lambert, Doucette and Bickman (2001) have noted, children and adolescents, their parents, and treating clinicians are most interested in outcomes (and we would add, *mechanisms*) at the *individual* level. Nonetheless, investigators and funding agencies have to this point been interested in outcomes and mechanisms at the *aggregated group* level. In other words, individuals who are directly involved in delivering interventions and individuals who are responsible for assessing the effectiveness of interventions currently represent two very different constituencies. The former constituency is most concerned with the drivers of individual behavior in specific situations, and the latter is most concerned with factors linked to patterns of behavior manifesting in groups and net of situation-specific or person-specific determinants. The functional-contextualist framework we advance in this chapter has the potential to satisfy the needs of both constituencies. In doing so, it has the potential to promote an important innovation in HIV/STI behavior change research and practice.

REFERENCES

Adimora, A.A., Schoenbach, V.J., Bonas, D.M., Martinson, F.E.A., Donaldson, K.H., and Stancil, T.R. (2002). Concurrent sexual partnerships among women in the United States. *Epidemiology, 13,* 320-327.

Agocha, V.B. and Cooper, M.L. (1999). Risk perceptions and safer-sex intentions: Does a partner's physical attractiveness undermine the use of risk-relevant information? *Personality and Social Psychology Bulletin, 25,* 746-759.

Ajzen, I. (1991). The theory of planned behavior. *Organizational Behavior and Human Decision Processes, 50,* 179-210.

Aldridge, D. and Pietoni, P. (1987). Research trials in general practice: Towards a focus on clinical practice. *Family Practice, 4,* 311-315.

Alexander, C.S. Young, J.K., Ensminger, M., Jounson, K.E., Smith, B.J., and Dolan, L.J. (1990). A measure of risk taking for young adolescents: Reliability and validity assessments. *Journal of Youth and Adolescence, 19,* 559-569.

Bajos, N. and Durand, S. (2001). *Teenage sexual and reproductive behavior in developed countries: Country report for France.* NY: Guttmacher Institute.

Barta, W., Portnoy, D., Kiene, S.M. Tennen, H., Abu-Hasaballah, K.S. and Ferrer, R. (2008*).* A Daily Process Investigation of Alcohol-Involved Sexual Risk Behavior Among Economically Disadvantaged Problem Drinkers Living with HIV/AIDS. *AIDS and Behavior,* electronic pre-print, DOI 10.1007/s10461-007-9342-

Bechtel, W. (2005). The challenge of characterizing operations in the mechanisms underlying behavior. *Journal of the Experimental Analysis of Behavior, 84,* 313-325.

Becker, M.H. (1974). The health belief model and personal health behavior. *Health Education Monographs, 2,* 324-508.

Bem, D. (1967). Self-perception: An alternative interpretation of cognitive dissonance phenomena. *Psychological Review, 74,* 183-200.

Bronfenbrenner, U. (1979). *The ecology of human development.* Cambridge: Harvard University Press.

Brown, J.D., L'Engle, K.L., Pardun, C.J., Guo, G., Kenneavy, K. and Jackson, C. (2005). Sexy media matter: Exposure to sexual content in music, movies, television and magazines predicts black and white adolescents' sexual behavior. *Pediatrics, 117*, 1018-1027.

Bryan, A., Fisher, J.D., and Fisher, W.A. (2002). Tests of the mediational role of preparatory safer sexual behavior in the context of the Theory of Planned Behavior. *Health Psychology, 32*, 71-80.

Carney, M.A., Tennen, H., Affleck, G., Del Boca, F.K., and Kranzler, H.R. (1998). Levels and patterns of alcohol consumption using timeline follow-back, daily diaries, and real-time "electronic interviews." *Journal of Studies on Alcohol, 59*, 447-454.

Cattell, R.B. and Johnson, R.C. (1986). *Functional psychological testing.* NY: Brunner/Mazel.

Cengiz, C., Park, J.S., Saraf, N. and Dieterich, D.T. (2005). HIV and liver diseases: Recent clinical advances. *Clinics in Liver Disease, 9*, 647-666.

Chapman, L. J. (1967). Illusory correlation in observational report. *Journal of Verbal Learning and Verbal Behavior, 6*, 151-156.

Charo, R.A. (2007). Politics, parents, and prophylaxis – Mandating HPV vaccination in the United States. *New England Journal of Medicine, 356*, 1905-1908.

Cole, D.A. and Maxwell, S.E. (2003). Testing mediational models with longitudinal data: Questions and tips in the use of structural equation modeling. *Journal of Abnormal Psychology, 112*, 558-577.

Crosby, R.A., DiClemente, R.J., Wingood, G.M., Salazar, L.F., Harrington, K., Davies, S.L. and Oh, M.K. (2003). Identification of strategies for promoting condom use: A prospective analysis of high-risk African American female teens. *Prevention Science, 4* (4), 263-270.

Danielsson, M., Rogala, C. and Sundström, K. (2001). *Teenage sexual and reproductive behavior in developed countries: Country report for Sweden.* NY: Guttmacher Institute.

Darroch, J.E., Singh, S., and Frost, J.J. (2001). Differences in teenage pregnancy rates among five developed countries: The roles of sexual activity and contraceptive use. *Family Planning Perspectives, 33* (6), 244-250 and 281.

Demmer, C. (2003). HIV prevention in the era of new treatments. *Health Promotion Practice, 4*, 449-456.

Donovan, B. and Ross, M.W. (2000). Preventing HIV: Determinants of sexual behaviour. *Lancet, 355*, 1897-1901.

Dye, C. and Upchurch, D.M. (2006). Moderating effects of gender on alcohol use: Implications for condom use at first intercourse. *Journal of School Health, 76*, 111-116.

Edgardh, K. (2002). Adolescent sexual health in Sweden. *Sexually Transmitted Infections, 78*, 352-356.

East, L., Jackson, D., O'Brien, L., and Peters, K. (2007). Use of the male condom by heterosexual adolescents and young people: Literature review. *Journal of Advanced Nursing, 59*, 103-110.

Fergusson, Y.O., Quinn, S.C., Eng, E. and Sandelowski, M. (2006). The gender ratio imbalance and its relationship to risk of HIV/AIDS among African-American women at historically black colleges and universities. *AIDS Care, 18*, 323-331.

Fishbein, M. and Ajzen, I. (1975). *Belief, attitude, intention, and behavior: An introduction to theory and research*. Reading, MA: Addison-Wesley.

Fisher, W.A., Fisher, J. D., and Byrne, D. (1977). Consumer reactions to contraceptive purchasing. *Personality and Social Psychology Bulletin, 3*, 293-296.

Flora, D.B., Khoo, S.T. and Chassin, L. (2007). Moderating effects of a risk factor: Modeling longitudinal moderated mediation in the development of adolescent heavy drinking. In T.D. Little, J.A. Bovaird, and N.A. Card (Eds.) Modeling contextual effects in longitudinal studies (p. 231-254). Mahwah, NJ: Erlbaum.

Futterman, D. (2005). HIV in adolescents and young adults: Half of all new infections in the United States. *Topics in HIV Medicine, 13*, 101-105.

Gallup, A.M. (2003). *The Gallup Survey*. Lanham, MD: Rowman and Littlefield.

Gullickson, A. (2006). Education and black-white interracial marriage. *Demography, 43*, 673-689.

Guttmacher Institute (2006). *Facts on sexually transmitted infections in the United States*. NY: Guttmacher Institute.

Hallett, T.B., Gregson, S., Lewis, J.J.C., Lopman, B.A., and Garnett, G.P. (2007). Behaviour change in generalized HIV epidemics: Impact of reducing cross-generational sex and delaying age at sexual debut. *Sexually Transmitted Infections, 83*, 50-54.

Halpern-Felsher, B.L., Kropp, R.Y., Boyer, C.B., Tschann, J.M. and Ellen, J.M. (2002). Adolescents' self-efficacy to communicate about sex: Its role in condom attitudes, commitment, and use. Adolescence, 39 (155), 443-456.

Halpern, C.T., Campbell, B., Agnew, C.R., Thompson, V. and Udry, J.R. (2002). Associations between stress reactivity and sexual and nonsexual risk taking in young adult human males. *Hormones and Behavior, 42*, 387-398.

Halpern, C.T., Hallfors, D., Bauer, D.J., Iritani, B., Waller, M.W. and Cho, H. (2004). Implications of racial and gender differences in patterns of adolescent risk behavior for HIV and other sexually transmitted diseases. *Perspectives on Sexual and Reproductive Health, 36*, 239-247.

Haynes, S.N. and O'Brien, W.H. (2000). *Principles and practice of behavioral assessment*. NY: Kluwer.

Hill, A.B. (1965). The environment and disease: Association or causation? *Proceedings of the Royal Society of Medicine, 58*, 295-300.

Hoyert, D.L., Kochanek, K.D., and Murphy, S.L. (1999). Deaths: Final data. *National Vital Statistics Reports, 47* (19). Hyattsville, MD: National Center for Health Statistics.

Kaestle, C.E., Halpern, C.T., Miller, W.C. and Ford, C.A. (2005). Young age at first sexual intercourse and sexually transmitted infections in adolescents and young adults. *American Journal of Epidemiology, 161*, 774-780.

Kahneman, D. (1999). Objective happiness. In D. Kahneman, E Diener, and N. Schwarz (Eds.), *Well-being: The foundations of hedonic psychology* (pp.85-105). NY: Russell Sage.

Kaiser Family Foundation (2004). *Sex Education in America*. Accessed online, http://www.kff.org/kaiserpolls/pomr012904oth.cfm

Kates, J., Sorien, R., Crowley, J.S. and Summers, T.A. (2002). Critical policy challenges in the third decade of the HIV/AIDS epidemic. *American Journal of Public Health, 92*, 1060-1063.

Kelly, J. (1995). *Changing HIV risk behavior: Practical strategies.* NY: Guilford.

Khan, M.R., Wohol, D.A., Weir, S.S., Adimora, A.A., Moseley, C., Norcott, K., Duncan, J., Kaufman, J.S. and Miller, W.C. (2007). Incarceration and risky sexual partnerships in a Southern U.S. city. *Journal of Urban Health*, DOI 1007/s11524-007-9237-8.

Kinsman, S.B., Romer, D., Furstenberg, F.F., and Schwarz, D.F. (1998). Early sexual initiation: The role of peer norms, *Pediatrics, 102*, 1185-1192.

Kongnyuy, E.J. and Wisonge, C.S. (2007). Alcohol use and extramarital sex among men in Cameroon. *BMC International Health and Human Rights, 7*, DOI: 10.1186/1472-698X-7-6.

Koutsky LA. Epidemiology of genital human papillomavirus infection (1997). *American Journal of Medicine, 102*, 3-8.

Krueger, R.F. and Piasecki, T.M. (2002). Toward a dimensional and psychometrically-informed approach to conceptualizing psychopathology. *Behaviour Research and Therapy, 40*, 485-499.

Lambert, E.W., Doucette, A., and Bickman, L. (2001). Measuring mental health outcomes in pre-post designs. *Journal of Behavioral Health Services and Research, 28,* 273-286.

Lane, S.D., Keefe, R.H., Rubinstein, R.A., Levandowski, B.A., Freedman, M., Rosenthal, A., Cibula, D.A., and Czerwinski, M. (2004). Marriage promotion and missing men: African American women in a demographic double bind. *Medical Anthropology Quarterly, 18*, 405-428.

Lescano, C.M., Hadley, W.S., Beausoleil, N.I, Brown, L.K., D'eramo, D., et al. (2007). A brief screening measure of adolescent risk behavior. *Child Psychiatry and Human Development*, 37, 325-336.

Liau, A., DiClemente, R.J., Wingood, G.M., Crosby, R.A., Williams, K.M., Harrington, K. et al. (2004). Associations between biologically confined marijuana use and laboratory-confirmed sexually transmitted diseases among African American adolescent females. *Sexually Transmitted Diseases, 29*, 387-390.

Mackie, J.L. (1974). *The cement of the universe: A study of causation.* Oxford: Clarendon.

Manlove, J., Ryan, S. and Franzetta, K. (2003). Patterns of contraceptive use within teenagers' first sexual relationships. *Perspectives on Sexual and Reproductive Health, 35*, 246-255.

Manlove, J., Terry-Humen, E., and Ikramullah, E. (2006). Young teenagers and older sexual partners: Correlates and consequences for males and females. *Perspectives on Sexual and Reproductive Health, 38*, 197-207.

Marlatt, G.A. and Gordon, J.R. (1985). *Relapse prevention: Maintenance strategies in the treatment of addictive behaviors.* NY: Guilford.

Miniño, A.M., Heron, M.P., Murphy, S.L., and Kochankek, K.D. (2007). Deaths: Final data. *National Vital Statistics Reports, 55* (19). Hyattsville, MD: National Center for Health Statistics.

Nock, M.K. (2007). Conceptual and design essentials for evaluating mechanisms of change. *Alcoholism: Clinical and Experimental Research, 31* (s3), 4s-12s.

Osmond, D.H. (2003). Epidemiology of HIV/AIDS in the United States. HIV InSite Knowledge Base Chapter. Accessed online, http://hivinsite.ucsf.edu.

Parsons, J.T., Halkitis, P.N., Bimbi, D., and Borkowski, T. (2000). Perceptions of the benefits and costs associated with condom use and unprotected sex among late adolescent college students. *Journal of Adolescence, 23*, 377-391.

Reiss, I.L. (1990). *An end to shame: Shaping our next sexual revolution.* NY: Prometheus Books.

Robinson, M.D., and Clore, G.L. (2002). Belief and feeling: Evidence for an accessibility model of emotional self-report. *Psychological Bulletin, 128,* 934-960.

Ross, M., and Wilson, A.E. (2003). Autobiographical memory and conceptions of self: Getting better all the time. *Current directions in Psychological Science, 12,* 66-69.

Staats, A.W. (1996). *Personality and behavior: Psychological behaviorism.* NY: Springer.

Stall, R. and Leigh, B.C. (1994). Understanding the relationship between drug or alcohol use and high risk sexual activity for HIV transmission: Where do we go from here? *Addiction, 89,* 131-134.

Steffensmeier, J.J.G., Ernst, M.E., Kelly, M., and Hartz, A.J. (2006). Do randomized controlled trials always trump case reports? A second look at propranolol and depression. *Pharmacotherapy, 26* (2), 162-167.

Stone, A. A., Shiffman, S., and DeVries, M. W. (1999). Ecological Momentary Assessment. In D. Kahneman, E. Diener, and N. Schwarz (Eds.), *Well-Being: The foundations of hedonic psychology* (pp. 26-39). New York, NY: Russell Sage.

Stokols, D. (1987). Conceptual strategies of environmental psychology. In D. Stokols and I. Altman (Eds), *Handbook of environmental psychology* (p. 41-70). NY: Wiley.

Tennen, H., Affleck, G., Armeli, S., and Carney, M.A. (2000). A daily process approach to coping. Linking theory, research, and practice. *American Psychologist, 55,* 626-636.

Todd, M., Armeli, S., Tennen, H., Carney, M. A., Ball, S. A., Kranzler, H.. R., and Affleck G. (2005). Drinking to cope: A comparison of questionnaire and electronic diary reports. *Journal of Studies on Alcohol, 66,* 1121-1129.

Tremblay, L. and Frigon, J.-Y. (2004). Biobehavioural and cognitive determinants of adolescent girls' involvement in sexual risk behaviours: A test of three theoretical models. *Canadian Journal of Human Sexuality, 13,* 29-43.

Wapner, S and Demick, J. (2002). The increasing contexts of context in the study of environment behavior relations. In R.B. Bechtel and A. Churchman (Eds.) *Handbook of environmental psychology.* NY: Wiley.

Weinberg, M.S., Lottes, I., and Shaver, F.M. (2000). Sociocultural correlates of permissive sexual attitudes: A test of Reiss's hypotheses about Sweden and the United States. *Journal of Sex Research, 37,* 44-52.

Weinhardt, L.S. and Carey, M.P. (2000). Does alcohol lead to sexual risk behavior? Findings from event-level research. In J.R. Heiman, C.M. Davis, and S.L. Davis (Eds.), *Annual review of sex research* (vol. 11, p. 125 -157). Society for the Scientific Study of Sexuality.

Weinstein, N.D. (2007). Misleading tests of health behavior theories. *Annals of Behavioral Medicine, 33* (1), 1-10.

Weiser, S.D., Leiter, K., Heisler, M., McFarland, W., Korte, F.P., DeMonner, S.M., Tlou, S., Phaladze, N., et al. (2006). A population-based study on alcohol and high-risk sexual behaviors in Botswana. *Public Library of Science Journal, 3*, 1940-1948.

Wight, D., Williamson, L., and Henderson, M. (2006). Parental influences on young people's sexual behaviour: A longitudinal analysis. *Journal of Adolescents, 29*, 473-494.

Woodsong, C. (2004). Covert use of topical microbicides: Implications for acceptability and use. *International Family Planning Perspectives, 30* (2) 94 -98.

Wulfert, E., Biglan, A. (1994). A contextual approach to research on AIDS prevention. *The Behavior Analyst, 17*, 353-363.

In: Life Style and Health Research Progress
Editors: A. B. Turley, G. C. Hofmann

ISBN: 978-1-60456-427-3
© 2008 Nova Science Publishers, Inc.

Chapter III

The Role of Procedural vs. Chronic Stress and Other Psychological Factors in IVF Success Rates

Hillary Klonoff-Cohen[*]
Department of Family and Preventive Medicine
University of California, San Diego

ABSTRACT

Background: Assisted reproductive technology (ART) including in vitro fertilization (IVF), intracytoplasmic sperm injection (ICSI), gamete intrafallopian transfer (GIFT), and zygote intrafallopian transfer (ZIFT) are universally available for infertile couples. Currently, 123,200 ART cycles are performed each year in the US, and >99% of these are IVF treatments. It is well documented that live birth success rates decrease significantly with advancing age, from 37% (<35 years), to 29% (35-37 years), to 20% (38-40 years), and finally 11% (41-42 years). Female and male lifestyle habits such as psychological stress could additionally influence IVF success rates, although there is no conclusive experimental evidence that lower stress levels result in better fertility treatment outcomes. Inconsistent and contradictory findings on the effects of psychosocial stress on IVF outcomes could be explained by the lack of distinction made between acute (i.e., procedural) and chronic (i.e., lifetime) emotional stress responses. This discrepancy could also pertain to anxiety, depression, and coping styles. Hence, the purpose of this chapter is to assess the impact of procedural and chronic psychological factors on IVF endpoints.

Methods: An exhaustive computerized search of the published literature was conducted using 8 databases and employing strict eligibility criteria. A total of 372 abstracts were retrieved, and 322 were excluded. Only a smattering of articles (n=50) met the inclusion criteria. Studies that examined the effects of chronic and procedural

---

[*] Hillary Klonoff-Cohen: 9500 Gilman Drive, 0607, La Jolla, CA 92093-0607; email: hklonoffcohen@ucsd.edu; phone: (858) 822-2966

anxiety, depression, coping styles, marital satisfaction, and stress on IVF outcomes were evaluated. Gender effects were also considered.

Results: Higher levels of anxiety and ineffective coping at the time of the procedure were both associated with decreases in pregnancy, implantation, and fertilization rates in women. In addition, higher procedural stress negatively impacted pregnancy. In contrast, chronic depression and negative mood were associated with lower pregnancy rates. Marital satisfaction and gender related stress differences had no effect on any IVF endpoints. Thus, procedural anxiety, coping, and stress (i.e., hormones) appeared to affect pregnancy success rates, whereas the effects of depression and mood on pregnancy were found at baseline. Consequently, different psychological factors may have diverse effects at various IVF endpoints.

Summary: The field of reproductive endocrinology requires more prospective studies that simultaneously evaluate the relationship among multiple psychological factors, and the time points at which these factors are measured (i.e., baseline vs. procedural), on the array of IVF endpoints (i.e., live births). If the results suggested in this chapter are confirmed in subsequent studies, then reducing stressors at the time of the procedure may diminish the number of treatment cycles and increase pregnancy and live birth delivery success rates after undergoing IVF. Similarly, treatment of existing depression and negative mood prior to beginning the IVF cycle may be beneficial.

INTRODUCTION

Overview

Assisted reproductive technology (ART) has been life transforming for couples with longstanding female-factor or male-factor infertility. Currently, 123,200 ART cycles are performed each year in the US, and >99% of these are in vitro fertilization (IVF) treatments. It is well documented that live birth success rates decrease significantly with advancing age, from 37% (<35 years), to 29% (35-37 years), to 20% (38-40 years), and finally 11% (41-42 years) (SART, 2005). Female and male lifestyle habits such as psychological stress could additionally influence IVF success rates. In 2003, the former President of the American Society for Reproductive Medicine commented, "While no one has elucidated the physiological relationship between women's stress and their IVF outcomes, it is known that stress has a number of negative effects."

Daily hormone injections, frequent blood tests and ultrasounds, undergoing a laparoscopic surgical procedure to extract oocytes, and awaiting fertilization and pregnancy results may all precipitate stress. Other concerns include missing work and the financial cost of repeated attempts, since most insurance policies in the US do not cover IVF (Klonoff-Cohen and Natarajan, 2004). Most importantly, because ART is perceived as the treatment of last resort, if it fails, the couple must dismiss their dream of producing a genetic child. Therefore, it is imperative to determine the role that stress plays to maximize success rates (i.e., a healthy live birth).

Currently, there is no conclusive experimental evidence that lower stress levels result in better fertility treatment outcomes. However, inconsistent and contradictory results concerning the effects of psychological stress on IVF outcomes may be explained by the lack of distinction drawn between acute (i.e., procedural) and chronic (i.e., lifetime) emotional stress responses. Moreover, a plethora of terms and definitions plague the psychological and reproductive literature, which further compounds the problem. In this chapter, acute (procedural) stress will refer to stress produced by or during fertility treatments, while chronic (baseline) stress will indicate pre-existing lifetime stress, due to infertility or other problems. Mood state, anxiety, and depression will also be presented, since they represent further obstacles to a successful IVF outcome.

Primary Objective

The purpose of this chapter is to assess the impact of procedural and lifetime stress and other psychological factors on IVF endpoints. In addition, a proposed underlying mechanism, limitations, and future recommendations will be presented.

IVF Procedure

In vitro fertilization was the first assisted reproductive technique developed and is the most commonly performed procedure in the US. It is effective in overcoming a variety of infertility problems, including tubal factors or marked sperm deficiencies. IVF is a four-stage procedure that consists of: STAGE I -ovarian stimulation; STAGE II-egg retrieval; STAGE III-fertilization; and STAGE IV-embryo transfer (Seibel, 1980).

The IVF procedures consist of the following steps: [I] the woman undergoes a baseline ultrasound; [a] medications are given, independently or in combination, to induce multiple eggs to simultaneously mature (e.g., the main protocol for ovarian stimulation is pituitary down-regulation with a gonadotropin releasing hormone (GnRH) agonist, followed by stimulation with gonadotropin; human chorionic gonadotropin (hCG) is used for the final phase of oocyte maturation); [b] follicular development is monitored using two modalities, ultrasound and estradiol levels; [II] oocytes are retrieved from the follicle by transvaginal aspiration with ultrasound guidance; [a] the oocyte then matures in a culture medium for 5–8 hours; [b] the sperm sample is collected and added to the oocytes approximately 6 hours after oocyte collection; [III] fertilization is confirmed by microscopic examination for two pronuclei 16–20 hours later; and [IV] embryos are transferred to the uterus either 48 or 72 hours after oocyte aspiration.

Study Outcomes

IVF endpoints: oocyte aspiration, sperm parameters, fertilization, embryo transfer, implantation, spontaneous abortion, and achievement of a pregnancy and live birth delivery.

Psychological measures: stress, anxiety, mood, depression, marital status, coping, and stress-related gender differences

METHODS

Sources of Information

An intensive computerized search of the published literature was conducted on a total of 8 databases, specifically PubMED (MEDLINE) (beginning in 1953); Biosis previews (from 1969); Web of Science (from 1975); PsychINFO (beginning in 1840); LexisNexis Academic (from 1981); Expanded Academic ASAP (from 1980); Ovid Medline (from 1966).

Study Selection

Criteria for inclusion consisted of human studies, case-control (retrospective) and prospective studies, with detailed methods and statistical analyses sections. General exclusion criteria consisted of case-reports, meeting abstracts, expert opinions, newspaper articles, magazines, and comments, all of which had insufficient information on psychosocial stress and/or ART endpoints. Articles not written in English were also excluded.

The emotional aspects of IVF treatment, and the effects of stress-related infertility were not included. Intervention studies were also beyond the scope of our review. Frozen embryos and oocyte donation studies were excluded because of the inability to determine the effect of psychological stress on IVF outcomes. Furthermore, those studies involving general infertility and animal studies were discarded. Rather, this chapter focused on the effects of stress on IVF outcomes.

The criteria for selecting studies consisted of: 1) an appropriate study design, 2) description of the selection and characteristics of subjects and comparison group with a sample size of >25, 3) the existence of standardized IVF outcome measures, 4) the use of standardized instruments and/or hormone measures to verify psychological stress, and 5) the existence of multivariate analysis. Two independent reviewers reviewed the publications to be included in accordance with the above-mentioned criteria.

Search Results

A total of 372 abstracts were retrieved from the eight databases, and 322 abstracts were excluded based on the eligibility criteria (e.g., animal studies, case-reports, opinions, and meeting abstracts with limited data, not written in English, intervention studies, infertility-related stress, general IVF related stress with no endpoints, and stress related to discontinuation or dropouts from IVF). This resulted in a total of 50 studies that will be discussed in this chapter.

RESULTS

The sample sizes of the studies ranged from 37 patients (Reading *et al.*, 1989; Yong *et al.*, 2000) to 500 subjects (Harrison *et al.*, 1987) (table 7). All studies recruited couples attending IVF clinics at university-affiliated or private clinics.

The 50 studies used a variety of standardized self-report instruments to assess anxiety (i.e., State Trait Anxiety Inventory), depression (i.e., Beck, Lubin and Zung Depression Scales), mood (i.e., Bipolar Profile of Moods State and Multiple Affect Adjective Checklist), coping (i.e., Ways of Coping scale), and marital satisfaction (i.e., Marital Adjustment scale and Maudsley Marital questionnaire) on a variety of IVF endpoints, but primarily "achievement of a pregnancy."

State Trait Anxiety Inventory (STAI) and Fertilization, Implantation and Pregnancy

State-Trait Anxiety Inventory consists of two 20-item scales. The State scale measures the degree of anxiety at a particular given time and the Trait scale assesses a stable personality trait, examining a person's "anxiety proneness."

Among the 21 studies that used STAI, 9 found a significant correlation between anxiety and IVF outcomes (Ardenti *et al.*, 1999; Demyttenaere *et al.*, 1991; Demyttenaere *et al.*, 1992; Eugster *et al.*, 2006; Facchinetti *et al.*, 1997; Gallinelli *et al.*, 2001; Johnston *et al.*, 1987; Kee *et al.*, 2000; Smeenk *et al.*, 2001). Six of these 9 studies found an effect with STAI on IVF pregnancy outcomes. Demyttenaere *et al.* (1991,1992) used a Dutch translation, administering it in the early follicular phase, as well as during oocyte retrieval and embryo transfer, and found that procedural anxiety increased among women with unsuccessful pregnancies. Kee *et al.* (2000) used a Korean version of STAI and also confirmed that the level of anxiety at the time of the procedure was significantly less in pregnant compared to non-pregnant women. Facchinetti *et al.* (1997) reported that procedural anxiety increased in the pregnancy failure group, but found no difference in baseline anxiety between the two groups. Smeenk *et al.* (2001) stated that women with higher anxiety at baseline (pre-ovulation) had a decreased risk of achieving a pregnancy, albeit anxiety was not measured during the procedure. The independent effects of anxiety on pregnancy are unclear, because depression and anxiety were highly correlated,

In a prospective study of 47 women undergoing a second IVF attempt, increased episodic anxiety, defined as a prolonged stress response with high state anxiety both before and after treatment (measured with the Dutch version of STAI), resulted in lower pregnancy rates (Eugster *et al.*, 2006). Episodic anxiety was described as a superior measure to acute anxiety (i.e., a high state anxiety at one assessment point). In this study, acute anxiety had no predictive value for successful pregnancies.

Three studies reported a relationship between anxiety and implantation or fertilization. One study (Gallinelli *et al.*, 2001) determined that anxiety (based on STAI completed the evening before oocyte retrieval) was significantly correlated with decreased implantation rates. Finally, two studies (Ardenti *et al.*, 1999; Johnston *et al.*, 1987) found that fertilization failure was associated with a significant increase in procedural anxiety.

A further 12 studies reported non-significant findings (Boivin and Takefman, 1995; Csemiczky *et al.*, 2000, Harlow *et al.*, 1996; Lovely *et al.*, 2003; Merari *et al.*, 1992; Merari *et al.*, 2002; Milad *et al.*, 1998; Sanders and Bruce, 1999; Slade *et al.*, 1997; Stoleru *et al.*, 1997, Thiering *et al.*, 1993; and Verhaak *et al.*, 2001) for anxiety and pregnancy. Among these studies: 1) all conceptualized anxiety as a generalized state rather than specifying procedural or chronic and 2) several were based on small sample sizes (e.g., Lovely *et al.*, 2003; Milad *et al.*, 1998; Stoleru *et al.*, 1997).

Summary

Based on a limited number of studies, it may be that procedural anxiety is more important than baseline anxiety in predicting pregnancy, implantation, and fertilization successes or failures.

Depression Scales and IVF Associated Pregnancy

The Beck Depression Inventory is a 21-item self-report questionnaire used for assessing the presence and severity of depressive symptoms and concerns. The Zung Self-Rating Depression Scale is a 20-item self-report questionnaire that is widely used as a screening tool, covering affective, psychological and somatic symptoms associated with depression. The Depression Adjective Check List (Lubin, 1981) is a set of seven alternate lists that has been widely employed as a self-report measure of transient depressive mood in adult populations.

A total of three studies (Kee *et al.*, 2000; Smeenk *et al.* 2001; Verhaak *et al.*, 2001) investigated the effects of baseline depression on IVF outcomes using the Beck Depression Inventory, while 2 additional studies used the Zung Depression Scale (Demyttenaere *et al.*, 1992; Demyttenaere *et al.*, 1998) (table 2). All 5 studies reported that baseline depression (over the past few days and past month) was lower in women who became pregnant than in those who did not achieve a pregnancy. Demyteenaere *et al.* (1992) also reported a further relationship of baseline depression and higher spontaneous abortion rates.

Furthermore, 2 studies (Merari *et al.*, 1992; Merari *et al.*, 2002) revealed that procedural depression appeared to have no effect on pregnancy outcome, using Lubin's Depression Adjective Check List.

In contrast, a final prospective study on 166 women (Anderheim *et al.*, 2005) found no effect of baseline or procedural depression on pregnancy outcome using the Psychological General Well-Being Index (a 22 item measure of psychological well being) during the first IVF treatment.

Summary

The three depression scales (i.e., Beck, Zung, and Lubin) had fairly consistent results, specifically women who reported higher levels of baseline depression were less likely to achieve a successful pregnancy. These instruments were not ideal for measuring dispositional or more life long depression, since the Beck Depression Inventory and Zung Depression

Scale were designed to measure depression over the past few days and past month, respectively, rather than over a longer period of time. In addition, depression was only measured once at baseline for every study, except one (Verhaak *et al.*, 2001). Finally, all studies chose "achievement of a pregnancy" as the sole endpoint, apart from one study (Demyttenaere *et al.*, 1992) that used number of oocytes, embryo transfer, miscarriage, and pregnancy.

Table 1. STAI and IVF outcomes

Specific end-points	Significant	Non-significant
Total	9	12
Fertilization	2	-
Implantation	1	-
Pregnancy	6	12

Table 2. Studies on depression and IVF outcome

Scale	# of studies (n=8)	
IVF end-points	Significant	Non-significant
Beck Depression Inventory		
Pregnancy	3	
Zung (Von Zerssen) Depression		
Miscarriage	1*	-
Pregnancy	2	-
Lubin's Depression Adjective Check List (DACL)		
Pregnancy	-	2
Psychological General Well Being Index		
Pregnancy	-	1

* Miscarriage and pregnancy measured in the same study by Demyttenaere *et al.*, 1992.

Bipolar Profile of Moods State and Mean Affect Adjective Checklist and Number of Embryos Transferred, Fertilization, and Pregnancy, and Live Birth Delivery

The Profile of Mood States is a 65-item test designed to assess six dimensions of mood or affect. A total of 4 studies used Bipolar Profile of Mood States (POMS). Two studies reported a significant effect of baseline negative mood on pregnancy (table 3). Sanders and Bruce in 1999 reported that lower scores on POMS (specifically, measures of agreeable-hostile) at baseline and 1-3 months prior to treatment were associated with lower pregnancy rates. Verhaak *et al.* (2001) determined that non-pregnant women showed an increase in negative mood, measured by POMS 3-12 days prior to the IVF cycle and 3-4 weeks after the pregnancy test.

Contrary to this, Klonoff-Cohen *et al.* (2001) reported that procedural negative mood (i.e., anxiety, hostility, depression, and total POMS score) was associated with decreased fertilization rates and fewer embryos transferred. Nevertheless, an older study by Reading *et al.* (1989) found no effect of mood on pregnancy. Finally, Klonoff-Cohen *et al.* (2001)

reported that higher baseline negative mood (anxiety scale) was associated with an increased risk of no live birth delivery.

Yong *et al.* (2000) administered the Multiple Affect Adjective Checklist (MAACL), consisting of 132 adjectives under two standardized test sets, "in general" (trait) and "today" (state). The MAACL scores for anxiety, depression, and hostility were highest before pregnancy compared to baseline and embryo transfer.

Table 3. Other psychological scales and IVF outcome

Scale	# of studies (n=13)	
	Significant	Non-significant
Bipolar profile Mood Status (POMS)		
Fertilization	1*	-
Embryo transfer	1*	-
Pregnancy	2	1
Live birth delivery	1*	-
Multiple Affect Adjective Checklist		
Before Pregnancy	1	-
Ways of Coping Scale		
Fertilization	1	-
Implantation	1	-
Spontaneous Abortion	1	-
Pregnancy	2	1
Marital Adjustment scale and Maudsley Marital Questionnaire		
Pregnancy	0	2

* Same study by Klonoff-Cohen et al, 2001.

Summary

Data on mood affect and IVF endpoints are inadequate. Two studies confirmed that procedural mood had a negative effect on fertilization rates and number of embryos transferred (Klonoff-Cohen *et al.*, 2001) and prior to pregnancy (Yong *et al.*, 2000). Three additional studies incriminated baseline negative mood with decreased pregnancy rates (Sanders and Bruce, 1999; Verhaak *et al.*, 2001) and no live births (Klonoff-Cohen *et al.* 2001). Based on an exceedingly small number of studies, it appears that there may be a relationship between baseline negative mood and pregnancy rates.

Ways of Coping Scale and Fertilization, Spontaneous Abortions, Implantation, and Pregnancy

The Ways of Coping scale measures 7 categories of coping: 1) self-controlling, 2) cognitive escape avoidance, 3) behavioral escape avoidance, 4) distancing, 5) problem solving, 6) seeking social support and 7) positive reappraisal. The Stroop Color Word test is a test of mental (attentional) vitality and flexibility. The task tests the ability to read words more quickly and automatically than naming colors.

There were a total of 5 studies that focused on coping styles, and 4 (Demyttenaere *et al.*, 1992; Demyttenaere *et al.*, 1998; Gallinelli *et al.*, 2001; Stoleru *et al.*, 1997) were statistically significant (table 3). The Ways of Coping Checklist "blamed self" (measured 1 day before oocyte retrieval) was higher in women with unsuccessful fertilizations than in women with successful fertilizations (Stoleru *et al.*, 1997). Gallinelli *et al.* (2001) reported that better coping skills lowered systolic blood pressure and heart rate in response to the Stroop Color Word test (measured 1 day before oocyte retrieval) in patients achieving implantation. Demyttenaere *et al.* (1992) found women with higher active coping, avoidance, and expression of emotion scores (using the Dutch Westbrook Coping scale), had significantly lower pregnancy and higher abortion rates after the first clinic visit. Interestingly, a later study by Demyttenaere *et al.* (1998) determined that better coping occurred in women who became pregnant. In contrast, Boivin and Takefman (1995) found no relationship between measures of coping during treatment and pregnancy outcome.

Summary
Coping style measured at the time of the procedure had an effect on pregnancy, spontaneous abortion, fertilization, and implantation.

Marital Satisfaction and Pregnancy

There were 2 studies by Boivin and Takefman (1995) (who used the Marital Adjustment scale during IVF treatment) and Verhaak *et al.* (2001) (who used the Maudsley Marital Questionnaire at baseline and post-IVF) which both reported no relationship between marital satisfaction and pregnancy (table 3).

Summary
The limited data on the role of marital satisfaction measured at the time of the procedure, suggests that it has no effect on pregnancy rates.

Stress Hormones and IVF Outcomes

Seven studies investigated the effect of stress hormones in conjunction with psychological scales on IVF endpoints (table 4).

Serum
Three studies measured prolactin and cortisol hormones in serum (Demyttenaere *et al.*, 1992; Merari *et al.*, 1992; Csemiczky *et al.*, 2000). All studies used radioimmunoassay methods (RIA) apart from one (Csemiczky *et al.*, 2000), which used fluoroimmunoassay methods. Samples were collected ≥3 times in all studies.

Only one study (Demyttenaere *et al.*, 1992) found a significant effect of stress hormones on pregnancy outcome, whereby women with higher serum cortisol concentrations measured at oocyte aspiration and embryo transfer had lower pregnancy rates. Two additional studies refuted these findings (Csemiczky *et al.*, 2000; Merari *et al.*, 1992).

Table 4. Studies using hormones

Hormones	# of studies (n=7)	
IVF endpoints	Significant	Non-significant
Prolactin and cortisol		
Pregnancy	1	3
Cortisol, 6-sulphatoxy-melatonin		
Pregnancy	-	1
Cortisol, Adrenaline, Noradrenaline		
Pregnancy	1	-
Cortisol, prolactin, allopregnanolone		
Miscarriage		1

Urine

Lovely *et al.* (2003) measured cortisol and 6-sulphatoxy-melatonin in urine, once at baseline with RIA methods. Neither stress hormone had an effect on pregnancy outcome. Smeenk *et al.* (2005) evaluated urinary adrenaline, noradrenaline, and cortisol on 3 occasions (i.e., the day before treatment, before oocyte retrieval and embryo transfer) using RIA methods. They found significant effects of adrenaline and noradrenaline during oocyte retrieval and embryo transfer on pregnancy outcome, but no association with cortisol. Harlow *et al.* (1996) measured cortisol and prolactin with fluoroimmunoassay and found no effect on pregnancy outcome.

Saliva

Finally, Milad *et al.* (1998) used salivary cortisol, prolactin, allopregnanolone collected at 3 occasions (day 13, 20, 27 after ET) with RIA methods. Prolactine and cortisol had no effects on miscarriage.

Summary

There was a paucity of studies combining physiologic and psychological stress measures. Among the small number of studies that addressed this issue, there were different body fluids (i.e., serum, urine, saliva) and techniques (e.g., RIA and fluoroimmunoassay methods), different numbers of measures, and different time periods. This lack of consistency makes the interpretation of these studies difficult.

Nevertheless, two studies, respectively, found that serum cortisol (Demyttenaere *et al.*, 1992) and urinary adrenaline and noradrenaline (Smeenk *et al.*, 2005) measured during the time of the procedure negatively affected pregnancy outcome. Serum cortisol is a measure of acute stress evaluated at the time of the procedure (Demyttenaere *et al.*, 1992).

In contrast, Smeenk *et al.* (2005) measured urinary noradrenaline and adrenaline, markers of chronic stress, once nocturnally after midnight at three time points. Traditionally, 24-hour urine samples are used in studies of chronic stress. In addition, adrenaline and noradrenaline are very sensitive to movement and activity (i.e., standing up from a seated position), as well as caffeinated beverages, alcohol, and smoking. These concerns were never discussed in Smeenk *et al.* (2005).

Traditional biological stress markers do not necessarily reflect perceived stress (Campagne, 2006), and several attenuating interactions may occur between stress hormones relevant to fertility. Some studies found no effects of psychological stress hormones on IVF success rates (Harlow *et al.*, 1996; Milad *et al.*, 1998), possibly because they relied on "traditional" general biological stress markers that were not relevant, instead of using more specific sensitive markers (Czemiczky *et al.*, 2000). In the future, stress should be measured before and during IVF treatment, with a combination of biologic and psychological measures.

Male Stress and Sperm Parameters

A total of 7 studies investigated the effects of male stress on sperm parameters. Three (Kentenich *et al.*, 1992; Clarke *et al.*, 1999; Ragni and Caccamo, 1992) found a relationship between increased male stress and decreased semen quality (morphology), while the fourth study (Harrison *et al.*, 1987) reported lower sperm density, sperm count, and sperm motility (table 6).

Conversely, three studies reported no difference in semen quality (Drudy *et al.*, 1994), or sperm motility (Tarabusi *et al.*, 2000; Pellicer and Ruiz, 1989) as a function of male stress. Finally, in a meta-analysis, sperm density and count decreased from baseline to the time of the procedure, while the proportion of abnormal sperm increased (Klonoff-Cohen and Natarajan, 2007).

Summary
Male stress may have an impact on sperm morphology.

Gender-Related Stress Differences and Pregnancy Outcome

There were a total of 13 statistically significant studies comparing female and male stress during ART treatment (table 5). Eleven studies (Beutel *et al.*, 1999; Chan *et al.*, 1989; Collins *et al.*, 1992; Edelmann *et al.*, 1994; Hsu and Kuo, 2002; Laffont and Edelmann, 1994; Lee *et al.*, 2001; Merari *et al.*, 2002; Newton *et al.*, 1990; Phromyothi and Virutamasen, 2003; Stoleru *et al.*, 1997) reported higher stress in women regardless of whether it was measured at the time of baseline or the time of the procedure. There were no studies in which men reported higher stress than women. The remaining two studies found no gender related-stress differences at baseline (Freeman *et al.*, 1985) or during the procedure (Boivin *et al.*, 1998).

Summary
Women had higher stress than men at baseline and at the time of the procedure.

Table 5. Gender comparison studies on stress and IVF

	Number of studies
A total number of studies	13
Higher stress in women	11
Baseline:	(3)
Procedural:	(7)
After Treatment:	(1)
Higher stress in men	0
No differences between women and men	2
Baseline:	(1)
Procedural:	(1)

All findings are statistically significant.

Table 6. Studies of male stress on sperm parameters and IVF/ICSI

	Number of Studies	
	Significant	Non-significant
Total number of studies	7	
Decrease in semen quality	3	1
Decreased sperm density, count, and motility	1	2*

*Motility only.

Mechanism for Stress and IVF Endpoints

Early research on stress and reproduction was plagued with methodological problems. However, recent experimental, clinical, and population-based research provides new evidence and suggests novel biological mechanisms, Three super-systems, the endocrine, immune and nervous system are involved in multiple interactions during acute and chronic stress (Nepomnaschy et al., 2007).

It has been proposed that a cascade of stress related hormones may negatively influence sexual function by interfering with the hypothalamic-pituitary-gonadal (HPG) axis at all three of its levels: the hypothalamus (to inhibit GnRH secretion), the pituitary gland (to interfere with GnRH-induced luteinizing hormone (LH) and follicle stimulating hormone (FSH) release) and the gonads (to alter the stimulatory effects of LH and FSH on sex steroid secretion) (Rivier and Rivest, 1991). Although it is clear that both the hypothalamic-pituitary-adrenal axis (HPA) and HPG systems exist in humans, the physiological link between them has not been clinically proven in human trials. Further research is currently being conducted in humans and relevant animal species to understand the physiological mechanisms behind the proposed HPA-HPG link and psychosocial stress and IVF endpoints.

Stress acts through different mechanisms, not only by inhibiting the HPA axis but also by altering the concentration of fertility hormones including FSH, GnRH, and LH, as well as substances such as cortisol, opioids, and melatonin. It also alters the follicular levels of glucocorticoid hormones, 11-beta hydroxysteroid dehydrogenase (11B-HSD), and affects semen quality. To differentiate acute stress from chronic stress in the future will require the collaboration of multi-disciplinary fields including gynaecology, biology, and psychology (Campagne, 2006).

CONCLUSION

In the ART literature, there is a lack of sophistication when measuring stress and other related psychological factors (e.g., anxiety, coping). Interviews (Boivin *et al.*, 1998), daily record keeping (Boivin *et al.*, 1998), and unstandardized questionnaires (Callan and Hennessey, 1988, Collins *et al.*, 1992) were used to elicit psychological information. Additionally, stress or other psychological factors were frequently measured only once (Bringhenti *et al.*, 1997; Callan and Hennessey, 1988; Chan *et al.*, 1989; Freeman *et al.*, 1985; Lee *et al.*, 2001). Furthermore, the type and timing of stress was overwhelmingly unspecified as acute or chronic.

There were multiple definitions for acute stress including "situational", "anticipatory", "treatment-related", and "procedural", all of which implied rather than specified exact time periods (e.g., oocyte retrieval or embryo transfer). "Baseline", "lifetime", "persistent", "pre-treatment", "predisposed", "pre-IVF", and "pre-existing" all described chronic stress, which was typically measured at the first visit, but allegedly inferred underlying stress in the past (e.g., 1 year ago, 1 month prior, during their lifetime). Timing of stress was altered depending on when the questionnaires were administered versus actually completed (particularly when patients filled them out at home). Finally, psychological instruments did not specify the appropriate time periods related to the questions, particularly "right now" "currently" or "today".

Taking these issues into account, we tried to advance the field by compiling, summarizing, and categorizing the studies by the effects of acute (i.e., procedural) vs. chronic stress and other psychological factors on IVF success rates (table 7). The overall major findings from the 50 studies were:

1. In women, anxiety, coping, and physiologic stress hormones measured at the time of the procedure negatively impacted IVF pregnancy success rates.
2. State (i.e., procedural) anxiety could eventually be a predictor for better pregnancy rates.
3. Men's stress could also be important to the ART process, but there were a paucity of studies on sperm parameters.
4. The effects of depression and mood at baseline negatively affected IVF-associated pregnancy rates.
5. The true contribution of chronic (i.e., lifetime) depression is unknown because of the lack of appropriate scales. Currently, depression is not measured as a long-term state, and no questionnaire asks about depressive symptoms over a very long time period. There are, standardized procedures for establishing the diagnosis of a long-term depressive disorder (e.g., Structured Clinical Interview for DSM Disorders) that use current and historical information (e.g., treatment, hospitalization) to establish a depression diagnoses.

6. One cannot rely solely on physiologic measures (e.g., adrenaline, noradrenaline, or cortisol) to determine the negative effects of stress on fertility treatment success rates, without standardization of: i) which specific or groups of hormones, ii) in what . body fluids, iii) when (e.g., during procedure vs. pre-treatment), and iv) how these indices should be measured.

The heterogeneity of these studies was primarily due to: 1) differences in study populations; 2) quality of self-reporting; 3) observing different IVF endpoints; and 4) types of stress instruments.

There is no consensus regarding the most appropriate measure of stress for infertile couples undergoing IVF. A final study employed seven instruments to provide a comprehensive evaluation of stress (i.e., Positive Affect Negative Affect Scale (PANAS), POMS, Perceived Stress Scale (before and after hormones), Expected Likelihood of Achieving a Pregnancy Scale, Infertility Reaction Scale, Ways of Coping Scale, and Network Resource Scale) at baseline and at the time of the procedure. They determined that both baseline acute and chronic stress affected biologic endpoints (i.e., the number of oocytes retrieved and fertilized), as well as pregnancy, live birth delivery, birth weight and multiple gestations, whereas procedural stress only influenced biological endpoints (Klonoff-Cohen *et al.*, 2001) (table 7). This study is not comparable because it focused on all the biologic and reproductive endpoints of IVF, prior to and at the time of treatment, using multiple measures of stress, which underscores the importance of replicating this inclusive approach.

Potential limitations of the studies that evaluated the effect of stress on IVF include: 1) using psychological measures that are general and not specific to ART; 2) not having a comparison group, apart from 7 studies that had a comparison group of fertile women that achieved pregnancy naturally (Baluch *et al.*, 1993; Bringhetti *et al.*, 1997; Csemiczky *et al.*, 2000; Harlow *et al.*, 1996; Hjelmstedt *et al.*, 2003; Kee *et al.*, 2000; Van Balen *et al.*, 1996); 3) having small sample sizes, high dropout rates, and retrospective or cross-sectional designs that measure stress at one time point, 4) recruiting only one race; 5) not examining IVF endpoints beyond pregnancy, specifically live birth deliveries and neonatal outcomes.

For future studies, there is a need for methodologically sound studies that identify markers for stress that are relevant to both acute and chronic stress and IVF outcomes. To achieve this, studies should: 1) consider baseline vs. procedural stress and all endpoints of IVF in the same study; 2) include a wider array of psychological factors; 3) assess both male and female roles; 4) include a comparison group; 5) adjust for potential confounders, including type of ovarian stimulation, number of embryos transferred, and other lifestyle habits, 6) collect multiple samples of stress hormones throughout the procedure, 7) obtain an adequate sample and good follow-up rates; 8) employ a longitudinal design to follow patients throughout the IVF procedure, pregnancy, and delivery; 9) investigate the impact of anti-depressant, anti-anxiety, and anti-stress medications on IVF outcomes; and 10) identify underlying mechanisms attributable to stress on IVF endpoints.

If the results suggested in this chapter are confirmed in subsequent studies, then reducing stressors at the time of the procedure may diminish the number of treatment cycles and increase pregnancy and live birth delivery success rates after undergoing IVF. Similarly, treatment of existing depression (as well as for other stressors such as negative mood) prior to beginning the IVF cycle may be beneficial.

Table 7. Summary of Psychological stress on IVF endpoints*

Endpoints	Authors	Sample	Type of stress
↓ Fertilization	Ardenti et al., 1999	n=200	Anxiety (P)
	Harrison et al., 1987	n=500	Stress (both B and P)
	Johnston et al., 1987	n=49	Anxiety (P)
	Klonoff-Cohen et al., 2001	n=151	Mood (anxiety, hostility, depression total score) (P), optimism (P)
	Stoleru et al., 1997	n= 48	Coping (P)
↓ Embryo Transfers	Klonoff-Cohen et al., 2001	n=151	Mood (depression and hostility) (P)
↓ Implantation	Gallinelli et al., 2001	n=40	Anxiety (P), Coping (P)
↓ Pregnancy rate	Demyttenaere et al., 1991	n=40	Anxiety (P)
	Demyttenaere et al., 1992	n=40	Depression (B), Anxiety (P), Coping (P), Cortisol (P)
	Demyttenaere et al., 1998	n=98	Depression (B), Coping (P)
	Boivin & Takefman, 1995	n=40	Stress (P)
	Eugster et al., 2006	n=47	Anxiety (E**)
	Facchinetti et al., 1997	n=49	Anxiety (P)
	Kee et al., 2000	n=216	Anxiety (P), Depression (B)
	Merari et al., 1992	n= 113	Depression (P)
	Merari et al., 2002	n=113	Depression (P)
	Sanders & Bruce, 1999	n=90	Mood (hostility) (B)
	Smeenk et al., 2001	n=291	Anxiety (B), Depression (B)
	Smeenk et al., 2005	n=168	Adrenaline/noradrenaline (P)
	Tarabusi et al., 2000	n=45	Heart rate (P)
	Thiering et al., 1993 (repeaters only)	n=330	Depression (Both B and P)
	Verhaak et al., 2001	n=207	Depression (B), Negative Mood (B)
	Yong et al., 2000	n=37	Mood/Affect (+)
↑ Spontaneous abortion	Demyttenaere et al., 1992	n=40	Depression (B), Coping (P)
No live birth delivery	Klonoff-Cohen et al., 2001	n=151	Negative Mood (anxiety) (B)

* Only statistically significant studies are presented
** E= Episodic Anxiety (defined as a prolonged stress response with high state anxiety both before and after treatment)
+ Before Pregnancy.

ACKNOWLEDGMENTS

The author would like to thank Ms. Angie Ghanem, BA for all her time and assistance in editing the chapter and compiling the tables. In addition, the author would like to express her gratitude to Dr. Elizabeth Klonoff for her suggestions regarding the psychological interpretations.

This chapter was supported by The University of California, Office of the President, Tobacco Related Disease Research Program, Grant # 4RT0032.

REFERENCES

Anderheim L, Holter H, Bergh C, Möller A (2005) Does psychological stress affect the outcome of in vitro fertilization? *Hum. Reprod.* 20(10):2969-75,

Ardenti R, Campari C, Agazzi L, La Sala GB. (1999) Anxiety and perceptive functioning of infertile women during in-vitro fertilization: exploratory survey of an Italian sample. *Hum. Reprod.* 14(12):3126-32.

Baluch B, Manyande A, Aghssa MM, Jafari R (1993) Failing to conceive with in vitro fertilization. *Psychol. Rep.* 72, 1107-1110.

Beutel M, Kupfer J, Kirchmeyer P, Kehde S, Kohn FM, Schroeder-Printzen I, Gips H, Herrero HJ, Weidner W (1999) Treatment-related stresses and depression in couples undergoing assisted reproductive treatment by IVF or ICSI. *Andrologia.* 31, 27–35.

Boivin J and Takefman JE (1995) Stress level across stages of in vitro fertilization in subsequently pregnant and nonpregnant women. *Fertil. Steril.* 64, 802–810.

Boivin J, Andersson L, Skoog-Svanberg A, Hjelmstedt A, Collins A, Bergh T (1998) Psychological reactions during in-vitro fertilization: similar response pattern in husbands and wives. *Hum. Reprod.* 13, 3262-3267.

Bringhenti F, Martinelli F, Ardenti R, La Sala GB (1997) Psychological adjustment of infertile women entering IVF treatment: differentiating aspects and influencing factors. *Acta Obstet. Gynecol. Scand.* 76, 431–437.

Callan VJ and Hennessey JF (1988) Emotional aspects in in-vitro fertilization and embryo transfer. J In Vitro Fert Embryo Transf 5, 290–295.

Campagne DM. (2006) Should fertilization treatment start with reducing stress? *Hum. Reprod.* 21(7):1651-8. Epub 2006 Mar 16.

Chan YF, O'hoy KF, Wong A, So WK, and Ho PC (1989) Psychosocial evaluation in an IVF/GIFT program in Hong Kong. *J. Reprod. Infant. Psych.* 7, 67–77.

Clarke RN, Klock SC, Geoghegan A, Travassos DE. (1999) Relationship between psychological stress and semen quality among in-vitro fertilization patients. *Hum. Reprod.* 14(3):753-8.

Collins A, Freeman EW, Boxer AS Tureck R (1992) Perception of infertility and treatment stress in females as compared with males entering in vitro fertilization treatment. *Fertil. Steril.* 57, 350–356.

Csemiczky G, Landgren BM, Collins A (2000) The influence of stress and state anxiety on the outcome of IVF-treatment: psychological and endocrinological assessment of Swedish women entering IVF-treatment. *Acta Obstet. Gynecol. Scand.* 79, 113–118.

Demyttenaere K, Nijs P, Evers-Kiebooms G, Koninckx PR. (1991) Coping, ineffectiveness of coping and the psychoendocrinological stress responses during in-vitro fertilization. *J. Psychosom. Res.* 1991;35(2-3):231-43.

Demyttenaere K, Nijs P, Evers-Kiebooms G, Koninckx PR (1992) Coping and the ineffectiveness of coping influence the outcome of in vitro fertilization through stress responses. *Psychoneuroendocrinology.* 17, 655–665.

Demyttenaere K, Bonte L, Gheldof M, Vervaeke M, Meuleman C, Vanderschuerem D, D'Hooghe T. (1998) Coping style and depression level influence outcome in in vitro fertilization. *Fertil. Steril.* 69(6):1026-33.

Drudy L, Harrison R, Verso J, Cottell E, Kondaveeti U, Barry-Kinsella C, Gordon A. (1994) Does patient semen quality alter during an in vitro fertilization (IVF) program in a manner that is clinically significant when specific counseling is in operation? *J. Assist. Reprod. Genet.* 11(4):185-8.

Edelmann RJ, Connolly KJ, Bartlett H. (1994) Coping strategies and psychological adjustment of couples presenting for IVF. *J. Psychosom. Res.* 38(4):355-64.

Eugster A, Vingerhoets AJJM, van Heck GL, and Merkus JMWM. (2004) The effect of episodic anxiety on an in vitro fertilization and intracytoplasmic sperm injection treatment outcome: A pilot study. *J. Psychosom. Obstet. Gynaecol.* 25(1):57-65

Facchinetti F, Matteo ML, Artini GP, Volpe A, Genazzani AR (1997) An increased vulnerability to stress is associated with a poor outcome of in vitro fertilization-embryo transfer treatment. *Fertil. Steril.* 68, 384-385.

Freeman EW, Boxer AS, Rickels K, Tureck R, Mastroianni L Jr. (1985) Psychological evaluation and support in a program of in vitro fertilization and embryo transfer. *Fertil. Steril.* 43, 48–53.

Gallinelli A, Roncaglia R, Matteo ML, Ciaccio I, Volpe A, Facchinetti F (2001) Immunological changes and stress are associated with different implantation rates in patients undergoing in vitro fertilization-embryo transfer. *Fertil. Steril.* 76, 85-91.

Harlow CR, Fahy UM, Talbot WM, Wardle PG, Hull MGR (1996) Stress and stress-related hormones during in-vitro fertilization treatment. *Hum. Reprod.* 11, 274–279.

Harrison KL, Callan VJ, Hennessey JF (1987) Stress and semen quality in an in-vitro fertilization program. *Fertil. Steril.* 48, 633-636.

Hjelmstedt A, Widstrom AM, Wramsby H, Hatthiesen AS, Collins A (2003) Personality factors and emotional responses to pregnancy among IVF couples in early pregnancy: a comparative study. *Acta Obstet. Gynecol. Scand.* 82, 151-161.

Hsu YL, Kuo BJ (2002) Evaluations of emotional reactions and coping behaviors as well as correlated factors for infertile couples receiving assisted reproductive technologies. *J. Nurs. Res.* 10, 291-302.

Johnston M, Shaw R, and Bird D (1987) Test-tube baby procedures: stress and judgments under uncertainty. *Psychol. Health.* 1, 25–38.

Kee BS, Jung BJ, Lee SH (2000) A study on psychological strain in IVF patients. *J. Assist. Reprod. Genet.* 17, 445-448.

Kentenich H, Schmiady H, Radke E, Stief G, Blankau A. (1992) The male IVF patient--psychosomatic considerations. *Hum. Reprod.* 7 Suppl 1:13-8.

Klonoff-Cohen H, Chu E, Natarajan L, Sieber W (2001) A prospective study of stress among women undergoing in vitro fertilization or gamete intrafallopian transfer. *Fertil. Steril.* 76,675-87.

Klonoff-Cohen H, and Natarajan, L. (2004) The concerns during assisted reproductive technologies (CART) scale and pregnancy outcomes. *Fertility and Sterility.* 81(4):982-988.

Klonoff-Cohen HS, Natarajan L. (2007) The impact of stress on pre- and post-sperm parameters among men undergoing IVF. Andrology Update. In press.

Laffont I, Edelmann RJ. (1994) Psychological aspects of in vitro fertilization: a gender comparison. *J. Psychosom. Obstet. Gynaecol.* 15(2):85-92.

Lee TY, Sun GH, Chao SC (2001) The effect of an infertility diagnosis on treatment-related stresses. *Arch. Androl.* 46, 67-71.

Lovely LP, Meyer WR, Ekstrom RD Golden, RN (2003) Effect of stress on pregnancy outcome among women undergoing assisted reproduction procedures. *South Med.* J 96, 548-551.

Lubin B. (1981) Additional data on the reliability and validity of the brief lists of the Depression Adjective Check Lists. *J. Clin. Psychol.* 37(4):809-11.

Merari D, Chetrit A, Modan B (2002) Emotional reaction and attitudes prior to in vitro fertilization: an inter-spouse study. *Psychol. Health.* 17, 629-640.

Merari D, Feldberg D, Elizur A, Goldman J, Modan B (1992) Psychological and hormonal changes in the course of in vitro fertilization. *J. Assist. Reprod. Genet.* 9, 161–169.

Milad M, Klock S, Moses S, Chatterton R (1998) Stress and anxiety do not result in pregnancy wastage. *Hum. Reprod.* 13, 2296–2300.

Nepomnaschy PA, Sheiner E, Mastorakos G, Arck PC. (2007) Stress, immune function, and women's reproduction. *Ann. N. Y. Acad. Sci.* 1113:350-64.

Newton CR, Hearn MT, Yuzpe AA (1990) Psychological assessment and follow-up after in-vitro fertilization: assessing the impact of failure. *Fertil. Steril.* 54, 879-886.

Pellicer A, Ruiz M. (1989) Fertilization in vitro of human oocytes by spermatozoa collected in different stressful situations. *Hum. Reprod.* 4(7):817-20.

Phromyothi V, Virutamasen P (2003) The determinant factors and the anxiety level of infertile couples during the treatment of in vitro fertilization and embryo transfer at Chulalongkorn Hospital. *J. Med. Assoc. Thai.* 86, 425-429.

Reading AE, Chang LC, Kerin JF (1989) Psychological state and coping styles across an IVF treatment cycle. *J. Reprod. Infant. Psychol.* 7, 95-103.

Ragni G, Caccamo A. (1992) Negative effect of stress of in vitro fertilization program on quality of semen. *Acta Eur. Fertil.* 23(1):21-3.

Rivier C, Rivest S (1991) Effect of stress on the activity of the hypothalamic-pituitary-gonadal axis: Peripheral and central mechanisms. *Biol. Reprod.* 45:523-32.

Sanders KA and Bruce NQ (1999) Psychosocial stress and treatment outcome following assisted reproductive technology. *Hum. Reprod.* 14, 1656–1662.

Seibel, M., ed. *Infertility: A Comprehensive Text.* 1980, Appleton and Lange: East Norwalk.

Slade P, Emery J, Lieberman BA. (1997) A prospective, longitudinal study of emotions and relationships in in-vitro fertilization treatment. *Hum. Reprod.* 12(1):183-90.

Smeenk JM, Verhaak CM, Eugster A, van Minnen A, Zielhuis GA, Braat DD (2001) The effect of anxiety and depression on the outcome of in-vitro fertilization. *Hum. Reprod.* 16, 1420-3.

Smeenk JM, Verhaak CM, Vingerhoets AJ, Sweep CG, Merkus JM, Willemsen SJ, van Minnen A, Straatman H, Braat DD. (2005) Stress and outcome success in IVF: the role of self-reports and endocrine variables. *Hum. Reprod.* 20(4):991-6. Epub 2005 Jan 21.

Society for Reproductive Technology (SART) (2005) National Clinic Summary Report. Accessed November 27, 2007. Available from: http://www.sart.org/

Stoleru S, Cornet D, Vaugeois P, Fermanian J, Magnin F, Zerah S, Spira A (1997) The influence of psychological factors on the outcome of the fertilization step of in vitro fertilization. *J. Psychosom. Obstet. Gynaecol.* 18, 189-202.

Tarabusi M, Matteo ML, Volpe A, Faccinetti F (2000) Stress-response in male partners of women submitted to in vitro fertilization and embryo transfer. *Psychother. Psychosom.* 69, 275-279.

Thiering P, Beaurepaire J, Jones M, Saunders D, Tennant C. (1993) Mood state as a predictor of treatment outcome after in vitro fertilization/embryo transfer technology (IVF/ET). *J. Psychosom. Res.* 37(5):481-91.

Verhaak CM, Smeenk JM, Eugster A, van Minnen A, Kremer JA, Kraaimaat FW (2001) Stress and marital satisfaction among women before and after their first cycle of in vitro fertilization and intracytoplasmic sperm injection. *Fertil. Steril.* 76, 525-531.

Yong P, Martin C, Thong J. (2000) A comparison of psychological functioning in women at different stages of in vitro fertilization treatment using the mean affect adjective check list. *J. Assist. Reprod. Genet.* (10):553-6.

In: Life Style and Health Research Progress
Editors: A. B. Turley, G. C. Hofmann

ISBN: 978-1-60456-427-3
© 2008 Nova Science Publishers, Inc.

Chapter IV

Use and Effectiveness of Three Modalities of Emotion Regulation After Negative Life Events: Rumination, Distraction and Social Sharing

Olimpia Matarazzo
Department of Psychology, Second University of Naples, Italy[1]

ABSTRACT

This study assessed the extent and efficacy of three regulatory modalities of the emotions elicited by negative life events: rumination, distraction and social sharing. Despite the wide literature existing on this subject, to my knowledge this is the first study comparing these regulatory modalities, from adolescence to old age, in order to estimate their use and their effectiveness in function of the significance of the negative event and of the participants' gender and age.

Eight hundred persons (400 female, 400 male) participated in this study: 200 adolescents (13-19); 200 young people (20-29); 200 adults (30-59); 200 old people (60-89). They were randomly assigned to two research conditions: very significant vs. not very significant negative life events.

Participants were asked to describe a very important negative life event or a not very important one and assess on 7-point scales when the event occurred, its appraisal, perceived importance and impact upon their beliefs, emotional intensity, the extent of rumination, distraction and social sharing, along with their relative frequency and duration, and their effectiveness to re-establish cognitive equilibrium and modulate the negative emotional burden; finally, the recovery from the event was assessed.

Qualitative data were treated through log-linear analyses. Quantitative data were first reduced by performing principal component analyses and then submitted to mediational regression analyses to evaluate the incidence of event significance on the three regulatory

[1] This research was supported by the Italian Ministry for University and Scientific Research: Grant FIRB RBAU017KNF_002 to Olimpia Matarazzo.

modalities through mediator variables (referred to the perceived cognitive and emotional event impact), controlling for gender and age. Finally, multiple regression analysis was performed to assess the effectiveness of rumination, distraction and social sharing in recovering from the event.

In brief, results showed that the significant events produced a higher cognitive and emotional impact than the less significant ones. Such impact, in turn, elicited a greater use of rumination and social sharing, a more consistent sense of pervasiveness of rumination and paradoxical effect of distraction. Instead, a suppression effect emerged on the use and perceived effectiveness of distraction.

The recovery from the event was positively predicted by the temporal distance from the event and the perceived effectiveness of rumination and social sharing, whereas it was negatively predicted by the use and extent of rumination, the cognitive impact of the event and the paradoxical effect of distraction. Females were more affected by the event impact and resorted to rumination and social sharing more than males. With age the use of social sharing and distraction grew.

The theoretical implications of these results are discussed.

INTRODUCTION

Emotion Regulation

Emotions play an important role in human (and in non-human) life. Since they arise as a sudden and whole-body response to an external or internal event appraised as relevant for the person's goals and well-being, they serve primarily a twofold communicational function: at the intrapersonal level, they inform the individuals whether or not the current state of affairs conforms to their concerns; at the interpersonal level, they signal to others the person's affective reaction through their physical manifestations. Emotions provide also a motivational function: they mobilise the organism's resources in order to activate cognitive and behavioural reactions able to maintain or modify the relationship between the individual and the environment (Arnold, 1960; Frijda, 1986; Lazarus, 1991; Stein, Trabasso, & Liwag, 1993). According to this point of view, rather than as feeling states, emotions are conceived as a multicomponential process unfolding over time, generated by the appraisal of an event, which develops into a set of physiological, experiential, expressive and behavioural reactions showing a temporal "dynamics" (Thompson, 1990), i.e. latency, increase, magnitude, duration and recovery. All the phases of the emotion genesis and deployment can be consciously or unconsciously, intrinsically or extrinsically monitored, evaluated and modified, so that the resulting explicit emotional reaction is mediated by the regulative action of these processes that can increase its adaptive value (Campos, Frankel, & Camras, 2004; Frijda, 1986, 2006, 2007; Thompson, 1994).

The concept of emotion regulation encompasses the whole of the processes by which emotions are shaped by individuals or by individual-environment transactions, that is the processes involving the cognitive, neurophysiological and behavioural level of the organism's functioning and the process managing inter-individual changes. The motives for regulation are supposed to be generally in the service of the individual's goals, such as promoting well-being and improving social interactions by showing a circumstance-appropriate emotional reaction. From this latter point of view, emotion regulation serves a similar function to display rules (Ekman & Friesen, 1969), while the function of restoring well-being by reducing the emotional impact generated by stressful events had already been highlighted by the studies on coping, especially as regards the role of emotion-focused coping (Lazarus & Folkman, 1984).

Although a wide agreement exists about the aforementioned inclusive definition of emotion regulation, many divergent positions persist regarding its origin, extension, loci, and effectiveness. For instance, some scholars see emotion regulation as coextensive with emotion, as part and parcel of it, often experientially and structurally indistinguishable (Campos *et al.*, 2004; Frijda, 1986, 2006, 2007); others hold a two-factors approach, according to which it would be worthy to distinguish, methodologically or ontologically, emotion and emotion regulation as two separate phenomena, the latter indicating the changes in emotion dynamics and in its hedonic valence once the emotion has been elicited, or the proactive measures activated in order to prevent or modify the insurgence of unwanted emotions (Cole, Martin, & Dennis, 2004; Gross, 1999; Gross & Thompson, 2007; Thompson, 1994). Other researchers take an intermediate position: Eisenberg and colleagues (Eisenberg, Fabes, Guthrie, & Reise, 2000) assume that some aspects of emotion regulation are an inherent part of the emotion genesis and manifestation, while others occur after the emotion onset or deployment. They also differentiate, for heuristic purposes, emotion regulation from emotion-related behavior regulation (or behavioral regulation), the former concerning the manipulation of "internal feeling states and emotion-related physiological processes" (Eisenberg *et al.*, 2000 p. 137), the latter concerning the management of the emotional expressions and actions. Emotion regulation is thought to involve attentional and cognitive processes (e. g. antecedents selection, appraisal), as well as neurophysiological processes. Behavioral regulation is assumed to encompass the effortful attempts to modulate the manifestations of emotional reaction (often in conformity with the display rules) and modify the emotion-inducing situations.

This distinction partially overlaps with Frijda's (1986) differentiation between regulation related to stimulus processing and regulation concerning output generation: the former is kept to encompass the means by which antecedents and appraisal are managed, the latter is thought to imply the control or modulation of the action readiness and explicit behavior. Both regulation processes can be conscious or unconscious: the stimulus processing can be regulated through the voluntary manipulation of attention and of approach towards the emotional stimuli (e.g. diverting from or focusing on them), through the aware modification of appraisal, or by means of defence mechanisms (Freud, 1926; A. Freud, 1946), such as denial, detachment, intellectualization, rationalization, isolation and so on. The output regulation can be produced by the voluntary inhibition, attenuation or enhancement of the emotional impulse, manifestation and related behavior, or by means of the homeostatic processes that act to keep a dynamic balance among the various physiological aspects of the affective reaction.

Gross and colleagues (Gross, 1998, Gross & Thompson, 2007; John & Gross, 2004) posit a large bipartition between antecedent-focused and response-focused regulation, but distinguish four modalities[2] within the first type of regulation: situation selection, situation modification, attentional deployment, cognitive change. The first two modalities refer to avoiding or altering the circumstances supposed to generate negative emotions and broadly correspond to the construct of proactive coping (Aspinwall & Taylor, 1997), that is the efforts activated to prevent the occurrence or alter the form of a potentially stressful event. Attentional deployment is reputed to encompass two major modalities: distraction and concentration. Distraction refers to averting the attention from taxing situations or from negative internal states and turning it to more positive aspects of the situation or to more agreeable thoughts and memories. Instead, concentration refers to focusing upon the features and thoughts concerning the emotional situation; when such concentration is reiterated and uncontrollable, it is termed rumination. Later, I will further discuss these two modalities, distraction and rumination, which represent, together with social sharing, the core of this study. Cognitive change regards modifying the emotional meaning of an event in order to alter its emotional impact. This modality largely corresponds to the well known reappraisal process (Lazarus, 1991; Folkman & Lazarus, 1988), by which the original appraisal of a stressful event is fashioned in a more positive way in order to reduce its burden, or the initial evaluation of one's own ability to cope with the event is reappraised in a more empowered way. According to Gross and colleagues, the response-focused regulation, which occurs after the onset of the emotional reaction, concerns the attempts to change or modulate the physiological, experiential and behavioral manifestations of the emotion, by means of medicaments, drugs, relaxation, suppression or ventilation of emotion expressivity, control of actions etc.

The construct of emotion regulation largely intersects, and overlaps with, the previous construct of coping, definable as the whole of the attempts and strategies that individuals activate in order to master stressful situations, i.e. situations that are appraised as exceeding one's own resources, in case of major stressors, or as taxing one's functioning, in case of daily hassles (Carver, Scheier, & Weintraub, 1989; Lazarus & Folkman, 1984, Lazarus, 1991). The coping tradition, however, does not typically comprise in its domain processes such as modulating positive emotions, or manifesting emotions in conformity with the display rules, and it has mainly focused on the conscious aspects of dealing with negative events, leaving out the unconscious and the automatic ones. Therefore, some scholars envisage emotion regulation as the wider domain encompassing the research in the coping area (Garnefski, Kraaij, & Spinhoven, 2001), whereas others (Compas, Connor-Smith, Saltzman, Thomsen & Wadsworth, 2001) have a different perspective and see emotion regulation as emotion-focused coping (i.e., coping referred to the cognitive or behavioral attempts to manage the emotions elicited by the stressor; Lazarus & Folkman, 1984); and others still prefer to conceive the two domains as separate but partially overlapping (Gross, 1999; Gross & Thompson, 2007).

I need to state that in this study that I assume a two-factor approach to emotion regulation, in the sense that I do not examine the short-time emotional dynamics but, I am

---

[2] Although the term generally used in literature to indicate all that people activate to cope with stressful events and regulate emotional experience is "strategies", I prefer to use the more neutral entry "modalities" because a "strategy" denotes planned actions aimed at a goal, whereas in my opinion the way of dealing with emotional events and experiences is often lacking planning and deliberateness.

interested in the long-term emotion regulation that is the manipulation of a negative emotion after its insurgence in order to reduce its aversive impact. This capacity is a form of meta-emotion (Gottman, Katz, & Hooven, 1997), supposing a level of cognitive development such that it can allow an individual to be aware and reflective of his/her internal states and able to deal with them. As Campos *et al.* (2004) admit, this "canonical" instance of two-factor emotion regulation can be observed only from teenagers onwards, i.e., the age groups examined in this study.

Besides, it is worthy to specify that the object of this study, that is dealing with negative life events after their occurrence, leads into the domain where emotion regulation and coping largely overlap: therefore, in this chapter I will use the terms 'coping' and 'emotion regulation' interchangeably[3].

ADAPTIVE AND NONADAPTIVE INSTANCES OF EMOTION REGULATION

Since emotion regulation implies that individuals are able to assess the environment's requests and their own resources and react in a flexible and adaptive way, this ability is seen as a central component of emotional competence (Saarni, 1990) and emotional intelligence (Salovey & Mayer, 1990) constructs. On a general level, both of them indicate the individual's capability of identifying, understanding, and managing emotions in effective and socially adequate ways.

Nevertheless, not all the means of regulating one's emotions are always helpful. For instance, the numerous studies that Gross and colleagues performed on reappraisal and suppression (e.g. Gross & John, 2003; Gross & Levenson, 1993, 1997; John & Gross, 2004) showed that the first strategy is by far more effective than the second. Since reappraisal – i.e., the modification in a more positive (or, according to the circumstance's requests, in a more negative) way of the emotional meaning of an event – occurs before the emotional response has been deployed, it is able to mutate the full emotional process without significantly entailing physiological, cognitive or relational charges. These results confirm the findings coming from the early studies on coping (Lazarus & Alefert, 1964; Lazarus, 1966), showing that preventive information useful to reappraise the meaning of cruel or disgusting films led to a decrease of the negative emotional experience without a concomitant increase of the arousal. They substantiate also the results of the correlational studies between emotion regulation styles and well-being showing that the habitual use of reappraisal is positively correlated with high tolerance to stressful events and is negatively correlated with depression, anxiety and other psychological diseases (Garnefski & Kraaij, 2006, 2007; Garnefski *et al.*, 2001).

On the contrary, suppression operates directly on the emotional reaction, after it has been deployed, by mitigating, abolishing or emphasizing its expression but without influencing the subjective experience. Since suppression demands effortful attempts in order to control

---

[3] I will use also the terms 'emotion', 'affect', and 'mood' interchangeably, because the distinction between them is not relevant to purposes of this study.

emotion manifestations, it entails a waste of cognitive resources otherwise employable and, according to John & Gross (2004), its habitual use is positively correlated with negative emotions, depression, and memory troubles. Other ineffective regulatory modalities include self-blame, rumination, catastrophizing (Garnefski & Kraaij, 2006, 2007; Garnefski *et al.*, 2001), venting, focusing on negative feelings (Blanchard-Fields, Stein & Watson, 2004; Gratz & Roemer, 2004; Tice & Bratslavsky, 2000) – all of which have been found positively correlated with depression and anxiety – and, on the opposite side, avoidance, denial, withdrawal (Gosling, Denizeau & Oberle, 2006; Skinner & Edge, 1998; Tice & Bratslavsky, 2000), which involve a sort of *emotional blindness* preventing individuals from acknowledging their negative emotions as well as their informational value about their own interactions with the environment. Finally, two general manners of dysfunctional emotional regulation are represented, respectively, by the incapability of tolerating emotional distress (Tice & Bratslavsky, 2000) and by the naive conception of emotions as fixed and overwhelming entities impossible to control or to modulate (Tamir, John, Srivastava & Gross, 2007). Being unable to tolerate bad feelings can lead to prefer the short-term regulation of negative emotions and neglect the long-term objectives involving negative states in the short term: for example, the incapability of tolerating the anxiety felt before an important performance can lead to an avoidant strategy of regulation and to procrastinate or abandon the performance. On the other hand, conceiving emotions as irrational or not modifiable "things" prevent people from engaging in whatever attempt to manage them.

EMOTION REGULATION ACROSS LIFESPAN AND GENDERS

During the development from infancy to adulthood, emotion regulation processes become increasingly intrinsic. Even if infants and children are endowed with innate regulatory resources, like temperament (e.g. positive mood, sleeping and eating regular patterns, approach tendencies) and cognitive skills (e.g. attention direction, such as shifting the gaze from unpleasant stimuli or focusing it on the pleasing ones), it is especially through the relationships with caregivers, (as well as with siblings) that they acquire and develop the capability of regulating their emotional states, e.g. how to modulate the experience and the expression of distress, how to show emotional expressions adequate to contextual cues, how to tolerate the delay of satisfaction and so on. According to the large number of studies performed on this topic (e.g. Campos *et al.*, 2004; Cole *et al.*, 2004; Eisenberg *et al.*, 2000; Spinrad, Eisenberg, & Gaertner, 2007; Thompson, 1994), thanks to the development of cognitive skills, mainly the language, regulatory abilities grow and are internalized in such a way as to prefigure a personal style of regulation that will constitute the basis of adult dealing with emotional events (Compas, Connor-Smith, Saltzman, Thomsen & Wadsworth, 2001).

During late childhood and adolescence, parental relationships still represent an important source of emotional regulation - e.g. their specific quality has been found associated to individual differences in regulatory styles or modalities (see Fox & Calkins, 2003, for a review) – but other social factors become increasingly important, such as school, peers, cultural and media models. Nevertheless, the extension of extrinsic influences is counterbalanced by the exponential growth of sophisticated cognitive abilities that allow more complex forms of emotion regulation, such as reframing, rationalisation, putting into perspective, placing affect regulation in the self-regulating context etc. Besides, the increased ability to choose, resulting from augmented cognitive and behavioral skills, means that teenagers and adolescents become progressively more able to modify their environment through the selection of school, friends, activities and way of life. This ability interacts, in turn, with the construction of the sense of self that is one of the principal development tasks (Bosma & Jackson, 1990; Havighurst, 1952) of this phase, including the building of a personal style of emotion regulation. This style can be adaptive or maladaptive. The numerous studies carried out upon coping and emotion regulation in adolescence (Abela, Vanderbilt & Rochon, 2004; Boekaerts, 2002; Compas *et al.,* 2001; Connor-Smith, Compas & Wadsworth, 2000; Kuyken, Howell & Dalgleish, 2006; Olah, 1995; Skinner & Edge, 1998) have highlighted that adaptive styles are characterized by a high level of flexibility and appropriateness to the nature of stressful situations enabling the use of active strategies (planning, problem solving, seeking instrumental social support etc.) when faced with modifiable events, and more passive or emotion-focused strategies (reappraisal, acceptance, seeking affective social support etc.) when faced with unmodifiable circumstances. Adaptive styles imply also the congruence between emotion experience and contextual cue, and the capability of inhibiting or controlling the expressive or behavioral manifestations of emotion when excessive or not pertinent.

On the contrary, maladaptive styles are rigid and stereotyped, and entail ineffective modalities such as self- or other-blaming, catastrophizing, focus on negative states, ventilation, avoidance, under- or overcontrol of emotional experiences and expressions, use of drugs and psychoactive substances to the point of addiction and so forth. The lack and the ineffectiveness of emotional regulatory modalities have been found related to diverse forms of adolescent psychopathology, like depression, anxiety, impulsivity, aggressive behavior, bipolar disorders etc. (Garber & Dodge, 1991; Kraaij, Garnefski, Jan de Wilde, Dijkstra, Gebhardt, Maes, & ter Doest, 2003; Kuyken et al., 2006; Silk, Steinberg, & Morris, 2003).

The personal style of emotion regulation is assumed to become internal and stable in young and middle-life adults, when the sense of self gets structured thanks to the maturation and the integration of the neural, cognitive and executive systems of the organism. Until a decade ago there were only few studies upon emotion regulation in this time of life from a developmental perspective: research had been rather focused on the function, motives, features and effectiveness of different regulatory strategies, on individual differences related to personality characteristics and to gender, on the weight of contextual and personality factors on the selection of a specific type of coping or regulatory modality. Since the full maturation of cognitive, physiological and executive skills may allow to consider adulthood as the acme of individual development - even at the emotional level - one could believe that the style of adult emotional regulation is the best that people can achieve during their life, after the asperities and immaturities of adolescence have been mitigated and before the old age decline begins. For example, one of the earliest developmental theories in the coping literature, put forward by Pfeiffer (1977), posits that with aging individuals regress to previous and poorer modalities of coping.

Subsequently, the increasing interest in development-based theoretic approaches (Baltes, 1987, 1997; Labouvie-Vief, DeVoe, & Bulka, 1989) led researchers to acknowledge that (1) moving to adulthood and old age, emotion conceptions change from an adolescent extrinsic, physical image to an inner, mental, symbolic direction, and the emotional language reflects this modification; (2) the specific life tasks of adulthood – engagement in work, in stable relationships or in marriage, in parenthood and so forth – which entail in turn different types of potential challenges and stressors, affect coping or emotion regulation demanding the use of appropriate strategies in order to deal with them; (3) the specific life tasks of older age – preserving physical health and cognitive skills or adjusting daily life goals to their decline – call for the use of regulatory ways aiming at preserving emotional well-being through minimizing losses.

In the frame of the Selection, Optimization, and Compensation model, Baltes and colleagues (Baltes,1997; Ebner, Freund, & Baltes, 2006) posit that the development across life span is directed towards growth, maintenance and losses prevention of cognitive and psychophysiological functioning: in order to preserve the equilibrium between gains and losses, individuals tend to select age-appropriate goals, moving from growth to maintenance and to losses prevention while shifting from young to adult and old age. An analogous point of view is put forward by the Socioemotional Selectivity Theory (Carstensen, 1995; Carstensen, Fung, & Charles, 2003), according to which lifetime perception affects the definition and the pursuit of individual goals. While young people tend to perceive time as "open-ended" (Carstensen et al., 2003) and pursue expansive, knowledge-based, and long-term objectives, with age time is increasingly perceived as restricted and, consequently, middle-aged and old people tend to pursue more limited, emotion-based, and short-term goals, which, being easier to achieve, imply, in turn, less stress and less negative emotions than striving goals.

Presumably this changed perspective from the future to the present and to everyday life contributes to explaining what the growing number of studies performed in recent years on the emotional life of adult and elderly people (Blanchard-Fields, Stein, & Watson, 2004; Blanchard-Fields, 2007; Carstensen et al. 2003; Diener & Suh, 1997; Garnefski & Kraaij, 2006; Gross, Carstensen, Pasupathi, Tsai, Gottestam, & Hsu, 1997; Labouvie-Vief & Medler, 2002; Kliegel, Jäger, & Phillips, 2007; Thomsen, Mehlsen, Viidik, Sommerlund & Zachariae, 2005) have found out: they show that, in spite of the general decline of health, cognitive skills, and vital resources, old people reveal (1) a good sense of well-being, (2) a level of life satisfaction similar to young people's, (3) a decrease in negative emotions whereas the positive ones remain stable, (4) a recovery from previous psychopathology, (5) a shorter duration of negative feelings than among younger people, (6) less intense aversive reactions when faced by interpersonal problems. These findings allow to infer that the elderly show better emotion regulation and more self-control than young and adult people.

According to the Socioemotional Selectivity Theory (Carstensen, 1995), the perception of their life limit leads old people to concentrate on the present and pursue emotionally significant goals representing a valued aim in se and not in the light of potential future achievements: therefore, the elderly use proactive strategies in order to promote positive emotions and avoid negative ones (e.g. cultivating interactions with family and friends rather than promoting new social encounters; maintaining their habits, avoiding potentially stressful situations etc.) and, when negative events nonetheless happen, older people tend to use both problem solving and emotional regulatory strategies in a more flexible manner than the younger (Blanchard-Fields, Chen, & Norris,1997). However, according to Blanchard-Fields and colleagues (Blanchard-Fields *et al.*, 2004; Blanchard-Fields, 2007), when dealing with interpersonal problems or significant negative events, the elderly prefer more passive strategies (i.e. emotion-focused strategies, especially positive reappraisal, but also downward comparison, acceptance, withdrawal etc.), while young and middle-aged adults are more prone to employ instrumental-strategies (i.e. problem solving, upward comparison, seeking active social support, reflecting on emotional experience etc), coherently with their respective available resources of lifetime, health, physical and cognitive skills. Their increasing decline puts older people in the condition of having to make "a virtue of necessity".

In older age gender differences related to emotion regulation seem to diminish or have been less investigated, whereas they are more prominent during adolescence and adulthood. Although the results of the copious studies examining this topic are not univocal, some findings can be considered by now acquired. Independently of their age and of the type of emotional events, females tend to seek emotional social support and use rumination more than males (Compas *et al.*, 2001; Eschenbeck, Kohlmann, & Lohaus, 2007; Nolen-Hoeksema, 2002; Nolen-Hoeksema & Jackson, 2001; Nolen-Hoeksema & Morrow,1993; Nolen-Hoeksema, Parker, & Larson, 1994; Papadakis, Prince, Jones, & Strauman, 2006; Tamres, Janicki, & Helgeson, 2002), who, in turn, seem more prone to use distraction (Nolen-Hoeksema, 1994, 2002; Nolen-Hoeksema, Larson, & Grayson, 1999; Nolen-Hoeksema & Morrow, 1993). Other findings are more controversial or age- and event-related: female adolescents are more prone to use problem solving than males (Eschenbeck, *et al.*, 2007; Griffith, Dubow, & Ippolito, 2000), who, in turn, tend to use avoidance more than their counterpart (Eschenbeck, *et al.*, 2007; Hampel & Petermann, 2005). But Griffith *et al.*, 2000 found that females also scored high in avoidant coping. Among adults, the meta-analytic review carried out by Tamres *et al.* (2002) upon fifty Anglophone studies performed between 1990 and 2000 showed that, independently of the type of stressful events, women were more likely than men to utilize active coping and positive self-talk (i.e. encouraging oneself to feel better in aversive events), besides seeking social support and rumination. They also tended to use more than men avoidance in achievement and personal health, venting and wishful thinking in personal and others' health. Men have been found more prone than women to use avoidance in relationships and others' health, venting in relationships and achievement. Nolen-Hoeksema and colleagues (Nolen-Hoeksema, Larson, & Grayson, 1999) reported higher use of distraction by males compared to females. Others studies (Birditt & Fingerman, 2003, Fischer & Manstead, 2000; Nolen-Hoeksema *et al.*,1999; Thomsen *et al.*, 2005) have highlighted that women reported more intense and long-lasting negative emotions than men, leading researchers to infer that they are less effective than their counterpart in emotion regulation, but no gender difference in emotional duration and intensity has been found in an Italian study (Matarazzo, 2001).

THREE MODALITIES OF EMOTION REGULATION AFTER NEGATIVE LIFE EVENTS: RUMINATION, SOCIAL SHARING, DISTRACTION

Negative events represent a discrepancy between the wished state of affair and the actual one. They can be seen either as a challenge if individuals perceive their own resources able to cope with them, or as a threat and/or a loss in case of the opposite appraisal (Lazarus & Folkman, 1984). According to stress response theories (Horowitz, 1986, 2003; Janoff-Bulman, 1992; Tait & Silver, 1989), self- regulation theories (Carver & Scheier, 1981, 1990; Endler & Parker, 1990), and the I-D (Immediate-Delayed) compensation theory (Martin, 1999), major negative life events (bereavement, severe illness, rape, violence, divorce, dismissal etc.) constitute threats to the maintenance of the system of assumptions about oneself and the world or to the attainment of people's relevant goals: therefore, they require the establishment of wide-ranging coping processes in order to (1) master their emotional impact, (2) reorganise pre-existing schemata to integrate new information, (3) reduce the divergence between their objectives and the current state of affair, (4) modify or renounce their goals if this divergence is unbridgeable.

Within the context of such processes, rumination, distraction, and social sharing have an important place.

Thinking back frequently or repetitively to a negative event immediately after its occurrence represents a widespread and generalized phenomenon (Rimé, Philippot, Boca, & Mesquita,1992). I assume that, firstly, it constitutes the cognitive content of the emotional experience related to the event and that its degree of presence is an effect of the perceived importance of the emotional event: therefore, it should be considered a cognitive aspect of emotion as well as an emotional regulatory modality. In this latter perspective, however, repetitive thoughts serve a variety of functions, some of which are adaptive while others are maladaptive. More generally, I posit that one of the most important functions of backward repetitive thoughts is to make the past present in one's minds and prolong its virtual existence, in order to (1) take the mental time to accept the (actual) state of affair, (2) envisage the strategies to modify it, (3) refute or deny what happened.

In a functional perspective, repetitive thoughts can contribute to processing and *working through* what happened in order to give it a meaning and integrate it into the individual's cognitive system by means of the assimilation-accommodation processes (Horowitz, 1986, 2003; Janoff-Bulman, 1992; Wells, 2000). They can indicate people's tendency to persist towards their goals and mentally plan the useful steps to attain them (Carver & Scheier, 1990; Martin & Tesser, 1996), according to the process that Taylor & Schneider (1989) called *mental simulation.* This process can be directed towards the future and can consist of imagining the possible different range of actions which could be taken in order to attain the prefixed goals. It can be directed also towards the past and can consist of imagining the alternative event outcomes which could have happened, if only one had changed something in the causal or temporal chain of steps leading to the real conclusion. In this case, the adaptive function of counterfactual thinking (Roese, 1997) can help people find reasons for what happened, envisage different behaviour to pursue in case of future analogous situations, and also cultivate the illusion of undoing the past and rebuilding it in the wished manner, an illusion that can lead to gradually accept the actual state of affair.

Some studies showed the beneficial cognitive effects of repetitive thoughts, at least in giving meaning to negative events or processing them as maturational experience (Bower, Kemeny, Taylor, & Fahey, 1998; Davis, Nolen-Hoeksema, & Larson, 1998; Horowitz, 2003; Janoff-Bulman, 1992; Taylor & Schneider, 1989; Ullrich & Lutgendorf, 2002; Wells, 2000). Nevertheless, the necessary conditions for them to provide a recovery function appear related to their duration and controllability: repetitive thoughts can be effective if restricted to the period immediately following the negative event and somehow under personal control (Compas, Connor, Osowiecki, & Welch, 1997; Davis & Nolen-Hoeksema, 2001; Greenberg, 1995; Segerstrom, Stanton, Alden, & Shortridge, 2003).

When repetitive thoughts last for a lengthy period and become intrusive, unintended, uncontrollable and overwhelming, they assume the features of rumination. This can be seen as a sign of the failed attempts to process what happened and assumes a clearly dysfunctional character: by preventing individuals from distancing themselves from the source of their suffering, rumination prolongs and exacerbates the dysphoric effects of the event and adds a sense of personal helplessness deriving from feeling at the mercy of their thoughts (Horowitz, 1986, 2003; Janoff-Bulman, 1992; Lyubomirsky & Nolen-Hoeksema, 1993; Martin & Tesser, 1996; Nolen-Hoeksema, 2004; Segerstrom et al., 2003; Tait & Silver, 1989).

As soon as rumination develops into a specific response style, i.e. the ruminative style – defined by Nolen-Hoeksema (1991; 2004) as the tendency to focus one's attention on one's dysphoric mood, its causes and consequences – its effects can result in psychopathology. A large number of evidence (for a review, see the meta-analysis carried out by Mor & Winquist, 2002) has shown that the ruminative style is strongly related to chronic negative affects (negative mood, depression and anxiety), poor problem solving (Lyubomirsky & Nolen-Hoeksema, 1995; Lyubomirsky, Tucker, Caldwell, & Berg, 1999; Watkins & Moulds, 2005), overgeneral autobiographical memory (Watkins & Teasdale, 2004), impoverished relationships and smaller capability to receive or perceive social support (Nolen-Hoeksema & Davis, 1999), rigid cognitive style, unmodifiable in spite of its ineffectiveness (Davis & Nolen-Hoeksema, 2000), behavioral avoidance (Moulds, Kandris, Starr, & Wong, 2007). As noted above, females are more prone than males to ruminate and, therefore, more susceptible to suffer the negative consequences deriving from the ruminative style.

Another general, well documented phenomenon following emotional experience is its sharing with other people. Rimé and colleagues (Luminet, Bouts, Delie, Manstead, & Rimé, 2000; Rimé, 2007; Rimé et al., 1992; Rimé, Finkenauer, Luminet, Zech, & Philippot, 1998; Rimé & Zech, 2001; Zech & Rimé, 2005) reported that 80 to 95% of people talk about their emotions in a recurrent and repetitive way for a time varying from minutes to weeks or months, in function of the emotional intensity. Social sharing appears largely independent of the emotional valence and the type of emotions: only shame and guilt tend to be communicated less than the others (Rimé & Zech, 2001). This has been observed both in studies based on recalled memories (Rimé et al., 1992) and in studies using experimental emotion induction (Luminet et al., 2000). Social sharing appears a cross-culturally extended (see Pennebaker, Zech, & Rimé, 2001, for a review) and not gender-related (Luminet et al., 2000; Rimé, 2007) phenomenon; however, some evidence indicates that it increases in old age (Rimé, Finkenauer, & Sevrin, 1995). The communication content regards both the circumstances and consequences of the emotional event and one's emotional experience (Luminet *et al.*, 2000; Rimé, 2007). Addressees are, above all, intimates and include parents, friends, spouse or companion; they vary in relation to the speakers' age and gender (Pennebaker *et al.*, 2001). The degree of social sharing seems to depend on the disruptiveness of the emotional event: in experimental studies (Luminet *et al.*, 2000), the emotional experience was communicated only after it had reached a high level of intensity.

The motives underlying emotional sharing after negative events appear similar to those which trigger repetitive thoughts, that is the cognitive need to find a meaning to what happened and re-establish or modify one's shattered goals (Luminet *et al.* 2000; Rimé *et al.*, 1998). Besides, they seem related to the need for affiliation induced by stressful events (Schachter, 1959, cit. in Luminet *et al.* 2000), according to which other people's presence is perceived as able to reduce stress-anxiety, and to the need to receive instrumental or emotional support by one's listeners (Davis & Nolen-Hoeksema, 2001; Lepore, Silver, Wortman, & Wayment, 1996). More generally, social sharing is related to the common sense belief that "putting outside" one's emotions is beneficial in se, since it represents a form of affective discharge allowing the individual to recover from their disrupting effect (Lepore *et al.*, 1996; Pennebaker *et al.*, 2001; Rimé & Zech, 2001). This belief, largely documented in a Belgian interview study (Zech & Rimé, 2005), is in some ways based on the cathartic conception underlying the "talking cure" for hysteria (Breuer & Freud, 1895).

Nevertheless, empirical findings accumulated by Rimé and his colleagues (Rimé *et al.*, 1992, 1998; Rimé & Zech, 2001; Zech & Rimé, 2005) tend to disconfirm rather than corroborate the idea that sharing negative emotions would serve a recovery function. Although people reported feeling better after sharing their emotions, objective indices of emotional recovery (e.g. emotional intensity of the memory, intensity of phenomenological manifestations of the remembered emotions etc.) did not differ either between shared and not shared emotions or between participants in emotional and neutral sharing conditions. Besides, the personal perception of un-recovered emotional episodes was accompanied by the need to keep sharing the emotional experience, whereas recovered episodes did not: therefore the length of social sharing can be seen as an index of the persistence of the event emotional impact.

However, compared to the people who habitually shared their emotions, those that had kept important emotional events secret presented higher level of illness and lower psychological well-being (Finkenauer & Rimé, 1998). These findings are consistent with the research tradition into emotional disclosure after traumatic events (Frisina, Borod, & Lepore, 2004; Lepore, 1997; Pennebaker, 1995; Pennebaker & Chung, 2007; Pennebaker *et al.*, 2001) showing that writing or talking about one's emotional reactions in laboratory setting produces large beneficial effects on health and psychological well-being, independently of social feedback. Instead, other findings emphasized the importance of social support – namely the readiness to listen and empathize on the recipient's part – in order to make social sharing effective: in this case, communicating the emotional experience seems to make it possible to mitigate its destructive impact, reduce rumination, and help identify problem-solving strategies or processes of acceptance and adaptation (Davis & Nolen-Hoeksema, 2001; Lepore *et al.*, 1996; Nolen-Hoeksema & Davis, 1999).

According to a considerable amount of studies (Lyubomirsky, Caldwell, & Nolen-Hoeksema, 1998; Morrow & Nolen-Hoeksema, 1990; Rusting & Nolen-Hoeksema 1998; Thayer, Newman, & McClain, 1994; Trask & Sigmon, 1999), distraction represents an effective modality of emotion regulation, especially when compared to rumination. Engaging oneself in pleasant or neutral activities and thoughts in order to divert one's attention away from memories of stressful events (Nolen-Hoeksema, 1991) appears to reduce their dysphoric effects both in the short and in the long term. The large corpus of experimental and correlational studies carried out by Nolen-Hoeksema and her colleagues in order to test the different effects of rumination and distraction on depression and other negative affects showed that, by shifting attention from the source of dysphoria to redirect it towards other actions or thoughts, distraction makes cognitive resources that can be employed for more adaptive goals available. Therefore, distraction was found to decrease the duration and severity of post-traumatic stress (Lyubomirsky & Nolen-Hoeksema, 1993; Lyubomirsky *et al.*, 1998; Nolen-Hoeksema, 1991); diminish sadness and depressed mood (Morrow & Nolen-Hoeksema, 1990); reduce angry response (Rusting & Nolen-Hoeksema, 1998); increase the capability of problem solving (Lyubomirsky & Nolen-Hoeksema,1995). Trask & Sigmon (1999), using a sequential task, found that distraction following a depressed mood induction reduced its degree and that rumination after the distraction task resulted in lower depressed mood than immediately after the mood induction.

Other findings are less encouraging about the beneficial effects of distraction: Fivush & Buckner (2000) highlighted that diverting the attention from one's feelings may result in externalizing disorders, such as alcoholism and violent behavior. Garnefski, Teerds, Kraaij, Legerstee, & van den Kommer (2004) did not found any evidence for the effectiveness of distraction-like strategies to recover from depressive symptoms. Martin & Tesser (1989, 1996) revealed that sometimes the positive effects of distraction are only temporary, while other researchers found that the attempt to avoid thinking of what happened may paradoxically increase the memory of it (Wegner, 1994; Wenzlaff, Wegner, & Roper, 1988). Moreover, not allowing the reflection on the event's repercussions on oneself, distraction risks to interfere with the process of cognitive reworking (Koole, Smeets, van Knippenberg, & Dijksterhuis, 1999).

OVERVIEW OF THE PRESENT STUDY

The general aim of this study was to investigate how people perceive and cope with negative life events. More specifically, my interest was to examine the use and effectiveness of the three long-term modalities of emotion regulation discussed above: rumination[4], distraction and social sharing.

As we have seen, although several studies have been carried out in order to investigate each modality or to evaluate the comparative effectiveness of rumination and distraction, to my knowledge this is the first study comparing these three regulatory modalities. Two

---

[4] It is needed to specify that by the term "rumination" , used for the sake of brevity, I refer both to repetitive thoughts and to rumination.

techniques of data collection were used: qualitative assessment (through narratives) and quantitative assessment (through evaluation scales). In this way, I aimed at gathering two broad types of information: an open account of one's personal experience of a negative life event and one's way to cope with it,, and a more constrained evaluation of this event and of the specific modalities of emotion regulation which had to be investigated. I aimed at testing whether such modalities and, more generally, the way people cope with negative events are affected by the significance of such events and by gender and age. Therefore, a cross-sectional research – from adolescence to old age – where the participants were asked to refer to an important or a not very important negative event, was performed.

The specific hypotheses I wished to test were the following:

- the more negative life events are appraised as important, the higher is their cognitive and emotional impact and the more they undermine the individuals' beliefs about themselves and the world;
- the particular modalities people spontaneously use to cope with aversive events vary in function of their significance: important negative events tend to mobilise emotion-focused coping rather than problem-focused coping (Lazarus & Folkman, 1984), because they are often perceived as irremediable (e.g. the death or mortal disease of a loved person) or going beyond one's resources to modify them; consequently, if it is not possible to alter the state of affairs, people's efforts should be directed to adapt their internal state. Less important negative events should mobilize both types of coping, according to individual differences;
- emotional regulatory processes aim at reducing the emotional impact produced by the event and at restoring psychological equilibrium. Rumination, social sharing and distraction are three different ways to accomplish this function. I assume they are based, respectively, on the attempt of "giving meaning" to the event and integrating it in one's own cognitive system, on the attempt of sharing the "weight" of one's own emotional experience and seeking other people's help, on the attempt of taking the distance from the negative event and preventing it from hindering one's own course of life. In my opinion, these ways of coping could be used together even if their respective use frequency would vary not only in function of interpersonal differences but primarily in function of the significance of the negative event. After significant events, rumination and social sharing should be used more than distraction since the event's salience might absorb a great amount of mental resources and make it difficult to divert one's attention from it. On the other hand, communicating one's experience could allow to keep the attention focused on it and, at the same time, share its weight and information relating to other people. After less significant events the respective use extent of such modalities should depend only on interpersonal differences;
- assuming that important events upset the individual's habitual life pattern and demand great efforts for bearing, understanding and accepting them, I suppose that the general impact of the event – which has been investigated in terms of its perceived importance, negative appraisal, repercussions on the personal beliefs system, and emotional response intensity - serves a mediational function between the

manipulated significance of the event and the use and subjective evaluation of the three regulatory modalities;

- as to the effects of the participants' gender and age on the frequency of these three regulatory modalities, I expected that, in accordance with what emerges in literature: (1) females would show a greater propensity to use rumination, while males would more frequently make use of distraction (Almeida & Kessler, 1998; Nolen-Hoeksema, 2002; Nolen-Hoeksema *et al.*, 1994; Nolen-Hoeksema *et al.*, 1999; Papadakis *et al.*, 2006; Tamres *et al.*, 2002); (2) no gender difference should be found concerning social sharing (Luminet *et al.*, 2000; Rimé *et al.*, 1992); (3) the elderly would share their emotional experience more often than other age groups (Rimé *et al.*, 1995). As regards rumination, there are contrasting findings in literature: some studies found no difference among age groups (Garnefski & Kraaij, 2006; Thomsen *et al.*, 2005), while other studies found that the elderly ruminated less than younger people (McConatha, Leone, & Armstrong, 1997; Phillips, Henry, Hosie, & Milne, 2006). To my knowledge, the differential use of distraction across life span has not been specifically investigated even if the well documented attempts of older people to avoid negative emotions and prevent their insurgence (Blanchard-Fields *et al.*, 2004; Blanchard-Fields, 2007; Carstensen *et al.* 2003; Labouvie-Vief & Medler, 2002) allow to expect that the elderly would use distraction more often than other age groups;

- with reference to the effectiveness of these modalities, I presumed that it would vary according to the quality of the communicative exchange realized during the social sharing, the length of time of rumination and the extent of distraction. Social sharing should be effective provided that the others are receptive and responsive, thus favouring the expression and exchange of one's emotional experience; immediately after the negative event, rumination could help the individual assimilate and re-integrate it within his/her cognitive reference framework, whereas its long-lasting persistence could reveal the incompleteness of the adaptive process and represent a further source of distress; distraction could reduce the dysphoric impact of the negative event but, if used massively and for a long period of time, it should hinder or weaken the cognitive reworking of the event. However, I supposed that the perceived usefulness of a regulatory modality could be a reliable predictor of its actual effectiveness.

METHOD

Participants

Eight hundred persons (400 female, 400 male) participated as unpaid volunteers in this study, after signing the informed consent. They came from the area of Naples (Italy) and belonged to four age-groups: 200 were adolescents aged between 13-19 (M = 15.58; DS = 1.75); 200 were young people aged between 20-29 (M = 24.76; DS = 2.88); 200 were adults aged between 30-59 (M = 43.26; DS = 8.31); 200 were elderly people aged between 60-89 (M = 69.21; DS = 5.98).

Adolescents were recruited at three high schools ("liceo", technical, and vocational schools); young people and adults were found at different faculties of Naples's Universities, in the workplaces (both employees and self-employed workers were recruited) and at home; the elderly were recruited at work, at home and at rest homes.

Participants were randomly assigned to two research conditions: very significant vs. not significant negative life event. Their gender was paired across age groups and across conditions.

Materials and Procedure

A paper-and-pencil questionnaire was created for this study and individually administered to participants, except for adolescents who had been grouped into classrooms. The questionnaire comprehension had been previously ascertained through a pilot study with 40 unpaid volunteers participants (10 for each age groups to investigate). Nobody found difficulties in comprehending the posed questions.

In the first part of the questionnaire participants were asked to describe a very significant or a not very significant negative life event occurred to them in the last 6 months to 6 years and specify the emotions they had felt, the consequences of the event on their life, their duration, and what they had done to cope with them.

The open account was followed by a second part, where participants were requested to assess, on thirty two 7-point scales, the following aspects of the described autobiographical experience: when the event occurred; its perceived importance (this question acted as manipulation check for the event relevance); to what extent it was perceived as unfair, painful, incomprehensible, unforeseeable, irremediable; its impact on their own beliefs about life, the others and themselves; the intensity of the emotions felt; to what extent rumination and social sharing were present (i.e. how much one thought back to /talked about the event) and their level of uncontrollability (to what extent they couldn't help thinking back to/ talking about the event), their relative dominance (i.e. how long the event memory was their dominant thought; how long speaking about the event was the dominant topic of conversation); and present frequency (how often they presently thought back to the event or talked about it); their perceived effectiveness to cope with the event and reduce its emotional impact; the pervasiveness of their thoughts about the event (i.e. to what extent thinking back to the event increased the perception of being overwhelmed and unable to overcome it; to what extent the wish to stop thinking back to the event was felt); the expected and the perceived help given from people with whom the event was shared; the perceived uncontrollability of talking about the event (i.e. feeling unable of not doing it); the attempts to distract their attention from the event and their outcome (i.e. to what extent the attempts of distraction were successful); the perceived effectiveness of distraction to cope with the event and reduce its emotional impact; the perception of the paradoxical effect of distraction (i. e. the difficulty of distraction with time, perceiving unexpectedly the event as a weight inside, the abrupt resurgence of the event's pain, a sense of extraneousness to the event); the perceived cognitive and affective persistence of the event and the recovery from it. For each question, score 1 of the scale indicated the minimum level of the presence of the considered dimension and score 7 indicated its maximum level. As to the temporal occurrence of the event, score 1 meant six months ago, score 7 six years ago. The order of presentation of the three regulatory modalities was randomized across participants, as well as the questions related to each modality, except for the question regarding their presence which was always presented as first.

Finally, the participants that felt to have at least partially recovered from the negative event were asked to indicate the most effective coping modality component out of a list of thirteen, or to specify any other component not included in the list. The listed components referred to thinking back to the event, social sharing, social support, distraction, reflection (i.e. examine what happened in order to understand it), problem-focused coping, beloved people's affection, emotional ventilation, passing of time[5].

It needs to be clarified that participants were requested to answer the questions about each of the three regulatory modalities only if they had employed it, otherwise, they were asked to omit the related responses. Participants were given no time limit to compile the questionnaire: on average, they took half an hour to complete it.

Classification of Narratives

For each area investigated (type of events, felt emotions, consequences and their duration, coping, current considerations[6]), narratives were analyzed by four independent judges, through a procedure of progressive abstraction of their content (Boucher, 1983) and summarized in a few general categories on the basis of their semantic resemblance. If one of the requested areas was not reported in the participants' account, the case was coded as "no response". The indices of agreement between the four judges, computed two at a time by means of the k of Cohen, varied from 0.73 to 0.87 with p always $<.001$. When there was disagreement between the judges, the opinion of a fifth judge was taken into account.

Narratives were analyzed without any reference to the event significance and to the participants' age and gender in order to prevent the creation of a semantic context that could affect their interpretation. Consequently, the construction of the categories did not consider the varying degree of seriousness of the events and of their effects, but only their semantic affinity. For example, the death of a beloved person and the death of a cat were both put in the category " death"; to be mocked and to be fired were both placed in the category "suffer harm, injustice, failure"; not having enough money to live on and having to repeat an examination, suffering from depression and feeling aloof after the event were all entered in

---

[5] More specifically, the thirteen coping modalities were: thinking back to the event for a long time, talking about it to other people, succeeding in thinking of something else, venting one's emotions, succeeding in remedying what happened, reflecting on what happened, loved person's affection, totally devoting to one's work or studies, time passing, made new projects for the future, psychological or medical support, traveling or other pleasant activities, other.

[6] Current considerations about the event were not required in the questionnaire; nevertheless, most participants included in their account the event conclusion and their opinions about what had happened, so this macro-category has been created post hoc.

the category "negative impact upon oneself and upon one's emotional state". Similarly, emotions were grouped into families based on their structural similarities, apart from their respective intensity. So, this narratives coding does not allow to identify the quantitative differences on the same semantic dimension between very significant and not very significant events, or between participants' age and gender, but only the qualitative differences concerning distinct semantic dimensions.

The general categories extracted for each area are listed below.

The types of events were classified into five categories: 1. death of a beloved person or pet[7]; 2. experience a dangerous or difficult situation (e.g. illness, accident, choice, exam, job admission test etc.); 3. loved person in a dangerous, unfair or difficult situation (the same cases as in the previous category but concerning other people); 4. suffer harm, injustice, failure (to be rejected, dismissed, humiliated, deceived, robbed, mocked, etc.); 5. conflictual relationships (end of relationships, unfaithfulness, quarrels, disputes, etc.).

The about fifty different emotional terms reported in narratives were grouped in the following emotion families: 1. SADNESS (sadness, sorrow, disappointment, pain, meaninglessness, bitterness, unhappiness, loneliness, despair, nostalgia, uneasiness etc.); 2. ANGER (anger, revengefulness, nervousness, irritation, hatred, contempt, sense of injustice etc.); 3. FEAR (fear, terror, anxiety, worry etc.); 4. HELPLESSNESS (discouragement, feeling useless, lack of self-confidence etc.); 5. CONFUSION (confusion, surprise, shock, disbelief etc.); 6. OTHER (i.e. emotions seldom mentioned such as guilt, shame, regret, feeling ridiculous, boredom, indifference, hope etc.). The 7th category was "no response". Participants could report all the felt emotions, but for each participant the emotions classified in the same family were computed only once[8].

The event consequences were organized into four categories: 1. negative impact upon oneself and upon one's emotional state (worsened living conditions, distrust about life and oneself, rumination[9], sleeping and eating disturbances, bad-temperedness, etc.); 2. changed attitudes in relationships and towards one's environment (modification of one's opinions and behavior about the others, work, study, relationships etc.); 3. loss of reference points (feeling alone, without affective and instrumental support; feeling unable to deal with life alone); 4. no response.

The duration of consequences was ranked as follows: 1. until one week after the event; 2. until one month after the event; 3. until one year after the event; 4. more than one year after the event. 5. no response.

The coping categories were the following: 1. problem-focused coping (i.e. behaviors allowing to modify the event or remediate its effects); 2. reflection/reappraisal (from now on, reappraisal; i.e. reflecting about the event in order to "give meaning" to it, modify its original meaning or reduce its impact); 3. social sharing/social support (i.e. talking to others about one's emotional experience or seeking family, friends, professional help); 4. distraction (i.e.

---

[7] The death of a pet was reported only in NVSEC while the death of a loved person was reported only in SEC.

[8] For example, if a participant cited sorrow, unhappiness, and anger, the first two emotions were computed only once as SADNESS and the third emotion was computed as ANGER.

[9] Rumination was placed in this category because it was not described alone but with other negative effects of the event. Since it was depicted by participants as unpleasant, unwanted and overwhelming , all the independent judges decided to put it among the event's consequences and not among the coping modalities.

taking the distance from the event by going out, travelling, working etc.); 5. time (waiting for time to pass); 6. avoidance (i.e. avoiding situations or places bringing the negative event to mind or conditions liable to produce a similar event); 7. suppression (i.e. controlling one's behavior in order to prevent emotional expression); 8. no response[10].

The current considerations were summarized in five categories: 1. maturational function of the experience (i.e. acknowledging that the event and its effects had contributed to personal maturation); 2. negative evaluation of the experience or persistence of its emotional impact (i.e. the experience was commented only in negative terms, or its impact was still present); 3. positive outcome of the event (i.e. at present, the described event was positively resolved without the individual's intervention); 4. recovery from the emotional experience or reduction of its impact (i.e. at present the event's pain or consequences had stopped or reduced); 5. no response.

RESULTS

The results concerning the narratives first and then the quantitative assessments were reported. Finally, the results related to the last query of the questionnaire, i.e. the selection of the most effective regulatory modality among those listed, were illustrated.

Narratives

The distribution of categories frequency for each area investigated is shown in table 1.

For each area, except for the emotions, data were treated by means of log-linear models[11] in order to assess the relationship between the event significance, the participants' gender and age group and the categories frequency. The "no response" categories were eliminated from the analyses. Since the log-linear models are based upon the same rationale as the chi square and require the occurrence of a limited number of cells with low frequencies, the "avoidance" and "suppression" coping categories were combined, as reported in table 1. Results were interpreted through the analysis of parameter estimates.

---

[10] In order to simplify subsequent statistical analyses, in the cases where more than one coping strategy was utilised, only the predominant one (i.e. the most extensively described strategy, or the most frequently referred to) was categorized.

[11] All the statistical analyses were performed using SPSS 12.0 package. As regards the log-linear analyses, it was first selected the best model using HILOG procedure and then tested it and other reduced models in GENLOG in order to obtain the best parsimonious one.

Table 1. Frequency distribution of narrative categories by event significance, age group, and gender

		Significant negative events								Not very significant negative events								Total
		adolescent		young		adult		elderly		adolescent		young		adult		elderly		
Type of events		M	F	M	F	M	F	M	F	M	F	M	F	M	F	M	F	
death	f	22	21	19	14	13	26	15	17	1	1	3	2	0	1	2	0	157
danger	f	11	1	10	9	8	3	15	13	19	10	10	13	9	14	23	20	188
others in danger	f	6	7	7	9	10	17	7	8	4	4	1	4	5	6	4	8	107
suffer harm	f	5	4	4	5	10	1	6	3	10	13	17	11	12	5	14	6	126
conflictual relationships	f	6	17	10	13	9	3	7	9	16	22	19	20	24	24	7	16	222
Total	f	50	50	50	50	50	50	50	50	50	50	50	50	50	50	50	50	800
Consequences																		
negative impact on oneself	f	39	34	25	30	25	21	33	33	30	22	24	27	27	29	31	29	459
loss of ref. points	f	2	5	5	2	5	9	4	4	2	1	0	0	0	0	0	0	39
changed attitude	f	7	11	11	15	7	6	12	12	16	26	17	19	10	11	17	20	217
no response	f	2	0	9	3	13	14	1	1	2	1	9	4	13	10	2	1	85
Total	f	50	50	50	50	50	50	50	50	50	50	50	50	50	50	50	50	800
Duration																		
up to 1 week	f	4	3	3	4	5	0	0	1	18	17	7	8	12	10	16	19	127
up to 1 month	f	8	3	4	2	0	1	2	1	10	9	4	9	5	3	9	15	85
up to 1 year	f	14	28	11	14	7	16	7	11	10	8	11	10	8	13	12	7	187
more than 1 year	f	12	13	10	13	11	10	39	34	3	0	3	4	0	1	5	9	167
no response	f	12	3	22	17	27	23	2	3	9	16	25	19	25	23	8	0	234
Total	f	50	50	50	50	50	50	50	50	50	50	50	50	50	50	50	50	800
Coping																		
problem-focused coping	f	3	5	8	9	10	4	10	6	16	17	10	10	27	18	17	14	183
reflection/ reappraisal	f	9	9	6	9	7	5	2	0	4	5	3	6	3	3	8	6	85

		Significant negative events								Not very significant negative events								Total
		adolescent		young		adult		elderly		adolescent		young		adult		elderly		
		M	F	M	F	M	F	M	F	M	F	M	F	M	F	M	F	
Coping																		
social sharing/support	f	10	19	12	17	14	17	13	26	8	7	7	6	6	13	10	18	203
distraction	f	5	2	5	2	6	8	12	7	9	4	1	1	1	4	12	9	88
time	f	5	2	0	2	2	4	8	10	2	3	4	2	2	3	0	3	52
avoidance/ suppression	f	3	2	8	4	0	0	5	0	2	7	11	1	5	3	3	0	54
no response	f	15	11	11	8	11	12	0	1	9	7	14	24	6	6	0	0	135
Total	f	50	50	50	50	50	50	50	50	50	50	50	50	50	50	50	50	800
Current considerations																		
matur. function	f	21	16	14	15	4	7	0	1	13	13	20	23	8	7	8	5	175
persistence	f	20	25	15	19	8	18	11	18	1	6	5	6	4	0	12	6	174
positive outcome	f	4	3	2	3	10	0	14	10	4	8	4	3	6	10	14	13	108
overcome or reduction	f	3	5	9	8	3	3	14	15	25	18	9	13	15	15	8	18	181
no response	f	2	1	10	5	25	22	11	6	7	5	12	5	17	18	8	8	162
Total	f	50	50	50	50	50	50	50	50	50	50	50	50	50	50	50	50	800
Emotion families																		
SADNESS	f	35	44	31	38	25	31	33	34	20	31	28	25	20	19	23	33	470
ANGER	f	8	12	16	12	10	11	23	8	23	24	25	19	26	28	20	22	287
FEAR	f	9	7	17	17	10	8	19	24	17	11	11	10	4	7	17	18	206
HELPLESSNESS	f	1	3	9	9	7	5	11	23	2	1	4	6	1	2	12	2	98
CONFUSION	f	7	3	2	1	4	5	12	9	0	3	14	5	4	1	3	3	76
other	f	2	5	4	8	3	4	17	19	3	6	3	3	5	3	16	14	115
no response	f	1	0	0	0	5	1	0	0	1	0	0	0	0	0	0	0	8
Total	f	63	85	79	85	64	65	115	117	66	76	85	68	60	60	91	92	1260

Note: M = males; F = females; f = frequency. Category labels have been shortened: e.g. others in danger = a loved person is in a dangerous, unfair or difficult situation; loss of ref. points = loss of reference points; matur. function = maturational function of the experience.

As regards the types of events, the most parsimonious model was the one implying a two-way association between event significance and type of event, and a three-way interaction between gender, age group and type of event (LR [d.f. 35] = 39.14, p = .289). In the significant event condition (SEC), the death of a beloved person and the dangerous or difficult situations for beloved persons were reported more often than in not very significant event conditions (NVSEC); the opposite ratio was found for "suffer harm, injustice, failure" and "conflictual relationships". As to the three-way interaction, compared to the reference categories (i.e. all the types of events reported by the elderly female participants), the young, adult and elderly males reported the "suffer harm, injustice, failure" events more often than theoretically expected, whereas the female adolescents and the adults of both genders described "experience a dangerous or difficult situation" less often.

As to the event consequences, the chosen model entailed the conditional independence between event significance and event consequences, and between age group and event consequences (LR [d.f. 33] = 26.28, p = .790). The "loss of reference points" category was cited more in SEC than in NVSEC, while it was the opposite for the "changed attitudes in relationships and towards one's environment" category. Given the "changed attitudes in relationships and towards one's environment" in the elderly as reference category, the "loss of reference points" category was mentioned less than theoretically expected by all the age groups, the "negative impact upon oneself and upon one's emotional state" category was cited more than expected by the adolescents and the elderly, and the "changed attitudes in relationships and towards one's environment" was quoted less by the adults. With regard to the consequences' duration, the selected model implied a three-way interaction between age group, event significance and duration (LR [d.f. 32] = 38.06, p = .213). Weighed against the reference category (i.e. the elderly in NVSEC evaluating that consequences had persisted "more than 1 year"), the categories contributing the most to that result were the following: the adolescents in SEC judging that the consequences lasted up to one year, the adolescents in NVSEC estimating that they lasted up to one week, the elderly in SEC evaluating that duration was more than one year, all of them being more numerous than expected in comparison with the reference category, and the adolescents and adults in NVSEC judging that the consequences persisted more than one year, the adults and elderly in SEC reporting that they lasted up to one week and up to one month, all of them being fewer than expected in comparison with the reference category.

As far as coping is concerned, the most parsimonious model entailed a two-way interaction between gender and coping and a three-way interaction between age group, event significance and coping (LR [d.f. 42] = 47.97, p = .244). Social sharing was mentioned more by females than by males; it was the opposite for avoidance/suppression. The reference categories for the three-way interaction were the six types of coping mentioned by the elderly in NVSEC, compared to which the parameter estimates highlighted the following ratios: in SEC, "problem-focused coping" mentioned by all the four age groups, reappraisal cited by the elderly, distraction reported by the adolescents and the young had less frequency than expected if compared to the corresponding types of coping of the reference categories, while "time" mentioned by the elderly and "avoidance/suppression" cited by the young had higher frequency; in NVSEC "social sharing/support" cited by the young, distraction mentioned by the young and the adults were less reported than expected in comparison with the corresponding types of coping of the reference categories, while "avoidance/suppression" cited by the young had the opposite direction.

In order to investigate whether the coping modalities varied in function of the type of negative events, a chi square test crossing the type of events with the coping modalities was performed[12], after excluding the "no response" for coping category (n = 135). Results were interpreted by means of adjusted standardized residuals. The frequency distribution of the responses is illustrated in table 2.

Table 2. Frequency distribution (f) of coping by type of events

Coping		Type of events					
		death	to be in danger	others are in danger	suffer harm	conflictual relationships	Total
problem solving	f	0	50	18	52	63	183
reappraisal	f	21	22	13	10	19	85
social sharing/support	f	55	38	36	25	49	203
distraction	f	24	28	3	11	22	88
time	f	17	6	9	3	17	52
avoidance/suppression	f	8	14	5	9	18	54
no response	f	32	30	23	16	34	135
Total	f	157	188	107	126	222	800

Results showed (χ^2 [d.f. 20] = 104.16, p<.001) that problem-focused coping was less used than theoretically expected for "death of a beloved person or pet" (it was never mentioned), while it was more frequently used than expected for "suffer harm, injustice, failure" and "conflictual relationships"; social sharing was more often used than expected for "death" and "loved person in a dangerous, unfair or difficult situation", while it was less often used for "experience a dangerous or difficult situation" and "suffer harm, injustice, failure"; distraction was more employed than expected for "death" and for "dangerous or difficult situation", while it was less utilized for "loved person in a dangerous unfair or difficult situation"; time was more mentioned for "death" and less mentioned for "dangerous or difficult situation" and for "suffer harm, injustice, failure". No significant differences were found for reappraisal and avoidance/suppression.

As to the current considerations, the saturated model emerged from analysis (i. e. a four-way interaction among all the variables) indicating a great variability among the participants' current opinions about what happened.

As far as the emotion families are concerned, since log-linear models imply the independence principle (i. e. the frequency in each cell is independent of frequencies in all other cells) while participants could report more than one emotion, data were coded in the following way: each family's occurrence or not occurrence for each participant was coded by 1/0. Then a 2 x 4 x 2 (gender x age group x event significance) MANOVA was carried out on the proportion of occurrences of six emotion families. In order to consider only robust effects

---

[12] The type of event was not put in log-linear models because the high number of variables with their respective values would have made the analysis not manageable.

I chose to set the significance level at $p< .01$. Results showed two main effects of age group (Pillai's trace $[18, 2343] = 12.09$, $p <.001$, $\eta^2 =.085$), and of event significance (Pillai's trace $[6, 779] = 14.13$, $p <.001$, $\eta^2 =.098$), a two-way interaction between age group and event significance (Pillai's trace $[18, 2343] = 3.66$, $p <.001$, $\eta^2 =.027$), and a three-way interaction between gender, age group and event significance (Pillai's trace $[18, 2343] = 2.24$, $p <.01$, $\eta^2 =.017$). The univariate tests, whose results were examined through Least Significant Difference *post hoc* test (LSD, $p< .01$), showed that the age group effect was due to SADNESS (F $[3, 784] = 5.20$, $p <.01$, $\eta^2 =.020$), less mentioned by adults than all other groups, FEAR (F $[3, 784] = 11.62$, $p <.001$, $\eta^2 =.043$), HELPLESSNESS (F $[3, 784] = 16.55$, $p <.001$, $\eta^2 =.060$), both cited most of all by the elderly, then by the young and finally by the adolescents and adults, and OTHER EMOTIONS (F $[3, 784] = 27.43$, $p <.001$, $\eta^2 =.095$), which the elderly cited more than all the other groups. The event significance effect emerged on SADNESS (F $[1, 784] = 28.37$, $p <.001$, $\eta^2 =.035$), on HELPLESSNESS (F $[1,784] = 18.65$, $p <.001$, $\eta^2 =.023$), both more cited in SEC than in NVSEC, and on ANGER (F $[1, 784] = 43.67$, $p <.001$, $\eta^2 =.053$), more mentioned in NVSEC than in SEC. The two-way interaction emerged on CONFUSION (F $[3, 784] = 10.62$, $p<.001$, $\eta^2 =.039$); the three-way interactions appeared on HELPLESSNESS (F $[3, 784] = 6.99$, $p<.001$, $\eta^2 =.026$).

In order to interpret the interactions, simple effect analyses upon the emotions where they occurred were performed. Once again, LSD ($p<.01$) was used as *post hoc* test. In SEC, CONFUSION (F $[3, 792] = 10.52$, $p <.001$, $\eta^2 =.038$) was more quoted by the elderly than by the young; in NVSEC it was quoted the most by the young. HELPLESSNESS (F $[10, 784] = 3.60$, $p <.001$, $\eta^2 =.044$) was reported in SEC more often by the elderly females than by all the other groups, and by the elderly males more than by the adolescent males; in NVSEC it was more cited by the elderly males than by the adult and adolescent males, whereas no difference was found among female age groups.

Quantitative Assessments

In order to reduce the number of items concerning the quantitative assessment of the emotional experience and of the three regulatory modalities, rumination, social sharing and distraction, six factorial analyses were performed on the items belonging to the same domain, with the principal components as factor extraction method and the scree test as criterion for the number of factors to extract. Except for the cases where only one component was extracted, the Varimax method was used for rotation, after controlling that the correlation coefficient between components was compatible with the orthogonal rotation. For each regulatory modality, analyses were carried out only on the participants that had actually used it, i.e. 722 participants for rumination (90.25 %), 676 for social sharing (84.5%), 566 for distraction (70.75%).

Results are depicted in table 3.

Table 3. Results of principal component analysis performed upon the below indicated dimensions

Dimensions	Components labels	Items	Loadings	Percent of Variance of each component	Cumulative Percent of Variance
Negative appraisal of the event	Negative appraisal of the event	to what extent the event was painful	.754		50.32
		to what extent the event was incomprehensible	.742		
		to what extent the event was irremediable	.728	50.32	
		to what extent the event was unfair	.670		
		to what extent the event was unforeseeable	.647		
Event impact upon one's beliefs	Event impact upon one's beliefs	how did the event affect one's beliefs about oneself	.883		64.83
		how did the event affect one's beliefs about the others	.796	64.83	
		how did the event affect one's beliefs about the life	.729		
Rumination (R)	Use and extent of rumination	present frequency of thinking back the event	.848		
		how much one had thought back to the event	.817	37.99	
		how long the event memory has been the dominant thought	.655		
		degree of uncontrollability of R	.628		69.50
	Pervasiveness of rumination	desire to interrupt R	.893	18.62	
		failure to deliver from R	.706		
	Effectiveness of rumination	emotional efficacy of R	.859	12.88	
		cognitive efficacy of R	.846		
Social sharing (SS)	Uuse and extent of social sharing	how long speaking about the event has been the dominant topic	.852		
		present frequency of talking about the event	.796	38.77	
		degree of uncontrollability of SS	.767		
		how much one had talked about the event	.617		58.92
	Effectiveness of social sharing and availability of social support	cognitive effectiveness of SS	.842		
		emotional effectiveness of SS	.787	20.15	
		listeners' supportiveness	.677		
		expected help from listeners	.580		

Table 3. Continued

Dimensions	Components labels	Items	Loadings	Percent of Variance of each component	Cumulative Percent of Variance
	Use and effectiveness of distraction	success of attempts of distracting	.827	31.63	
		cognitive effectiveness of D	.823		
		emotional effectiveness of D	.788		
		attempts of distracting	.673		51.95
Distraction (D)	Paradoxical effect of distraction	feeling the event as a weight inside	.788	20.32	
		difficulty to distract oneself with time	.709		
		abrupt resurgence of the event's pain	.645		
		sense of extraneousness to the event	.560		
		to what extent the event is still cognitively present (reverse scored)	.901		
Current impact of the event	Recovery from the event	to what extent the event is still emotionally present (reverse scored)	.881	75.08	75.08
		level of the perceived recovery from the event	.815		

Note: for each component, items were listed in function of their loadings.

The last component, "recovery from the event", was originally labelled "current impact of the event": since the three items loading on it (the degree of recovery from the event and of its cognitive and emotional persistence) were inversely correlated and this could create some confusion in the interpretation of the component, I decided to reverse the two scales referred to the event persistence and repeat the factor analysis. The component was then labelled "recovery from the event".

In order to establish the effects of event significance, gender, and age group upon the variables thought to mediate the relationship between the manipulated independent variable (i.e. event significance) and the three regulatory modalities, four 2x2x4 ANOVAs were performed on: perceived importance of the event, emotional intensity, negative appraisal of the event, and event impact upon one's beliefs. Further, a 2x2x4 ANOVA was run to ascertain the effect of the abovementioned variables on the temporal occurrence of the event, which was assumed as predictor in subsequent regression analysis on the recovery from the event. Once again the significance level was set at $p \leq .01$, the LSD was employed as *post hoc* test, and the interaction effects were interpreted by means of simple effects analyses, whose results are reported in the text.

In tables 4a and 4b means and standard deviations of all the dependent variables of this study are reported. All the further statistical analyses upon the components extracted from the factor analysis were carried out upon the factorial scores; however, in tables 4 (a and b) mean scores of the items loading on each component were reported in order to facilitate their reading. In table 5 the results of ANOVAs are summarized.

The main effect of event significance was found in all the fifth ANOVAs: in SEC scores were higher than in NVSEC. The main effect of gender emerged on the following variables: "negative appraisal of the event", "event impact upon one's beliefs", and "emotional intensity", on which females reported higher scores than males. The main effect of age group emerged in almost all the variables, in many of which it however interacted with the event significance. The two variables on which only the main effect of age group appeared were "temporal occurrence of the event", where scores ranked in decreasing order from the elderly to the adolescents, and "perceived importance of the event" that the adolescents perceived lower than all the other age groups. The interaction between age group and event significance was found on the remaining three variables: "negative appraisal of the event" (F [3.792] = 19.29 p <.001, η^2 =.068), where in SEC the elderly produced higher scores than all the other participants, whilst in NVSEC the young and adults gave higher scores than the adolescents and the elderly; "event impact upon one's beliefs" (F [3.792] = 8.22, p <.001, η^2 =.030), on which all groups were similar in SEC, while in NVSEC the elderly reported the lowest scores; "emotional intensity" (F [3.792] = 16.25, p <.001, η^2 =.058), where in SEC the elderly produced higher scores than the adolescents whilst in NVSEC young and adult scores over came those of the elderly and adolescents.

Table 4a. Significant negative events: Means and standard deviations of dependent variables

Variables		Significant negative events							
		adolescent		young		adult		elderly	
		male	female	male	female	male	female	male	female
Negative appraisal of the event	M	4.95	5.39	5.05	5.39	5.27	5.44	5.9	6.07
	SD	1.23	1.19	1.39	1.2	1.33	1.34	.89	.88
Event impact upon one's beliefs	M	4.63	5.04	4.5	4.92	4.25	4.77	4.51	5.19
	SD	1.77	1.7	1.52	1.57	1.66	1.89	1.72	1.71
Use and extent of rumination	M	4.56	5.36	4.81	5.41	4.41	5.58	5.1	5.86
	SD	1.56	1.4	1.63	1.36	1.66	1.36	1.38	1.09
Pervasiveness of rumination	M	4.26	4.67	3.62	4.41	3.48	3.57	5.18	5.31
	SD	2.07	1.64	2.01	2.09	2.2	2.01	1.69	1.66
Effectiveness of rumination	M	3.25	3.87	3.14	3.57	3.61	3.41	3.42	3.27
	SD	1.82	1.97	1.76	1.85	2.2	1.84	2.04	1.83
Use and extent of social sharing	M	3.93	3.62	3.23	3.91	3.59	4.06	3.3	4.43
	SD	1.59	1.86	1.84	2.07	2.07	1.76	2.24	2.28
Effectiveness of social sharing etc.	M	3.55	4.12	3.7	3.55	3.52	3.79	3.13	3.74
	SD	1.81	2.1	2.27	1.94	1.91	1.81	2.34	2.17
Use and effectiveness of distraction	M	4.09	3.89	3.69	2.95	3.74	2.83	3.29	2.38
	SD	1.66	1.96	1.76	1.99	2.04	2.02	2.38	2.22
Paradoxical effect of distraction	M	2.86	3.42	2.73	2.41	3.14	2.52	2.14	1.54
	SD	1.44	2.13	1.84	2.19	1.96	2.26	2.18	2.2
Recovery from the event	M	4.29	3.85	4.31	4	4.01	3.41	4.13	3.48
	SD	1.3	1.55	1.57	1.64	1.59	1.58	1.39	1.22
Temporal occurrence of the event	M	3.32	2.34	3.06	3	3.62	3.78	6.08	6.64
	SD	2.29	1.81	2.24	1.98	2.37	2.48	.76	1.26
Perceived importance of the event	M	6.32	6.6	6.54	6.66	6.52	6.76	6.8	6.78
	SD	.79	.61	.73	.66	1.23	.6	.4	.58
Emotional intensity	M	5.86	6.58	6.3	6.3	6.5	6.6	6.9	6.76
	SD	1.41	.97	1.63	1.54	1.23	1.05	.3	.59

Table 4b. Not very significant negative events: Means and standard deviations of dependent variables

Variables		Not very significant negative events							
		adolescent		young		adult		elderly	
		male	female	male	female	male	female	male	female
Negative appraisal of the event	M	3.26	3.25	3.91	4.03	3.43	4.05	3.08	2.94
	SD	1.32	1.33	1.07	1.14	1.33	1.26	1.27	.94
Event impact upon one's beliefs	M	2.78	2.74	3.01	3.51	2.32	2.73	1.74	1.95
	SD	1.54	1.54	1.53	1.52	1.54	1.66	.79	1
Use and extent of rumination	M	2.67	2.55	3.15	3.31	1.99	3.15	2.75	2.8
	SD	1.27	1.35	1.88	1.66	1.48	1.87	1.46	1.53
Pervasiveness of rumination	M	2.73	2.85	2.79	3.25	1.64	2.4	3.17	3
	SD	1.81	2.02	1.93	2.25	1.73	2.08	1.95	1.95
Eeffectiveness of rumination	M	2.84	2.76	2.8	2.84	2.32	2.52	2.8	2.66
	SD	1.59	1.8	1.69	1.97	1.82	2.5	2.1	2.3
Use and extent of social sharing	M	2.03	2.14	2.65	2.82	2.31	3.13	1.93	2.52
	SD	1.24	1.33	1.57	1.5	1.15	1.43	1.35	1.26
Effectiveness of social sharing etc.	M	2.54	2.76	2.8	3.47	3.37	3.83	3.33	4.04
	SD	1.72	1.85	1.76	2.12	1.79	1.91	2.28	2
Use and effectiveness of distraction	M	3.81	4	3.64	3.38	3.01	3.44	4.39	4.14
	SD	1.82	1.88	2.09	2	2.39	2.36	1.89	2.19
Paradoxical effect of distraction	M	2.11	2.11	2.09	1.91	1.43	1.85	2.38	1.8
	SD	1.36	1.35	1.51	1.59	1.47	1.8	1.37	1.26
Recovery from the event	M	6.05	6.01	5.69	5.79	5.99	5.65	6.21	6.32
	SD	.8	1	1.26	1.04	.98	1.04	.8	.8
Temporal occurrence of the event	M	1.7	1.38	1.98	2.5	1.94	2.18	4.6	4.32
	SD	1.29	1.16	1.45	2.1	1.83	1.99	2.52	2.59
Perceived importance of the event	M	3.02	2.92	3.46	3.6	3.14	3.5	3.22	3.34
	SD	.94	.9	.84	.76	1.07	.81	.82	.77
Emotional intensity	M	4.18	4.26	5.04	5.62	5	6	4.16	4.26
	SD	1.54	1.75	1.77	1.59	1.69	1.11	1.5	1.35

Table 5. Results of ANOVAs (pδ01)

Dependent Variables	Effects	F	df	η^2
Negative appraisal of the event	age group	4.55*	3. 784	.017
	gender	7.11*	1. 784	.009
	relevance	513.64**	1. 784	.396
	age group x relevance	19.45**	3. 784	.069
Event impact upon one's beliefs	age group	6.77**	3. 784	.025
	gender	12.64**	1. 784	.016
	relevance	380.59**	1. 784	.327
	age group x relevance	8.31**	3. 784	.031
Perceived importance of the event	age group	7.88**	3. 784	.029
	relevance	3458.1**	1. 784	.815
Emotional intensity	age group	13.01**	3. 784	.047
	gender	9.83*	1. 784	.012
	relevance	291.09**	1. 784	.271
	age group x relevance	16.6**	3. 784	.060
Temporal occurrence of the event	age group	83.89**	3. 784	.243
	relevance	77.91**	1. 784	.090

Note: * pδ.01; ** p<.001.

With regard to the three regulatory modalities, in order to test the effect of the event significance on them and establish the role of the variables assumed to mediate this relationship, seven regression analyses employing the macro made available by Preacher & Hayes (2007) for "estimating and comparing indirect effects in multiple mediator models"[13] were run. In the mediational model frame, this macro makes it possible to test simultaneously the effects of multiple mediational variables, in order to establish if the effect of the independent variable on the dependent one is partially or fully carried out through them or is independent of them. The dependent variables were the seven components related to rumination, social sharing and distraction extracted from the factor analysis. The mediational variables were: perceived importance of the event, emotional intensity, negative appraisal of the event, event impact upon one's beliefs. Event significance was coded as dummy variable (1 = significant event; 0 = not very significant event). Gender and age were put in the analyses as covariates: gender was coded as dummy variable (1 = female; 0 = male) and age was chosen instead of age group because the former was a continuous variable. For each modality, the analyses were performed only on the participants that had used it.

Since the effects of the event significance - together with those of gender and age group - on the mediational variables had been already tested by means of the ANOVAs (whose results showed that all these variables increased whit significant events), for each mediational regression analysis, only the effect of the mediators on the dependent variables, the total effect of the event significance on the dependent variable, and its direct effect were reported after controlling for the multiple mediational effects and the covariates effect. According to the assumptions of mediational model (e.g. Baron & Kenny, 1986; MacKinnon, Krull, & Lockwood, 2000), if the total effect is significant and the direct effect is not, there is a complete mediation; if the direct effect drops but still remains significant, there is a partial

---

[13] The macro is available on: http://www.comm.ohiostate.edu/ahayes/SPSS%20programs/ indirect.htm.

mediation; if the direct effect does not change, there is no mediational effect; finally, if the direct effect increases after controlling for mediational variables, a suppression effect has to be assumed, often due to the opposite direction of independent and mediational variables effects.

As to the model tested for the use and extent of rumination (R^2 = .519; F [7.714] = 110.09; p < .001), the following variables affected this component: importance of the event (ß = .279; p <.001), emotional intensity (ß = .106; p <.001), negative appraisal of the event (ß = .088; p <.05), event impact upon one's beliefs (ß = .090; p <.01), gender (ß = .201; p <.001). All the mediational variables increased with the significant events. Females scored higher than males. After controlling for mediational variables, the total effect of the event significance (ß = 1.23; p <.001) drops dramatically under the level of statistical significance when calculating its direct effect (ß = -.049; p =.703), indicating the presence of complete mediation. As regards the model tested for the pervasiveness of rumination (R^2 = .077; F [7.714] = 8.45; p < .001), the direct effect of mediators concerned the negative appraisal of the event (ß = .117; p <.05), the event impact upon one's beliefs (ß = .179; p <.001), and age (ß = .005; p <.01). Once again the complete mediation occurred, as the comparison between total effect (ß = .329; p <.001) and direct effect (ß = -.128; p = .468) of the event significance demonstrated. The model tested for the perceived effectiveness of rumination (R^2 = .016; F [7.714] = 1.68; p =.111) as well as the total (ß = .111; p =.137) and the direct (ß = .135; p =.458) effects of the event significance failed to reach statistical significance. However, the perceived effectiveness of rumination was affected by the negative appraisal of the event (ß = -.123; p <.05).

The use and extent of social sharing (R^2 = .351; F [7.668] = 51.69; p < .001) was affected by the following mediators: perceived importance of the event (ß = .136; p <.01), its negative appraisal (ß = .127; p <.01), its impact upon one's beliefs (ß = .214; p <.001), gender (ß = .134; p <.05), and age (ß = .003; p <.05). Also in this case, there was a complete mediation, as the comparison between total effect (ß = .995; p <.001) and direct effect (ß = -.123; p = .390) of the event significance showed. The only mediators which directly affected the perceived effectiveness of social sharing and availability of social support[14] (R^2 = .036; F [7,668] = 3.61; p < .001) were emotional intensity (ß = .059; p <.05) and age (ß = .008; p <.001). Neither did the total or the direct effect of the independent variable reach the statistical significance level.

The use and perceived effectiveness of distraction (R^2 = .054; F [7.558] = 4.57; p < .001) was affected negatively by the perceived importance of the event (ß = -.191; p <.001) and positively by age (ß = .008; p <.001). This opposite direction of the two mediational variables produced the suppression effect showed by the statistical significance level reached by the direct effect of independent variable (ß = .481; p <.001) only after controlling for the mediational variables, while its total effect did not. Finally, the paradoxical effect of distraction (R^2 = .340; F [7,558] = 40.98; p < .001) was affected by the following mediators: emotional intensity (ß = .058; p <.05), negative appraisal of the event (ß = .194; p <.001), event impact upon one's beliefs (ß = .222; p <.001), and age (ß = .005; p <.001). The total effect of the event significance (ß = .959; p <.001) dropped after controlling for the

---

[14] For the sake of brevity, this component will be from now on labelled only as "effectiveness of social sharing".

mediational variable but its direct effect on the paradoxical effect of distraction still was significant (β = .360; p <.05).

In order to assess whether and to what extent the regulatory modalities, along with the other variables considered in this study, had affected the recovery from the event, a standard multiple regression analysis was performed using as predictors: participants' gender and age, perceived importance of the event, its temporal occurrence, its negative appraisal, its impact upon one's beliefs, emotional intensity, use and extent of rumination and of social sharing, perceived effectiveness of the three regulatory modalities, perceived pervasiveness of rumination and of the paradoxical effect of distraction. The analysis was performed only on the participants that had used all the three regulatory modalities, i.e., 437 participants (54.63%). Once again, gender was coded as dummy variable (1 = female; 0 = male) and age, as continuous variable, was chosen instead of age group. The perceived importance of the event was used instead of the event significance so as to prevent multicollinearity, since the two predictors were highly correlated with each other (r of Pearson = .895; VIF = 6.76 for perceived importance and = 5.16 for event significance) and the previous analyses showed that the effect of event significance was totally or partially dropped out after introducing mediational variables, with the only exception of the suppression effect on the use and perceived effectiveness of distraction. Results are reported in table 6.

Table 6. Results of standard multiple regression analysis with recovery from the event as dependent variable

R = .773 ; R^2 = .597 ; F (14, 422) = 44.61; p< .001			
Predictors	β	t	p
gender	.023	.717	.474
age	-.051	-1.390	.165
perceived importance of the event	-.173	-3.431	.001
temporal occurrence of the event	.125	3.541	.000
emotional intensity	.031	.763	.446
negative appraisal of the event	-.067	-1.614	.107
event impact upon one's beliefs	-.098	-2.381	.018
use and extent of rumination	-.468	-9.256	.000
use and extent of social sharing	-.072	-1.770	.078
use and effectiveness of distraction	.032	.990	.323
perceived effectiveness of rumination	.071	2.111	.035
perceived effectiveness of social sharing and availability of social support	.072	2.128	.034
pervasiveness of rumination	.037	1.090	.276
paradoxical effect of distraction	-.098	-2.465	.014

The predictor showing the most positive relation with the recovery from the event was the temporal occurrence of the event, whilst the perceived effectiveness of rumination and of social sharing showed a weaker, even if still significant, positive relation. The perceived importance of the event, its impact upon one's beliefs, the paradoxical effect of distraction and, above all, the use and extent of rumination were negatively related to the criterion variable. The remaining variables did not affect it.

In order to investigate whether the variables not affecting directly the recovery from the event (i.e. gender, age, emotional intensity, negative appraisal of the event, pervasiveness of rumination, use and extent of social sharing, use and perceived effectiveness of distraction) had affected it indirectly through the mediation of the other variables examined in this study, seven regression analyses employing the macro made available by Preacher & Hayes (2007) for estimating and comparing indirect effects in multiple mediator models were carried out.

It is worthy to note that, in each analysis, all the variables considered in this study - except for the variable which, from time to time, was taken as the independent one - were included in the model as mediators or as covariates as a function of their logical position regarding the relationship between the independent and the dependent variables (e.g. in the analysis where age was the independent variable, only gender was included as covariate; in the analysis where the pervasiveness of rumination was the independent variable, gender, age, temporal occurrence of the event, its perceived importance, its negative appraisal, its impact upon one's beliefs and emotional intensity were included as covariates and the variables concerning the regulatory modalities were included as mediators) (please, add). In this way, the same model was tested both for the multiple regression and the seven mediational analyses; moreover, the reciprocal effects between the components of rumination, social sharing and distraction were assessed. (please, delete) The analyses were performed only on the participants that had used all the three regulatory modalities.

Results showed that neither gender nor age had had any total or direct effect on the recovery from the event. On the contrary, the comparison between the total (B = -.241; p <.001) and the direct (B = .018; p = .446) effect of emotional intensity highlighted that this variable affected the recovery from the event only indirectly trough the mediation of the following variables: perceived importance of the event (B = .628; p <.001), its negative appraisal (B = .315; p <.001), its impact upon one's beliefs (B = .243; p <.001), use and extent of rumination (B = .320; p <.001), its pervasiveness (B = .084; p <.01), its perceived effectiveness (B = .090; p <.01), use and extent of social sharing (B = .220; p <.001), its perceived effectiveness (B = .076; p <.05), paradoxical effect of distraction (B = .216; p <.001). Also the negative appraisal of the event affected the dependent variable only indirectly (total effect: B = -.450; p <.001; direct effect: B = -.064; p =.107), by means of all the mediators (with B going from .220 – pervasiveness of rumination – to 1.088 – perceived importance of the event - and p always <.001), except for gender, age, (please, delete) perceived effectiveness of social sharing, use and perceived effectiveness of distraction.

The pervasiveness of rumination did not affect the recovery from the event either directly or indirectly. Nevertheless it showed a positive relationship with use and extent of social sharing (B = .154; p <.01) and the paradoxical effect of distraction (B = .276; p <.001). The use and extent of social sharing affected indirectly the recovery (total effect: B = -.498; p <.001; direct effect: B = -.071; p =.078) and showed a positive relationship with use and extent of rumination (B = .611; p <.01), pervasiveness of rumination (B = .151; p <.01), paradoxical effect of distraction (B = .478; p <.001). perceived importance of the event (B = .933; p <.001), emotional intensity (B = .616; p <.001), temporal occurrence (B = .347; p <.01) and negative appraisal (B = .412; p <.001) of the event, and event's impact upon one's beliefs (B = .434; p <.001) (please, delete). Also the use and perceived effectiveness of distraction affected indirectly the dependent variable (total effect: B =.141; p <.01; direct effect: B = .031; p =.323) and showed a positive relationship with age (B = 2.677; p <.001) (please, delete) the perceived effectiveness of rumination (B = .159; p <.001) and of social sharing (B = .248; p <.001), while a negative relationship with the perceived importance of the event (B = -.237; p <.01) and (please, delete) the use and extent of rumination (B = -.133; p <.01) was found.

Selection of the Most Effective Regulatory Modality

Finally, the data referred to the participants' answers about the last query of the questionnaire, i.e. to indicate the most effective regulatory modality out of the proposed list of thirteen, were treated through three chi square tests for two independent samples, crossing the type of responses with, respectively, event significance, gender, and age group[15]. Results were interpreted by means of adjusted standardized residuals analysis. The frequency distribution of the responses is illustrated in table 7.

Table 7. Frequency distribution of perceived most effective coping modality by gender, age group, and event significance

	Gender		Age group				Event significance		
	Male	Female	Adolesc.	Young	Adult	Elderly	Very significant	Not very significant	Total
kept thinking back to the event	27	34	31	14	11	5	39	22	61
talked with others	34	57	24	28	33	6	34	57	91
thought of other things	31	29	27	14	10	9	21	39	60
emotional ventilation	37	42	23	22	17	17	33	46	79
remediate to what happened	59	36	15	15	25	40	24	71	95
reflection on the event	55	35	21	38	13	18	35	55	90
engaged in work or study	14	12	2	8	9	7	15	11	26
affection of beloved persons	42	53	24	18	29	24	71	24	95
passing of time	56	65	20	25	31	45	77	44	121
plans for the future	8	8	3	7	5	1	7	9	16
professional support/help	14	8	1	5	5	11	15	7	22
travel or plea sant activities	9	3	4	3	1	4	3	9	12
other modalities	4	11	1	3	2	9	9	6	15
Total	390	393	196	200	191	196	383	400	783

[15] Log linear analysis was not performed because the response modalities were too numerous and results would have been rather confusing. Note that only the participants who believed they had at least partially overcome the event were requested to answer this question.

As regards the event significance, results (χ^2 [d.f. 12] = 85.09, p<.001) showed that beloved people's affection, time passing, thinking back to the event for a long time, psychological or medical support were cited more than theoretically expected in SEC than in NVSEC; on the contrary, social sharing, distraction (succeeding in thinking of something else), succeeding in remedying what happened, reflecting on the event showed the opposite trend. The perceived efficacy of the remaining listed coping modalities did not vary in function of the event significance. As to gender effects, results (χ^2 [d.f. 12] = 27, p<.001) highlighted that females judged social sharing more effective than males, while the latter considered remedying what happened and reflecting on the event more helpful than the former did. No difference was found on the other coping modalities. As far as the age group is concerned, results (χ^2 [d.f. 36] = 136.14, p<.001) illustrated that thinking back to the event was mentioned the most by the adolescents and the least by the elderly, social sharing was cited the most by the adults and the least by the elderly; distraction was judged the most effective coping modality above all by the adolescents and least of all by the elderly; remedying what happened was reported the most by the elderly and the least by the adolescents and the young; reflecting on the event was quoted mainly by the young and the least by the adults; totally devoting themselves to their work or studies was reported the least by the adolescents; time passing and psychological support were both mentioned the most by the elderly and the least by the adolescents; finally the elderly cited other coping modalities, not contained in the list, more than the other participants. No difference was found on the remaining listed coping modalities.

CONCLUSION

This study aimed at investigating how people perceive, experience and deal with negative life events and whether event significance, gender, and age affected the above-mentioned processes. In this frame, the use and the perceived effectiveness of rumination, social sharing, and distraction as emotional regulatory modalities were specifically examined.

The two types of evidence deriving from narratives and quantitative assessments formed a composite but coherent plot from which some guidelines will be drawn.

The manipulation of the event significance was successful: it affected not only quantitative assessment of the emotional episodes reported in the two research conditions but also their qualitative features. The prototypical irremediable event, the death of a loved person, was the most remembered one in SEC, while conflictual relationships, that is foreseeable and often amendable events, were the most reported ones in NVSEC. Emotion families characterized by a low level of arousal and action readiness, such as SADNESS and HELPLESSNESS, were elicited more often by significant events than by not very significant ones, while the opposite happened with ANGER, that is an emotion family marked by a high level of arousal and action readiness. Although the most cited event consequences category, i.e. "negative impact upon oneself and upon one's emotional state", did not show frequency difference in function of the event significance, the sense of losing reference points, implying feeling alone and unable to deal with life, was reported almost only in SEC, whereas the perception of changed attitudes in relationships and towards one's environment, which entails changes in behavioral transactions with one's milieu, was referred more often in NVSEC than in SEC.

On the whole, these findings suggest that major negative events often involve perceiving active responses, i.e. any action aimed at changing environmental aspects in order to remediate, modify or undo what happened, as useless. The results also support the hypothesis put forward about the individuals' proneness to use emotion-focused rather than problem-focused coping in major negative events, given their frequently being irremediable. Both log-linear analyses and the chi square test on the type of coping by type of events showed that problem-solving strategies were more often used in minor than in major life events, even if in log-linear analysis results this tendency appeared somehow less clear because of the further interaction between event significance and age group. Nevertheless, it is worthy to note that social sharing/support, the most used coping category in SEC, encompassed episodes in which communicating one's emotional experience was motivated by a number of reasons, including emotional venting, need for empathy or affiliation, seeking of emotional or instrumental help, sometimes by professional caregivers. One can infer that after significant negative events participants needed others' contribution also for identifying problem-solving strategies which they could have found autonomously in less stressful situations. However, the general long-lasting duration of significant negative events consequences[16] suggests not only that significant negative events have had a persistent impact upon the participants' life, but also that the coping strategies employed to deal with them have been scarcely effective. On the contrary, the general shorter-lasting duration of not very important events suggests the opposite considerations. Nevertheless, since the efficacy of the coping modalities that participants reported to have used has not been assessed, it has not been possible to establish the respective weight of event impact and coping effectiveness on event consequences duration: therefore, the previous suggestion has only a speculative character.

The significant negative events were assessed in a clearly different way from the not very significant ones. This difference was found in all the variables assumed to capture the subjective evaluation of the reported emotional experience and to mediate the incidence of the manipulated variable on the three regulatory modalities specifically investigated. Compared to the less significant ones, significant events were perceived as consistently more important, were appraised more negatively, were felt to shatter more severely one's general beliefs and produced a higher emotional reaction. These findings corroborated the hypothesis based on response stress theories (Horowitz, 1986, 2003; Janoff-Bulman, 1992; Tait & Silver, 1989), according to which traumatic events threaten habitual routines and bring into question one's notions and expectations about oneself, the others and the world.

The variables by means of which the subjective effects produced by the manipulation of event significance have been evaluated, have proved to be able to clarify the processes through which the independent variable affected the three regulatory modalities. More specifically, these variables functioned as mediators between the event significance and the components which emerged from the factor analyses on items referring to rumination, social sharing and distraction.

---

[16] Also in this case such a tendency has to be disentangled from the somehow confusing three-way interaction of duration, event significance and age groups emerged from log-linear analysis.

Before commenting on these findings, it is worthy to observe that the components extracted by the factor analyses showed a theoretically explainable internal congruence. The three components emerged from items related to rumination – its use and extent, pervasiveness, and perceived effectiveness – reflect the conceptually relevant dimensions documented by literature and investigated in this study. The items loading on the first component denote the structural features of rumination, that is the frequency of repetitive thoughts after the event and at present, their level of uncontrollability and cognitive dominance; the items loading on the second component indicate the subjective perception of the rumination overwhelmingness, i.e., the desire to interrupt repetitive thoughts and its failure; items loading on the third component denote the perceived cognitive and emotional effectiveness of rumination. The two components referring to social sharing designate its structural features and its perceived effectiveness along with the expected and perceived level of social support. The fact that the items assessing the perceived effectiveness of social sharing and the degree of expected and received social support loaded on the same component corroborates the idea that the subjective efficacy of communicating one's emotional experience is connected with the need and the perception of others' responsiveness. Note that the items loading on the first component of social sharing are structurally similar to the items loading on the first component of rumination, i.e. the frequency of talking about the event after its occurrence and at present, its level of uncontrollability and cognitive dominance.

It must be said that the questionnaire included only two items aiming at testing the dysfunctional effects of social sharing: one concerning its level of uncontrollability (to what extent participants couldn't help talking about the event) and the other its level of dominance (how long speaking about the event was the dominant topic of conversation). Nevertheless, unlike my expectations, these items did not load on a specific component of factorial analysis: on the contrary, as we have seen, they loaded on the same component as the items designating the frequency of talking about the event after its occurrence and at present, i.e. the component labelled as "use and extent of social sharing". On the one hand, the structural analogy between this component and "use and extent of rumination" suggests that as the thoughts' repetitiveness and uncontrollability represent a definitional feature of rumination, so the reiteration and the uncontrollability of talking represent an intrinsic feature of social sharing. On the other hand, the absence in this questionnaire of further items aiming at testing the possible dysfunctional features of social sharing does not allow us to know whether the similarities between rumination and social sharing would have extended to this aspect as well.

The items loading on distraction components showed a grouping criterion somehow different from rumination and social sharing. The first component, which encompasses both the two items referring to the attempts of distracting oneself from the event and to their success and the two items related to the perceived efficacy of distraction, seems to indicate that distraction is considered *in se* an effective regulatory modality. In other terms, it is possible to infer that distraction from a negative event is an effortful process rather than a natural and somewhat automatic process like rumination and social sharing. As a result, the mere fact of being able to distract oneself from negative events indicates that one's efforts have been effective: this awareness is part of the overall assessment of the distraction effectiveness in dealing with negative events. The second component includes the items denoting the paradoxical effect of distraction which, as described in literature (e.g. Koole *et al.,*1999; Wegner, 1994; Wenzlaff *et al.*, 1988), in this study have been identified as the inner "weight" of the event in spite of diverting the attention from it, the difficulty to distract oneself with the passing of time, the abrupt resurgence of the event's pain, the sense of extraneousness to the event.

The structural similarity between rumination and social sharing shown by the results of factor analyses was further supported by the results of mediational analyses. Both the use and extent of rumination and social sharing were affected by the event significance only indirectly, i.e. through the complete mediation of the variables capturing the internal repercussions of the two different values of the independent variable. The increase of almost all the mediational variables enhanced the use and extent of rumination and social sharing, except for age as far as the first variable was concerned and for emotional intensity as far the second was concerned. Both the independent variable and the mediators failed to predict the efficacy of rumination, although such a component was affected negatively by the negative appraisal of the event. Quite similarly, the perceived effectiveness of social sharing was predicted only by emotional intensity and age.

Considered on the whole, these findings support the hypotheses about the function of rumination and social sharing based on assumptions and evidence from previous literature (e.g. Horowitz, 2003; Janoff-Bulman, 1992; Martin & Tesser, 1996; Rimé *et al.*, 1998; Rimé & Zech, 2001; Ullrich & Lutgendorf, 2002; Wells, 2000). Both work as "sense-seekers" to understand what happened, restore one's shattered beliefs and re-establish psychological balance. Rumination is based only on one's cognitive resources, whereas social sharing relies also on others' contribution, thus serving the supplementary function of increasing individuals' network and enhancing social relationships (Rimé, 2007).

The finding according to which only the use of rumination and not of social sharing is affected by emotional intensity leads to advance further considerations about their respective function.

As I said in the Introduction, I assume that rumination pertains first of all to the cognitive content of emotion and represents an intrinsic and somehow automatic modality of emotion regulation. In other terms, I posit that thinking of an event is a subjective manifestation of its importance for the individual's "concerns" (Frijda, 1986), i.e. a subjective reaction to its emotional meaning. The more important an event, the longer it occupies one's mind, independently of its hedonic valence: in fact, people keep thinking of positive emotional experiences as well. At the same time, this cognitive aspect of emotion serves an intrinsic regulatory function by producing a sort of habituation to emotional feelings, through which emotion intensity can be modulated. In my opinion, habituation is the primary – emotional – function of rumination. The search for meaning may be considered as a cognitive, more elaborate function, even though repetitive thoughts are often unwanted and uncontrolled.

On the contrary, the independence found between the use of social sharing and emotional intensity does not corroborate Rimé and colleagues' findings (Luminet *et al.*, 2000; Rimé *et al.*, 1998) about the incidence of the event's emotional salience on the onset of social sharing. As far as the participants in this study are concerned, communicating one's emotional experience seems to have been mainly motivated by the cognitive need for understanding why what happened had happened, thanks to the others' contribution, rather than by the need of reducing emotional intensity by sharing its weight with others. Nevertheless, the relationship between emotional intensity and social sharing becomes more complex when considering that – apart from the organism variable "age"- emotional intensity was the only mediational variable affecting – though rather weakly - the perceived effectiveness of social sharing. One might suppose that social exchange, although not motivated by emotional urge, involved the communication of the emotional experience and that the higher the emotional intensity, the more its sharing was perceived as effective.

However, it must be stressed that the perceived effectiveness of social sharing – and much more of rumination - remains substantially unexplained by the event significance and its subjective repercussions, as assessed by the mediational variables. This leaves the question of the potential predictors of the perceived efficacy of these regulatory modalities unsolved. The age incidence on the perceived effectiveness of social sharing suggests that, at least for this regulatory modality, a possible explanation criterion has to be found at the level of the individual differences in emotion regulation.

Instead, despite the apparently disturbing suppression effect, results concerning the use and perceived effectiveness of distraction conform to the hypotheses about the role of the event's perceived importance as negative predictor and of the age increase as positive predictor. As it was supposed, distracting oneself from negative events appeared to have been easier when they were perceived as less important. Since less important events demand less emotional and cognitive involvement than more important ones, the attempts of diverting one's attention from them probably were less difficult and more successful than in the case of more important events. The positive relationship between age increase and use and perceived effectiveness of distraction had been foreseen on the basis of previous evidence showing older people's tendency not to focus on negative feelings and use, among others, avoidant or proactive strategies of emotion regulation (Blanchard-Fields *et al.*, 2004; Blanchard-Fields, 2007; Carstensen *et al.* 2003). So, the effect of suppression, produced by the divergent direction of the influence of these two variables, is theoretically explicable.

As regards the pervasiveness of rumination and the paradoxical effect of distraction, i. e. the "dysregulation" effects of these two regulatory modalities, both were positively predicted by negative appraisal, event impact on one's beliefs, and age; the paradoxical effect of distraction was affected also by emotional intensity. Once again, these findings seem to conform to the hypotheses underlying this study. The more the event was perceived as disconfirming one's beliefs system, the more the modalities activated in order to cope with it were felt as producing an opposite outcome than the wished one. Moreover, the finding that the paradoxical effect of distraction was predicted also by emotional intensity leads to infer that diverting the attention from negative events and their internal repercussions does not appear to be an effective strategy for managing emotions.

As I have already noted, the dysfunctional effect of social sharing failed to be specifically assessed by this questionnaire.

The effectiveness of rumination, social sharing and distraction in recovering from the event has been evaluated together with the incidence of all the variables assessed in this study and assumed to affect, positively or negatively, the recovery from the reported emotional experience. The perceived effectiveness of rumination and social sharing and, above all, the time gone by from the event occurrence were the variables that directly predicted the recovery. On the contrary, the perceived importance of the event, its impact upon one's beliefs, the paradoxical effect of distraction, and, above all, the use and extent of rumination were the variables affecting negatively the recovery – so indicating the present persistence of the emotional experience.

The negative appraisal of the event and the use and extent of social sharing affected the current persistence of the event only indirectly through most mediational variables, except the perceived effectiveness of rumination and social sharing, the use and perceived effectiveness of distraction, gender and age. Also emotional intensity affected indirectly and negatively the recovery through almost all the mediators, except the perceived effectiveness of social sharing, the use and perceived effectiveness of distraction, gender and age. Instead, the use and perceived effectiveness of distraction affected positively the recovery but through the positive mediation of age and the perceived effectiveness of rumination and social sharing, and the negative mediation of event importance and use and extent of rumination.

Gender, age and pervasiveness of rumination did not affect either directly or indirectly the recovery.

The results related to the efficacy of three emotion regulation modalities – one of the most important aims of the research – need to be further commented on.

In accordance with the hypotheses, the more important and negatively featured an event is perceived and the stronger its cognitive and affective repercussions are felt, the more prolonged the event's internal permanence is. Note that the perceived importance and the impact of the event on one's beliefs continued to predict its current permanence, even after controlling for the other mediational variables, whereas the emotional intensity and the event's negative appraisal affected the outcome only through the mediators. This finding shows that it is not the emotional reaction *in se* to enable to predict the event's persistence in one's mind, but its positive relationship with the cognitive consequence of the event and the fact that it increases all the components of the emotion regulatory modalities, except the use and effectiveness of distraction. Conversely, this finding suggests that the recovery from the dysphoric emotional reaction to a negative event is somehow a side effect of the recovery from the cognitive consequences of an event.

The finding that the strongest predictor of the current permanence of the event is the use and extent of rumination corroborates the wide-ranging corpus of studies showing the dysfunctional effect of rumination and its incidence in extending the internal length of the event one is repetitively and compulsively focused on (Horowitz, 1986, 2003; Janoff-Bulman, 1992; Lyubomirsky & Nolen-Hoeksema, 1993; Martin & Tesser, 1996; Nolen-Hoeksema, 2004; Segerstrom *et al.*, 2003; Tait & Silver, 1989). Since the items loading on this component assessed - in decreasing weight order - the present and the past frequency, the cognitive dominance and the uncontrollability of rumination, the negative relationship between this component and recovery can be interpreted in a twofold way. On the one hand, it seems to indicate that the longer the rumination duration, the longer the mental persistence of the event - as most scholars state (Horowitz, 1986, 2003; Lyubomirsky & Nolen-Hoeksema, 1993; Lyubomirsky et al., 1998; Nolen-Hoeksema, 1991, 2004; Segerstrom *et al.*, 2003; Tait & Silver, 1989). On the other, it can point out that the un-recovered events still activate ruminative thoughts aiming at accomplishing the meaning-search process, as some authors posit (Martin, 1999; Martin & Tesser, 1996). As this study did not include an experimental manipulation of the rumination (and the other regulatory modalities) use degree, it was not possible to establish *a priori* a causal relationship between use of rumination and recovery, but only to advance a number of theoretical or logical considerations able to support an interpretation rather than another. The temporal direction between rumination and recovery should lead us to support the first of the two interpretations; however, in my opinion, the second – i.e. until it is un-recovered, an event is still ruminatively present in one's mind – is equally sustainable from a conceptual point of view. Anyway, this interpretation, like the other, leads us to admit that the use of rumination has been largely ineffective to cope with the event.

Similar considerations also apply as regards the negative function indirectly exerted by the use and extent of social sharing on the recovery. Even though the effect of this component is less noticeable than the effect of the use of rumination, nevertheless it signals once again that the outcome of a hypothetical emotion regulatory modality is the opposite of the desired effect. These results corroborate and further extend the findings about the ineffectiveness of social sharing for recovering from the event emerged from the wide corpus of research carried out by Rimé and colleagues (e.g. Rimé *et al.*, 1998; Zech & Rimé, 2005). They also confirm the similarity about rumination and social sharing found throughout this study, which is further strengthened by the observation that their perceived effectiveness positively and directly affected the recovery but remains substantially unexplained by most of the variables supposed to assess the event salience and its subjective repercussions.

It is worthy to repeat that, according to this study, while the use extension of rumination and social sharing predicts the persistence of the negative event, their perceived effectiveness predicts the recovery function. In my opinion, this apparent incongruence is due to the fact that the assessment of the use and the subjective effectiveness of the regulatory modalities have been carried *a posteriori,* from a backward perspective: the participants who felt they had recovered from the event assessed more positively the effectiveness of these modalities, and participants who still felt the event's mental burden still ruminated on it and talked about it.

The positive relationship between the perceived and actual effectiveness of the regulatory modalities has been found also for the use and effectiveness of distraction. This component affected indirectly the recovery through the positive relationship with age and the perceived effectiveness of rumination and social sharing, and through the negative relationship with the perceived importance of the event and the use and extent of rumination. On the one hand, this finding is analogous to the ones concerning the role played by the perceived effectiveness of rumination and social sharing on recovery: the subjective perception of the efficacy of the regulatory modality predicts – or corresponds to – the recovery. On the other hand, the negative relationship with the use and extent of rumination seems to corroborate the previous assumptions (e.g. Nolen-Hoeksema, 1991, 2004; Nolen-Hoeksema, & Morrow, 1993) about the process through which distraction is effective, that is to divert one's attention from the event, so preventing rumination. Nevertheless, the extent of this result is limited by the presence of the negative relationship between this component and the perceived importance of the event: the more important an event is perceived, the more difficult it is to distract one's attention. On the contrary, the paradoxical effect of distraction - which directly influences the current persistence of the event – is enhanced by the increase of the cognitive and emotional correlates of the salient negative event. Such a result further reduces the scope of the effectiveness of distraction and partially disconfirms the findings of a wide number of studies showing the beneficial effect of distraction in dealing with major life negative events (Lyubomirsky et al., 1998; Morrow & Nolen-Hoeksema, 1990; Rusting & Nolen-Hoeksema 1998; Thayer et al., 1994; Trask & Sigmon, 1999).

On the whole, these results highlighted that, in spite of their ample use (especially as far as rumination and social sharing are concerned), the three regulatory modalities seem, in fact, scarcely effective or, when they serve a recovery function, the processes by which this function acts remain unclear. Probably, this is largely due to individual differences, which have not been specifically investigated by this study, except for age and gender.

As regards these variables, it can be observed that the present findings showed fewer gender differences than age group differences.

The overall results emerging from qualitative and quantitative assessments and from the last query of the questionnaire - i.e. the selection of the most effective regulatory modality out of the proposed list of thirteen – seem to show that females and males are more similar than gender-role stereotypes suppose them to be, even though some differentiation lines clearly emerged from this study, too. Both genders perceived with equal intensity the event's importance, described quite similar event typologies and consequences, showed analogous emotional responses to negative events in terms of emotion families reported, and did not differ as far as the recovery from the event is concerned. Instead, the differences between genders were found in the quantitative assessment of the event features and in the coping modalities use or evaluation. Compared to males, females appraised the event more negatively and felt its emotional and cognitive impact more intensely, were more prone to use rumination and, above all, social sharing and social support, while males tended to use suppression and avoidance strategies and perceive problem solving-like strategies - as remediate to or reflect on what happened - as the most effective ones. No gender difference was found with regard to the rumination and social sharing effects evaluation and the distraction use and assessment. These results confirm the previous findings concerning female proneness to ruminate and seek social support (e.g. Eschenbeck et al., 2007; Nolen-Hoeksema, 2002; Nolen-Hoeksema & Morrow, 1993; Tamres et al., 2002) and male proneness to avoidant strategies use (Eschenbeck, et al., 2007; Hampel & Petermann, 2005). However they do not support either the gender difference about the distraction use (Nolen-Hoeksema, 1994, 2002; Nolen-Hoeksema et al., 1999) or the gender likeness about social sharing (Luminet et al., 2000; Rimé et al., 1992).

On the whole, these findings corroborate, at least as regards the areas investigated in this study, the theories of sex difference claiming that women are more prone to intensely felt and overtly expressed emotion (La France & Banaji,1992) and that they are biologically hard-wired to react to threat adopting a "tend-and-befriend" (Taylor, Klein, Lewis, Gruenewald, Gurung, & Updegraff, 2000) response rather than the "fight-or-flight" response proposed by Cannon (1932). Female susceptibility to feel negative events' impact and their preference for using social sharing and seeking social support to cope with them are predicted by these theories.

More numerous are the differences related to age, even though the frequent reciprocal interactions between the four age groups make it quite difficult to identify clear-cut differentiation lines. So, I will only summarize and comment on the most important and theoretically relevant findings, which concern especially the elderly and the adolescents. With regard to the emotions elicited by the event, the elderly tended to report more often the types of emotion involving a sense of threat and poor resources to cope with it, such as FEAR, HELPLESSNESS, CONFUSION, while adolescents and adults cited them less than the others. The elderly differentiated the frequency of coping modalities described in the function of the event significance, even though they tended to report distraction, social sharing/support and passing of time more often than the other participants. Adolescents attached less importance to the reported events than the other three groups and felt the emotions generated by them less intensely. The elderly evaluated the event's emotional and cognitive impact in a clearly differentiated manner in function of its significance: they were little involved in not very significant events and highly involved in significant ones. The temporal occurrence of the event reported varied according to the age group: the older the participants' age, the more the event was placed in the past.

With regard to the quantitative assessment of rumination, social sharing and distraction, with age the participants used more frequently social sharing and distraction and felt more intensely the dysfunctional effect of rumination and distraction, and the beneficial effects of social sharing. The age groups showed different judgements about the most effective coping modality believed to be the most helpful to recover from the event. For instance, adolescents judged more effective than the elderly "kept thinking back to the event" and "thought of other things", while the latter estimated "remediate to what happened", "professional support" and "passing of time" more effective than adolescents did.

On the whole, adolescents seem more detached and less emotionally involved than the other participants. This is perhaps due to the fact that they are rather unlikely to have already experienced major negative life events, such as the death of a loved person, divorces, separations, dismissals and so on. From this point of view, it would seem that adolescents are able to put in perspective the events concerning themselves and modulate their evaluations and emotional responses according to the events' seriousness. From another perspective, we could think that they adopt an avoidant-like emotional style, or a form of proactive coping (Aspinwall & Taylor, 1997), based on freezing emotional events before the emotional response is triggered. Since this aspect has not been specifically investigated in this research, the previous suppositions remain at a speculative level.

The research results seem to confirm the recent findings on emotional life in old age, showing that emotion regulation increases in this stage of life (Blanchard-Fields et al., 2004; Blanchard-Fields, 2007; Carstensen et al. 2003; Garnefski & Kraaij, 2006; Gross et al., 1997; Labouvie-Vief & Medler, 2002; Kliegel et al., 2007). They also corroborate the findings of Rimé et al. (1995), according to which social sharing grows in old age, and the findings (Garnefski & Kraaij, 2006; Thomsen et al., 2005) showing no difference among age groups with regard to the use of rumination. The age increase has been the only variable to show a clear effect on the perceived effectiveness of social sharing and on the use and effectiveness of distraction. This finding leads to infer that the current efficacy of these modalities in predicting the recovery depended, at least partially, on the proneness of old people to employ them and emphasize their positive aspects in the more general frame typical of this lifespan age, i.e. the awareness that one cannot but accept what cannot be changed. From this point of view, the fact that with age the perception of the dysfunctional effects of rumination and distraction increases does not contradict the previous assumption but, rather, signals that old people are more open to perceive (and perhaps, avoid) the negative repercussions of maladaptive modalities of dealing with negative events.

Finally, it needs to be remarked that the most robust predictor of the recovery is the time gone by from the event and that this finding is analogous to the one emerging from the selection of the most useful modality of coping – showing that the most effective ways to deal with important negative events were the passing of time and the affection of the loved persons.

Therefore, I would like to close this chapter quoting the famous line of the French singer-songwriter Léo Ferré: "*Avec le temps, va, tout s'en va*" [With time everything goes away].

ACKNOWLEDGMENTS

I am grateful to Simona Baldi, Anna Iadicicco, Nadia Petolicchio, and Filomena Tuccillo for their participation in this research. Particularly, I thank Nadia Petrolicchio and Filomena Tuccillo also for their contribution in preparing the tables and references for this chapter. Finally, I am very grateful to Luciana Pasqua, Vincenzo Paolo Senese, and Lucia Abbamonte for their valuable comments on an earlier version of this chapter.

REFERENCES

Abela, J. R. Z., Vanderbilt, E., & Rochon, A. (2004). A test of the integration of the response styles and social support theories of depression in third and seventh grade children. *Journal of Social and Clinical Psychology*, 23 (5), 653-674.

Almeida, D. M., & Kessler, R. C. (1998). Everyday stressors and gender differences in daily distress. *Journal of Personality and Social Psychology*, 75, 670-680.

Aspinwall, L. G., & Taylor, S. E. (1997). A stitch in time: Self-regulation and proactive coping. *Psychological Bulletin,* 121, 417-436.

Arnold, M. B. (1960). *Emotion and personality*, Vol.1: *Psychological aspects.* New York: Columbia University Press.

Baltes, P. B. (1987). Theoretical propositions of life-span developmental psychology: On the dynamics between growth and decline. *Developmental Psychology, 23,* 611–626.

Baltes, P. B. (1997). On the incomplete architecture of human ontogeny: Selection, optimization, and compensation as foundation of developmental theory. *American Psychologist, 52,* 366–380.

Baron, R. M., & Kenny, D. A. (1986). The moderator-mediator variable distinction in social psychological research: Conceptual, strategic, and statistical considerations. *Journal of Personality and Social Psychology, 51,*1173-1182.

Birditt, K. S., & Fingerman, K. L. (2003). Age and gender differences in adults' descriptions of emotional reactions to interpersonal problems. *Journal of Gerontology: Series B: Psychological Sciences*, 58B, 237-245.

Blanchard-Fields, F. (2007). Everyday problem solving and emotion: An adult developmental perspective. *Current Directions in Psychological Science*, 16, 26-31.

Blanchard-Fields, F., Chen, Y., & Norris, L. (1997). Everyday problem solving across the adult life span: Influence of domain specificity and cognitive appraisal. *Psychology and Aging, 12,* 684–693.

Blanchard-Fields, F., Stein, R., & Watson, T. L. (2004). Age differences in emotion-regulation strategies in handling everyday problems. *Journals of Gerontology: Series B: Psychological Sciences and Social Sciences, 59B*, 261-269.

Boekaerts, M. (2002). Intensity of emotions, emotional regulation, and goal framing: How are they related to adolescents' choice of coping strategies? *Anxiety, stress and coping*, 15, 401- 412.

Bosma, H., & Jackson, S. (eds.) (1990). *Coping and self concept in adolescence.* Berlin: Springer.

Boucher, J. D. (1983). Antecedents to emotions across cultures. Chapter 28. In: S. H. Irvine & J. W. Berry (eds.) *Human Assessment and Cultural Factors.* (pp. 407- 420). New York: Plenum Press.

Bower, J. E., Kemeny, M. E., Taylor, S. E., & Fahey, J. L. (1998). Cognitive processing, discovery of meaning, CD4 decline, and AIDS related mortality among bereaved HIV-seropositive men. *Journal of Consulting and Clinical Psychology, 66,* 979–986.

Breuer, J. & Freud, S. (1895/1957) *Studies on Hysteria.* New York: Basic Books.

Campos, J. J., Frankel, C. B., & Camras, L. (2004). On the nature of emotion regulation. *Child Development*, 75 (2), 377-394.

Cannon, W. B. (1932). *The wisdom of the body.* New York: Norton.

Carstensen, L. L. (1995). Evidence for a life-span theory of socioemotional selectivity. *Current Directions in Psychological Science, 4,* 151-156.

Carstensen, L. L., Fung, H. H., & Charles, S. T. (2003). Socioemotional selectivity theory and the regulation of emotion in the second half of life. *Motivation and Emotion*, 27 (2), 103-123.

Carver C.S., & Scheier M.F. (1981). *Attention and self-regulation: A control-theory approach to human behavior.* New York: Springer-Verlag.

Carver C.S., & Scheier M.F. (1990). Origins and functions of positive and negative affect: A control-process view. *Psychological Review*, 97, 19-35.

Carver, C. S., Scheier, M. F., & Weintraub, J. K. (1989). Assessing coping strategies: A theoretically based approach. *Journal of Personality and Social Psychology*, 56 (2), 267-283.

Cole, P. M., Martin, S. E., & Dennis, T. A. (2004). Emotion regulation as a scientific construct: Methodological challenges and directions for child development research. *Child Development*, 75 (2), 317-333.

Compas, B. E., Connor, J., Osowiecki, D., & Welch, A. (1997). Effortful and involuntary responses to stress: Implications for coping with chronic stress. In B. H. Gottlieb (Ed.), *Coping with chronic stress* (pp. 105–130). New York: Plenum Press.

Compas, B. E., Connor-Smith, J. K., Saltzman, H., Thomsen, A. H., & Wadsworth, M. E. (2001). Coping with stress during childhood and adolescence: Problems, progress, and potential in theory and research. *Psychological Bulletin*, 127 (1), 87-127.

Connor-Smith, J. K., Compas, B. E., Wadsworth, M. E., Thomsen, A. H., & Saltzman, H. (2000). Responses to stress in adolescence: Measurement of coping and involuntary stress responses. *Journal of Consulting and Clinical Psychology*, 68 (6), 976-992.

Davis, C.G., Nolen-Hoeksema, S., & Larson, J. (1998). Making sense of loss and benefiting from the experience: Two construals of meaning. *Journal of Personality and Social Psychology, 75,* 561-574.

Davis, C. G., & Nolen-Hoeksema, S. (2001). Loss and meaning: How do people make sense of loss? *American behavioral scientist*, 44, 726-741.

Davis, R. N., & Nolen-Hoeksema, S. (2000). Cognitive inflexibility among ruminators and nonruminators. *Cognitive Therapy and Research, 24,* 699–711.

Diener, E., & Suh, E. (1997). Measuring quality of life: Economic, social, and subjective indicators. *Social Indicators Research, 40,* 189-216.

Ebner, N. C., Freund, A. M., & Baltes, P. B. (2006). Developmental changes in personal goal orientation from young to late adulthood: From striving for gains to maintenance and prevention of losses. *Psychology and Aging*, 21 (4), 664-678.

Eisenberg, N., Fabes, R. A., Guthrie, I. K., & Reiser, M. (2000). Dispositional emotionality and regulation: Their role in predicting quality of social functioning. *Journal of Personality and Social Psychology*, 78 (1), 136-157.

Ekman, P., & Friesen, W. V. (1969). The repertoire of nonverbal behavior: Categories, origins, usage, and coding. *Semiotica*, 1, 49-98.

Endler, N. S., & Parker, J. D. A. (1990). Multidimensional assessment of coping: A critical evaluation. *Journal of Personality and Social Psychology*, 58, 844-854.

Eschenbeck, H., Kohlmann, C., & Lohaus, A. (2007). Gender differences in coping strategies in children and adolescents. *Journal of Individual Differences*, 28 (1), 18-26.

Finkenauer, C., & Rimé, B. (1998). Keeping emotional memories secret: Health and subjective well-being when emotions are not shared. *Journal of Health Psychology, 3,* 47-58

Fisher, A. H., & Manstead, A. (2000). The relation between gender and emotions in different cultures. In A. H. Fisher, (Ed.), *Gender and emotion: Social psychological perspectives* (pp. 71-94). New York: Cambridge University Press.

Fivush, R., & Buckner, J. P. (2000). Gender, sadness, and depression: the development of emotional focus through gendered discourse. In A. Fischer (Ed.), *Gender and emotion: social psychological perspectives* (pp. 232–253). Cambridge: Cambridge University Press.

Folkman, S., & Lazarus, R. S. (1988). *Manual for the ways of coping questionnaire.* Palo Alto, CA: Consulting Psychologists Press.

Fox, N. A., & Calkins, S. D. (2003). The development of self-control of emotion: Intrinsic and extrinsic influences. *Motivation and Emotion*, 27, 7-26.

Freud, A. (1946). *The ego and the mechanisms of defence.* New York : International Universities Press.

Freud, S. (1926/1959). *Inhibitions, symptoms, anxiety* (A. Strachey, Transl. and J. Strachey, Ed.). New York: Norton.

Frijda, N. H. (1986). *The emotions*. Cambridge: Cambridge University Press.

Frijda, N. H. (2006). *The laws of emotions*. London: Lawrence Erlbaum.

Frijda, N. H. (2007, January). The multifarious processes of emotion regulation. Paper presented at the *Meeting on Emotions and interactions: Emotion regulation in different contexts*, University of Parma, Italy.

Frisina, P. G., Borod, J. C., & Lepore, S. J. (2004). A meta-analysis of the effects of written emotional disclosure on the health outcomes of clinical populations. *Journal of Nervous Mental Disorders, 192,* 629-634

Garber, J., & Dodge, K. A. (1991). *The development of emotion regulation and dysregulation*. Cambridge: Cambridge University Press.

Garnefski, N., & Kraaij, V. (2006). Relationships between cognitive emotion regulation strategies and depressive symptoms: A comparative study of five specific samples. *Personality and Individual Differences*, 40, 1659-1669.

Garnefski, N., & Kraaij, V. (2007). The cognitive emotion regulation questionnaire: Psychometric features and prospective relationships with depression and anxiety in adults. *European Journal of Psychological Assessment*, 23, 141-149.

Garnefski, N., Kraaij, V., & Spinhoven, Ph. (2001). Negative life events, cognitive emotion regulation and emotional problems. *Personality and Individual Differences*, 30, 1311-1327.

Garnefski, N., Teerds, J., Kraaij, V., Legerstee, J., & van den Kommer, T. (2004). Cognitive emotion regulation strategies and depressive symptoms: differences between males and females. *Personality and Individual Differences, 36,* 267–276.

Gottman, J., Katz, L., & Hooven, C. (1997). *Meta-emotion: How families communicate emotionally*. Mahwah, NJ: Lawrence Erlbaum.

Gratz, K. L., & Roemer, L. (2004). Multidimensional assessment of emotion regulation and dysregulation: Development, factor structure, and initial validation of the difficulties in emotion regulation scale. *Journal of Psychopathology and Behavioral Assessment*, 26, 41-54.

Greenberg, M. A. (1995). Cognitive processing of traumas: The role of intrusive thoughts and reappraisals. *Journal of Applied Social Psychology, 25,* 1262–1296.

Griffith, M.A., Dubow, E.F., & Ippolito, M.F. (2000). Developmental and cross-situational differences in adolescents' coping strategies. *Journal of Youth and Adolescence, 29,* 183–204.

Gross, J. J. (1998). Antecedent- and response-focused emotion regulation: Divergent consequences for experience, expression and physiology. *Journal of Personality and Social Psychology*, 74, 224-237.

Gross, J. J. (1999). Emotion regulation: Past, present, future. *Cognition and Emotion*, 13, 551-573.

Gross, J. J., Carstensen, L. C., Pasupathi, M., Tsai, J., Gottestam, K., & Hsu, A. Y. C. (1997). Emotion and aging: Experience, expression, and control. *Psychology and Aging*, 12 (4), 590-599.

Gross, J. J., & John, O. P. (2003). Individual differences in two emotion regulation processes: Implications for affect, relationships, and well-being. *Journal of Personality and Social Psychology*, 85, 348-362.

Gross, J. J., & Levenson, R. W. (1993). Emotional suppression: Physiology, self-report, and expressive behavior. *Journal of Personality and Social Psychology*, 64, 970-986.

Gross, J. J., & Levenson, R. W. (1997). Hiding feelings: The acute effects of inhibiting negative and positive emotion. *Journal of Abnormal Psychology*, 106, 95-103.

Gross, J. J., & Thompson, R. A. (2007). Emotion regulation: Conceptual foundations. In J. J. Gross, (Eds.). *Handbook of Emotion Regulation* (pp. 3-24). New York: Guilford.

Hampel, P., & Petermann, F. (2005). Age and gender effects on coping in children and adolescents. *Journal of Youth and Adolescence, 34*, 73–83.

Havighurst, R. J.(1952). *Developmental tasks and education.* New York: Davis McKay.

Horowitz, M.J. (1986). *Stress response syndromes* (2nd ed.). New York: Jason Aronson.

Horowitz, M. J. (2003). *Treatment of stress response syndromes.* Washington, DC: American Psychiatric Publishing.

Janoff-Bulman, R. (1992). *Shattered assumptions: Towards a new psychology of trauma.* New York: Free Press.

John, O. P., & Gross, J. J. (2004). Healthy and unhealthy emotion regulation: Personality processes, individual differences, and life span development. *Journal of Personality*, 72, 1301- 1334.

Kliegel, M., Jäger, T., & Phillips, L. H. (2007). Emotional development across adulthood: Differential age-related emotional reactivity and emotion regulation in a negative mood induction procedure. *International Journal of Aging and Human Development*, 64 (3), 217-244.

Koole, S. L., Smeets, K., van Knippenberg, A., & Dijksterhuis, A. (1999). The cessation of rumination through self-affirmation. *Journal of Personality and Social Psychology*, 77, 111-125.

Kraaij, V., Garnefski, N., de Wilde, E. J., Dijkstra, A., Gebhardt, W., Maes, S., & ter Doest, L. (2003). Negative life events and depressive symptoms in late adolescence: Bonding and cognitive coping as vulnerability factors? *Journal of Youth and Adolescence*, 32 (3), 185-193.

Kuyken, W., Howell, R., & Dalgleish, T. (2006). Overgeneral autobiographical memory in depressed adolescents with, versus without, a reported history of trauma. *Journal of Abnormal Psychology*, 115 (3), 387-396.

Labouvie-Vief, G., DeVoe, M., & Bulka, D. (1989). Speaking about feelings: Conceptions of emotion across the life span. *Psychology and Aging*, 4 (4), 425-437.

Labouvie-Vief, G., & Medler, M. (2002). Affect optimization and affect complexity: Modes and styles of regulation in adulthood. *Psychology and Aging*, 17, 571-587.

La France, M., & Banaji, M. (1992). Toward a reconsideration of the gender–emotion relationship. In M. S. Clark (Ed.), *Review of personality and social psychology* (Vol. 14, pp. 178–201). Newbury Park, CA: Sage.

Lazarus, R. S. (1966). *Psychological stress and the coping process.* New York: McGraw Hill.

Lazarus, R.S. (1991). *Emotion and adaptation.* New York: Oxford University Press.

Lazarus, R. S., & Alefert, E. (1964). Short-circuiting of threat by experimentally altering cognitive appraisal. *Journal of Abnormal and Social Psychology*, *69*, 195-205.

Lazarus, R. S., & Folkman, S. (1984). *Stress, appraisal, and coping*. New York: Springer.

Lepore, S. J. (1997). Expressive writing moderates the relation between intrusive thoughts and depressive symptoms. *Journal of Abnormal and Social Psychology*, *73*, 1030-1037.

Lepore, S. J., Silver, R., C., Wortman, C. B., & Wayment, H. A. (1996). Social constraints, intrusive thoughts, and depressive symptoms among bereaved mothers. *Journal of Personality and Social Psychology*, 70 (2), 271-282.

Luminet, O., Bouts, P., Delie, F., Manstead, A. S. R., & Rimé, B. (2000). Social sharing of emotion following exposure to a negatively valenced situation. *Cognition and emotion*, 14 (5), 661-688.

Lyubomirsky, S., Caldwell, N. D., & Nolen-Hoeksema, S. (1998). Effects of ruminative and distracting responses to depressed mood on retrieval of autobiographical memories. *Journal of Personality and Social Psychology*, 75 (1), 166-177.

Lyubomirsky, S., & Nolen-Hoeksema, S. (1993). Self-perpetuating properties of dysphoric rumination. *Journal of Personality and Social Psychology*, 65, 339-349.

Lyubomirsky, S., & Nolen-Hoeksema, S. (1995). Effects of self-focused rumination on negative thinking and interpersonal problem solving. *Journal of Personality and Social Psychology*, 69, 176-190.

Lyubomirsky, S., Tucker, K. L., Caldwell, N. D., & Berg, K. (1999). Why ruminators are poor problem solvers: Clues from the phenomenology of dysphoric rumination. *Journal of Personality and Social Psychology*, 77 (5), 1041-1060.

MacKinnon, D. P., Krull, J. L., & Lockwood, C. M. (2000). Equivalence of the mediation, confounding, and suppression effect. *Prevention Science*, *1*, 173-181.

Martin, L. L. (1999). I-D compensation theory: Some implications of trying to satisfy immediate-return needs in a delayed-return culture. Psychological Inquiry, 10, 195-209.

Martin, L.L., & Tesser, A. (1989). Toward a motivational and structural theory of ruminative thought. In J.S. Uleman, & J.A. Bargh (Eds.), *Unintended thought* (pp. 306-326). New York: Guilford.

Martin L., & Tesser A. (1996). Some ruminative thoughts. In R. S. Wyer (Eds.), *Advances in social cognition*, Vol.9 (pp. 1-48). Hillsdale, NJ: Lawrence Erlbaum..

Matarazzo O. (2001). Eventi emozionanti in adolescenza e in età adulta [Emotional events in adolescence and in adulthood]. In O. Matarazzo (Ed.), *Emozioni e Adolescenza* (pp 33-86). Napoli: Liguori.

McConatha, J. T., Leone, F. M., & Armstrong, J. M. (1997). Emotional control in adulthood. *Psychological Reports*, 80, 499–507.

Mor, N., & Winquist, J. (2002). Self-focused attention and negative affect: A meta-analysis. *Psychological Bulletin*, 128, 638-662.

Morrow, J., & Nolen-Hoeksema, S. (1990). Effects of responses to depression on the remediation of depressive affect. *Journal of Personality and Social Psychology*, 58, 519-527.

Moulds, M. L., Kandris, E., Starr, S., & Wong, A. C. M. (2007). The relationship between rumination, avoidance and depression in a non-clinical sample. *Behaviour Research and Therapy*, 45 (2), 251-261.

Nolen-Hoeksema, S. (1991). Responses to depression and their effects on the duration of depressive episodes. *Journal of Abnormal Psychology*, 100, 569-582.

Nolen-Hoeksema, S. (1994). An interactive model for the emergence of gender differences in depression in adolescence. *Journal of Research on Adolescence, 4*, 519-534.

Nolen-Hoeksema, S. (2002). Gender differences in depression. In I. H. Gotlib & C. L. Hammen (Eds.), Handbook of depression, (pp. 492-509). New York: Guilford.

Nolen-Hoeksema, S. (2004). The response styles theory. In C. Papageorgiou & A. Wells (Eds.), Depressive rumination: Nature, theory, and treatment (pp. 107-124). New York: Wiley.

Nolen-Hoeksema, S. & Davis, C. G. (1999). "Thanks for sharing that": Ruminators and their social support networks. *Journal of Personality and Social Psychology, 77*, 801-814.

Nolen-Hoeksema, S. & Jackson, B. (2001). Mediators of the gender difference in rumination. *Psychology of Women Quarterly, 25*, 37-47.

Nolen-Hoeksema, S., Larson, J., & Grayson, C. (1999). Explaining the gender difference in depressive symptoms. *Journal of Personality and Social Psychology*, 77 (5), 1061-1072.

Nolen-Hoeksema, S., & Morrow, J. (1993). Effect of rumination and distraction on naturally occurring depressed mood. *Cognition and Emotion*, 7, 561-570.

Nolen-Hoeksema, S., Parker, L. E., & Larson, J. (1994). Ruminative coping with depressed mood following loss. *Journal of Personality and Social Psychology*, 67 (1), 92-104.

Olah, A. (1995). Coping strategies among adolescents: A cross-cultural study. *Journal of adolescence*, 18, 491-512.

Papadakis, A. A., Prince, R. P., Jones, N. P., & Strauman, T. J. (2006). Self-regulation, rumination, and vulnerability to depression in adolescent girls. *Development and Psychopathology*, 18 (3), 815-829.

Pennebaker, J. W. (1995). *Emotion, disclosure, and health.* Washington: American Psychological Association.

Pennebaker, J. W., & Chung, C.K. (2007). Expressive writing, emotional upheavals, and health. In H. Friedman & R. Silver (Eds.), *Handbook of health psychology*. New York: Oxford University Press. http://pennebaker.socialpsychology.org/

Pennebaker, J. W., Zech, E., & Rimé, B., (2001). Disclosing and sharing emotion: Psychological, social and health consequences. In M. S. Stroebe, W. Stroebe, R.O. Hansson, & H. Schut (Eds.). *Handbook of bereavement research: Consequences, coping, and care* (pp. 517-539). Washington DC: American Psychological Association.

Pfeiffer, E. (1977). Psychopathology and social pathology. In J. E. Birren & K. W. Schaie (Eds.), *Handbook of the psychology of aging* (pp. 650-671). New York: Van Norstrand Reinhold.

Phillips, L. H., Henry, J. D., Hosie, J. A., & Milne, A. B. (2006). Age, anger regulation and well-being. *Aging and Mental Health*, 10 (3), 250-256.

Preacher, K. J., & Hayes, A. F. (2007). Asymptotic and Resampling Strategies for Assessing and Comparing Indirect Effects in Multiple Mediator Models. Draft on: http://www.comm.ohio-state.edu/ahayes/SPSS%20programs/indirect.htm

Rimé, B. (2007). The social sharing of emotion as an interface between individual and collective processes in the construction of emotional climates. *Journal of Social Issues*, 63, 307-322.

Rimé, B., Finkenauer, C., Luminet, O., Zech, E. & Philippot, P. (1998). Social sharing of emotion: New evidence and new questions. In W. Stroebe, & M. Hewstone (Eds.), *European Review of Social Psychology*, Vol.9 (pp. 145-189). Chichester, UK: Wiley.

Rimé, B., Finkenauer, C., & Sevrin, F. (1995). *Les émotions dans la vie quotidienne des personnes âgées: Impact, gestion, mémorisation, et réevocation* [Emotions in everyday life of the elderly: Impact, coping, memory, and reactivation]. Unpublished manuscript, University of Louvain, Louvain-la-Neuve, Belgium, cit. in Rimé, B., Finkenauer, C., Luminet, O., Zech, E., & Philippot, P. (1998). *Op.cit.*

Rimé, B., Philippot, P., Boca, S., & Mesquita, B. (1992). Long-lasting cognitive and social consequences of emotion: Social sharing and rumination. *European Review of Social Psychology, 3*, 225–258.

Rimé, B., & Zech, E. (2001). The social sharing of emotion: Interpersonal and collective dimensions. *Boletin de Psicologia*, 70, 97-108.

Roese, N. J. (1997). Counterfactual thinking. *Psychological Bulletin*, 121, 133-148.

Rusting, C. L., & Nolen-Hoeksema, S. (1998). Regulating responses to anger: Effects of rumination and distraction on angry mood. *Journal of Personality and Social Psychology*, 74 (3), 790-803.

Saarni, C. (1990). Emotional competence: How emotions and relationships become integrated. In R. A. Thompson (Eds.), *Socioemotional development,* Vol. 36 (pp. 115-182). Lincoln: University of Nebraska Press.

Salovey, P., & Mayer, J. D. (1990). Emotional intelligence. *Imagination, Cognition and Personality*, 9, 185-211.

Schachter, S. (1959). *The psychology of affiliation.* Minneapolis, MN: University of Minnesota Press.

Segerstrom, S. C., Stanton, A. L., Alden, L. E., & Shortridge, B. E. (2003). A Multidimensional structure for repetitive thought: What's on your mind, and how, and how much? *Journal of Personality and Social Psychology*, 85 (5), 909-921.

Silk, J. S., Steinberg, L., & Morris, A. S. (2003). Adolescents' emotion regulation in daily life: Links to depressive symptoms and problem behaviour. *Child Devolpment*, 74 (6), 1869-1880.

Skinner, E., & Edge, K. (1998). Reflections on Coping and Development across the Lifespan. *International Journal of Behavioral Development, 22* , 357–366

Spinrad, T. L., Eisenberg, N., & Gaertner, B. M. (2007). Measures of Effortful Regulation for Young Children. *Infant Ment Health Journal,* 28 (6), 606-626.

Stein, N. L., Trabasso, T., & Liwag, M. (1993). The representation and organization of emotional experience: Unfolding the emotion episode. In M. Lewis, & J. M. Haviland (Eds.), *Handbook of emotions* (pp. 279-300). New York: Guilford.

Tait, R., & Silver, R.C. (1989). Coming to terms with major negative life events. In J.S. Uleman, J.A. Bargh (Eds.), *Unintended thoughts* (pp. 351-382). New York: Guilford.

Tamir, M., John, O. P., Srivastava, S., & Gross, J. J. (2007). Implicit theories of emotion: Affective and social outcomes across a major life transition. *Journal of Personality and Social Psychology*, 92 (4), 731-744.

Tamres, L. K., Janicki, D., & Helgeson, V. S. (2002). Sex differences in coping behavior: A meta-analytic review and an examination of relative coping. *Personality and Social Psychology Review, 6,* 2–30.

Taylor, S. E., & Schneider, S. K. (1989). Coping and the simulation of events. *Social Cognition, 7,* 174–194.

Taylor, S. E., Klein, L. C., Lewis, B. P., Gruenewald, T. L., Gurung, R. A. R., & Updegraff, J. A. (2000). Biobehavioral responses to stress in females: Tend-and-befriend, not fight-or-flight. *Psychological Review, 107,* 411–429.

Thayer, R. E., Newman, J. R., & McClain, T. M. (1994). Self-regulation of mood: Strategies for changing a bad mood, raising energy, and reducing tension. *Journal of Personality and Social Psychology, 67,* 910-925

Thompson, R. A. (1990). Emotion and self-regulation. In R. A. Thompson (Ed.), *Socioemotional development. Nebraska Symposium on Motivation* (Vol. 36, pp. 367–467). Lincoln: University of Nebraska Press.

Thompson R. A. (1994). Emotion regulation: A theme in search of definition. In N. A. Fox (Eds.), *The development of emotion regulation: Biological and behavioral considerations. Monographs of the Society for Research in Child development,* 59 (pp. 25-52).

Thomsen, D. K., Mehlsen, M. Y., Viidik, A., Sommerlund, B., & Zachariae, R. (2005). Age and gender differences in negative affect - Is there a role for emotion regulation? *Personality and Individual Differences,* 38, s. 1935-1946.

Tice, D. M., & Bratslavsky, E. (2000). Giving in to feel good: The place of emotion regulation in the context of general self-control. *Psychological Inquiry,* 11, 149-159.

Trask, P. C., & Sigmon, S. T. (1999). Ruminating and distracting: The effect of sequential tasks on depressed mood. *Cognitive Therapy and Research,* 23, 231-246.

Ullrich, P. M., & Lutgendorf, S. (2002). Journaling about stressful events: Effects of cognitive processing and emotional expression. *Annals of Behavioral Medicine, 24,* 244–250.

Watkins, E., & Moulds, M. (2005). Distinct modes of ruminative self-focus: Impact of abstract versus concrete rumination on problem solving in depression. *Emotion, 5,* 319–328.

Watkins, E., & Teasdale, J. D. (2004). Adaptive and maladaptive self-focus in depression. *Journal of Affective Disorders, 82,* 1–8.

Wegner, D. M. (1994). Ironic processes of mental control. *Psychological Review,* 101, 34-52.

Wells, A. (2000). *Emotional disorders and metacognition: Innovative cognitive therapy.* New York: Wiley..

Wenzlaff, R. M., Wegner, D. M., & Roper, D. W. (1988). Depression and mental control: The resurgence of unwanted negative thoughts. *Journal of Personality and Social Psychology,* 55 (6), 882-892.

Zech, E., & Rimé, B. (2005). Is talking about an emotional experience helpful? Effects on emotional recovery and perceived benefits. *Clinical Psychology and Psychotherapy, 12,* 270-287.

In: Life Style and Health Research Progress
Editors: A. B. Turley, G. C. Hofmann

ISBN: 978-1-60456-427-3
© 2008 Nova Science Publishers, Inc.

Chapter V

The Influence of Psychosocial Factors on Vaccination Response: A Review

Anna C. Phillips

School of Sport and Exercise Sciences, University of Birmingham, UK

ABSTRACT

Measuring the antibody response to medical vaccination is regarded as a useful model for studying the influence of psychological factors on immunity. It allows an assessment of the impact of psychosocial variables on an *in vivo* integrated immune response and within the context of other bodily systems. The response to vaccination is also clinically relevant in that it provides an estimation of protection against infectious disease. Positive psychosocial factors, such as support from close friends and family, are associated with a stronger antibody response. Negative psychosocial factors, on the other hand, have been shown to attenuate the response to vaccination. The chronic stress consequent on caregiving for a spouse with dementia has consistently been related to a poorer antibody response to a range of vaccinations and even more everyday stressful life events have been associated with a poorer antibody response in both young and older adults. In contrast, acute or short-term stress may actually potentiate the antibody response to vaccination. This review will discuss the scientific evidence regarding the impact of both chronic and acute stress and other behavioural and psychosocial variables on the antibody response to vaccination. Implications for interventions to improve immunity and protection against infectious disease will be suggested.

GLOSSARY

Antigen	Any molecule that generates, and binds to antibody.
B-lymphocytes	One of two major types of lymphocyte. When activated by antigen, B-lymphocytes differentiate into cells that produce antibody against the antigen.

Immunoglobulin	Also known as antibody. Immunoglobulins are secreted by B-lymphocytes, and help fight infection through various mechanisms.
In vitro	Experimental techniques where the experiment is performed outside a living organism. The conditions, and therefore results, may not represent *in vivo* function
In vivo	Research conducted within the whole organism.
Neuroticism	A trait-like, or stable, personality dimension consisting of emotional instability and maladjustment
Thymus-dependent	Antibody responses, usually against a protein antigen, that require the B-lymphocytes to get "help" from T-lymphocytes
Thymus-independent	Antibody responses, against a polysaccharide or lipopolysaccharide antigen, in which the B-lymphocytes do not require "help" from T-lymphocytes
T-lymphocytes	One of two major types of lymphocyte. One of their many functions include "helping" B-lymphocytes produce an antibody response.
Vaccination	The injection of a dead or attenuated pathogen (disease causing agent) in order to induce an adaptive immune response, and protect against disease.

INTRODUCTION

The field of psychoneuroimmunology examines the interactions between psychological and immunological parameters. Although historically the immune system has been thought to operate in a largely autonomous fashion, it is now known that it has close links with the central nervous system. Such links were originally suggested by results from research conducted by Ader and colleagues in the late 1970's and early 1980's. In an elegant series of studies that the immune system is susceptible to classical conditioning (see Ader and Cohen, 1993, for a review). For example, the repeated pairing of a neutral stimulus, saccharine, with an immunosuppressant drug in rats resulted in the animals showing immunosuppression in response to an antigen when presented solely with the neutral stimulus alone (N. Cohen, Ader, Green, and Bovbjerg, 1979). Subsequently, we have learned much from both animal and human studies about the intimate interactions between the nervous and immune systems and have increasingly come to appreciate the bidirectional nature of these links (Maier and Watkins, 1998; Petrovsky, 2001). Such interactions provide the biological foundations for psychological factors to influence immune function, and ultimately affect our susceptibility to disease and our health and well-being.

PSYCHOSOCIAL FACTORS AND IMMUNITY: ENUMERATIVE MEASURES

The relationship between psychosocial factors and immunity has received considerable attention over the past 30 years, with particular interest being directed at the association between psychological stress and the ability of the immune system to respond to infection. Early research focused especially on the influence of psychosocial stress on enumerative measures of immunity; individuals exposed to chronic stress showed reduced numbers of B-lymphocytes (McKinnon, Weisse, Reynolds, Bowles, and Baum, 1989; Schaeffer et al., 1985), helper T-lymphocytes (Futterman, Wellisch, Zighelboim, Luna-Raines, and Weiner, 1996; Kiecolt-Glaser, Glaser et al., 1987; McKinnon et al., 1989), cytotoxic T-lymphocytes (De Gucht, Fischler, and Demanet, 1999; McKinnon et al., 1989), natural killer (NK) cells (De Gucht et al., 1999; McKinnon et al., 1989) and lowered concentrations of secretory immunoglobulin A in saliva (Deinzer, Kleineidam, Stiller-Winkler, Idel, and Bachg, 2000; Jemmott et al., 1983; Jemmott and Magloire, 1988; McClelland, Alexander, and Marks, 1982) compared to matched controls. In addition, persons suffering the chronic stress of separation/divorce showed lower numbers of T-helper cells than married individuals (Kiecolt-Glaser, Fisher et al., 1987). However, it is difficult to determine the clinical significance of such enumerative changes, given that such changes lie within the range of normal variation for healthy participants (Vedhara, Fox, and Wang, 1999). Changes in cell number may simply reflect lymphocyte migration and recirculation rather than increased production of cells. Additionally, cell number changes could be a consequence of shifts in plasma volume and haemoconcentration; in such circumstances, changes in cell number would reflect increased density of a lymphocyte population rather than signal a true increase in absolute cell numbers. In addition, even absolute changes in cell number might not necessarily reflect alteration in the capacity of the immune system to mount an effective response to antigenic challenge (Vedhara, Fox et al., 1999). Consequently, measuring changes in cell number is perhaps not the optimal means of determining variations in the functional capacity of the immune system, and hence the likely clinical implications of psychosocial variables for disease resistance and susceptibility.

PSYCHOSOCIAL FACTORS AND IN VITRO IMMUNE FUNCTION

In vitro measures of immune function, such as lymphocyte proliferation to mitogen and NK cell cytotoxicity, have been argued to provide a better indication of the functional capacity of the immune system (Vedhara, Fox et al., 1999). These measures have been demonstrated to be susceptible to the influence of chronic stress (Arnetz et al., 1987; Bartrop, Luckhurst, Lazarus, Kiloh, and Penny, 1977; Esterling, Kiecolt-Glaser, and Glaser, 1996; Irwin et al., 1990; Kiecolt-Glaser, Glaser et al., 1987; Linn, Linn, and Klimas, 1988; Sabioncello et al., 2000; Schleifer, Keller, Camerino, Thornton, and Stein, 1983; Workman and La Via, 1987), and marital dissatisfaction (Kiecolt-Glaser, Fisher et al., 1987; Kiecolt-Glaser et al., 1997; Kiecolt-Glaser et al., 1993); both psychosocial exposures have been found to impair cell proliferation and/or NK cell cytotoxicity. Nevertheless, the isolated testing of any particular network of immune cells provides only limited information about the overall status of what is a highly integrated and complex system (Vedhara, Fox et al., 1999), and an imperfect understanding of the relationship between psychosocial factors and vulnerability to disease (Burns, Carroll, Ring, and Drayson, 2003).

THE ANTIBODY RESPONSE TO VACCINATION

A clinically relevant model which examines the impact of psychosocial factors on the integrated response of the immune system to a challenge would avoid many of these disadvantages. The antibody response to vaccination provides us with such a model. Vaccines act as real immune system challenges, albeit altered in such a way so not to induce disease. Therefore, by measuring the antibody levels in response to vaccination we can assess directly how well the immune system responds to infectious challenge. The antibody titre or level is the endpoint of a series of immunological events, starting with pathogen recognition and resulting in the production of antibodies highly specific to the particular challenging agent. Accordingly, the antibody response gives an overall measure of how well the immune system responds to antigenic challenge and reflects the integrated response. It is also clinically relevant in that antibody levels are directly related to susceptibility and resistance to the specific disease in question.

BASIC IMMUNOLOGY OF THE VACCINE RESPONSE

The immune response to vaccination involves the coordination of a wide variety of immune cells. The vaccine antigen is initially recognized and presented by professional antigen presenting cells, such as dendritic cells. The antigen is then recognized by specific T lymphocytes, which proliferate and differentiate into T-helper lymphocytes. Some vaccine antigen types are also recognized by B-lymphocytes without the necessity for antigen processing. When stimulated by an antigen, either alone or in conjunction with stimulation by T-helper lymphocytes, B-lymphocytes proliferate and mature into short lived plasma cells which produce the earliest antibody or immunoglobulin, IgM. In a primary response to an antigen not previously encountered, the peak IgM response occurs around five days after vaccination. Interaction between the activated T- and B-lymphocytes leads to the formation of germinal centers and then the production of high affinity IgG and IgA antibody. This response is slower than the IgM response, and reaches a peak around 28 days after vaccination. Secondary antibody responses, in which the immune system has been previously exposed to the antigen, are more rapid and of greater magnitude.

Psychosocial factors may alter both the quantity and quality of antigen-specific antibody present at different times after immunization by moderating a variety of processes within the immune response. These include the initial clonal expansion of T- and B-lymphocytes, long term maintenance of serum IgG levels against the specific antigen, or the speed and size of the antibody response to secondary antigen exposure via antigen-specific lymphocyte pool maintenance.

STRESS AND VACCINATION

The most commonly investigated psychological factor in the context of vaccination is psychosocial stress. This has been measured in various ways including: exposure to a particular chronic stressor, such as care-giving for a spouse with dementia; questionnaires measuring perceived stress levels; or checklists of the occurrence of negative stressful life events.

STRESS, MOOD, AND NON-PATHOGENIC INOCULATIONS

The earliest studies using the vaccination model used novel non-pathogenic antigens to examine the antigen-specific antibody response. On days when participants reported high negative mood and negative life events, antigen-specific sIgA antibody levels to an oral rabbit albumin capsule were reduced; these levels were elevated on days when relatively high positive mood and positive life events were reported (Stone, Cox, Valdimarsdottir, Jandorf, and Neale, 1987; Stone et al., 1994). The primary immune response has also been examined using a novel protein antigen, keyhole limpet hemocyanin (KLH), which elicits a thymus-dependent antibody response. In one study of young women, the KLH-specific IgG antibody response was lower at eight weeks, but not three weeks, post-vaccination in participants reporting fewer positive life events prior to vaccination (Snyder, Roghmann, and Sigal, 1990). In contrast, in a more recent study, distress was observed not to be related to the development of anti-KLH IgG three weeks post-vaccination (Smith et al., 2004). These data provide some evidence that the antibody response to a single antigenic exposure may be susceptible to psychosocial influence, although there is some inconsistency between studies.

PRIMARY AND SECONDARY VACCINATIONS

An advantage of using the response to vaccination as a model of immune function is that the variation in inoculation schedules for certain vaccinations can be used to examine which particular aspects of the immune response may be vulnerable to psychosocial influence. For example, vaccination with an antigen to which the participant has not been previously exposed induces a primary antibody response. In contrast, vaccination against more common pathogens such as influenza, induce a secondary immune response. By examining the effect of stress on both primary and secondary immune responses, we can begin to determine which aspects of the immune response are most susceptible to stress-induced modulation. Hepatitis B vaccination is useful in this context, as there is a low likelihood of prior naturalistic exposure to this pathogen, and the schedule consists of three inoculations over a six month period, thus incorporating an initial primary response and later secondary response to vaccination.

Two studies have examined the association between stress and the primary antibody response to hepatitis B, measured one month following the initial vaccination. In the earlier study, individuals reporting higher mean perceived stress and anxiety over the whole vaccination period, likely to indicate some trait or stable dispositional tendency, were less likely to have sero-converted by the time of the second inoculation (Glaser et al., 1992). In the second study, of an emotional disclosure intervention, the disclosure group did not differ from controls in antibody levels at the time of the second inoculation (Petrie, Booth, Pennebaker, Davison, and Thomas, 1995). However, the ongoing impact of the intervention on psychological stress levels was not measured, making it difficult to interpret the data from this study. Consequently, at this stage, the evidence that stress influences the primary antibody response to hepatitis B vaccination is inconclusive (Burns, Carroll, Ring et al., 2003; S. Cohen, Miller, and Rabin, 2001).

The secondary antibody response to hepatitis B vaccination has received more attention, again with mixed results. The largest of these studies examined the association between life events stress and the final antibody titre in two cohorts of students, vaccinated either in the past twelve months or at least thirteen months previously (Burns, Carroll, Ring, Harrison, and Drayson, 2002). Whereas life events exposure was not related to antibody response in the recently vaccinated cohort, participants in the earlier vaccinated cohort who reported higher life events over the past year were over twice as likely to show an inadequate antibody titre as those with lower life events exposure. This finding suggests that the immunogenicity of the hepatitis B vaccination may initially override the influence of life events stress, although there was also more power to detect effects in the earlier vaccinated cohort as more participants exhibited inadequate antibody titres (Burns, Carroll et al., 2002). Nevertheless, this study provides some evidence that psychosocial stress may have its principal effects on the rate of deterioration of antibody protection (Burns, Carroll, Ring et al., 2003). In a study where a low dose of hepatitis B vaccine was administered, a higher stress index, comprising life events exposure and psychological symptoms, at two months post-vaccination was associated with a poorer antibody response, and the stress index at six months also tended to relate negatively to antibody response (Jabaaij et al., 1993). However, since only the final antibody titre was measured, it is difficult to determine whether, in this instance, stress predominantly influenced initial sero-conversion or the maintenance of antibody levels. In addition, the inclusion of psychological symptoms in the composite stress index makes it difficult to ascribe this finding to any specific aspect of stress (Burns, Carroll, Ring et al., 2003). A similar study using the full dosage hepatitis B vaccination did not yield any significant stress effects (Jabaaij et al., 1996), although it is possible that this was due to the absence of a two-month assessment of stress, which was the main predictor of antibody response in the previous study by this group. In the study already mentioned above (Glaser et al., 1992), stress and anxiety were not associated with the secondary antibody response to hepatitis B. Similarly, life events stress and perceived stress were not related to antibody status five months following the initial inoculation in a more recent study (Marsland, Cohen, Rabin, and Manuck, 2001). Finally, one study reported a positive association between perceived life event stress, depression and anxiety over the vaccination period and hepatitis B antibody status nine months following the initial vaccination (Petry, Weems, and Livingstone, 1991). This anomalous result has been attributed to the relatively low levels of stress experienced by the participants in this study, suggesting that moderate levels of life change stress experienced during the initial stages of antibody formation may be beneficial to the antibody response, although high levels may be detrimental (Petry et al., 1991). Such an interpretation receives support from animal research where moderate stress at the time of vaccination has been associated with an enhanced antibody response, discussed below (see e.g. Dhabhar and McEwen, 1996). In summary, the data on stress effects on hepatitis vaccination response thus far are somewhat mixed, but there appears to be stronger evidence for a negative effect of psychological stress on the secondary response to this antigen (Burns, Carroll, Ring et al., 2003; S. Cohen et al., 2001).

STRESS AND THYMUS-DEPENDENT, THYMUS-INDEPENDENT, AND CONJUGATE VACCINES

A further advantage to the vaccination model is that there are different types of vaccination, which can be used to help elucidate which cells involved in the vaccination response are influenced by psychological factors. Most vaccinations, which consist of inactivated or dead viruses like influenza, induce what is known as a thymus-dependent antibody response. In this type of response, the B cells, the antibody "factories", require the help of T cells, in order to produce antibody. A few vaccinations, however, protect against bacterial infections, such as meningococcal A, or toxins, such as tetanus. The immune response against these pathogens does not require and cannot receive T-cell help in order to produce antibodies, and are thus termed thymus-independent vaccines. A third type of vaccine exists in which substances that elicit a T-cell response are conjugated to a thymus-independent pathogen in order to boost the efficiency of the antibody response against the thymus-independent pathogen. Conjugate vaccines like meningococcal C induce a thymus-dependent response. If psychological factors are consistently associated with the response to thymus-dependent and conjugate vaccinations but not with thymus-independent response, this would imply that it is T-cells that are particularly liable to psychological influence. Indeed, there is evidence to suggest that psychological factors like stress may exert their effects mainly on T-cells, as in one recent study higher frequency and intensity of stressful life events were associated with a poorer response to influenza and meningococcal C, but not to meningococcal A vaccination (Phillips, Burns, Carroll, Ring, and Drayson, 2005). In addition, no association was found between stress and antibody response to a pneumonia vaccination in pre-school children (Boyce et al., 1995). However, older care-givers for spouses with dementia have been reported to show poorer maintenance of antibody levels in the longer term following pneumonia vaccination than controls (Glaser, Sheridan, Malarkey, MacCallum, and Kiecolt-Glaser, 2000), although it is possible that other factors such as age, severity of stress, and a lack resources to deal with stress, such as social support, may interact to impair antibody-mediated immunity more generally than just the T-cell response.

VACCINATION IN YOUNGER ADULTS

Studies of student samples, in which stress is usually assessed using a range of life events checklists and perceived stress measures, comprise much of vaccination response literature. Such studies generally confirm that individuals reporting higher numbers of life events and/or greater perceived stress show poorer antibody status. This can be seen above for the hepatitis B (Burns, Carroll et al., 2002; Glaser et al., 1992) and meningococcal C (Burns, Drayson, Ring, and Carroll, 2002) vaccinations. The antibody response to the influenza vaccination has also received considerable attention in younger adults. In one study, students who did not achieve a four-fold increase in antibody titre to the A-strains of the vaccine at five months post-vaccination reported higher stressful life event exposures, and there was also a trend for those who were unprotected at five-weeks to report more stressful life events in the period following vaccination (Burns, Carroll, Drayson, Whitham, and Ring, 2003). In addition, participants reporting higher perceived stress showed inadequate antibody titres to the A/Panama influenza strain at five months (Burns, Carroll, Drayson et al., 2003). In a study of the effects of daily stress and feelings of being overwhelmed during the 10 days following vaccination, higher stress ratings were associated with lower antibody titres to the A/New Caledonia strain at both one and four months following vaccination (Miller et al., 2004). Further, students reporting higher numbers of negative life events and a greater severity of stressful events showed a poorer response to the B/Shangdong influenza strain at both five weeks and five months post-vaccination (Phillips, Burns et al., 2005). These studies provide evidence that stressful life events both preceding, and in the period immediately following vaccination can influence the antibody response. They also show that both the peak antibody response and the decay in antibody protection are influenced by stressful life events, although it is difficult at this stage to explain why antibodies against different influenza strains are associated with stress across the different studies. One possibility is that strain novelty influences the associations observed, with relatively novel vaccine strains being associated with life events stress and less novel strains being related to social support and other factors (Phillips, Burns et al., 2005). Novelty and prior exposure have also been cited by other authors to explain strain-specific associations (Vedhara, Cox et al., 1999).

VACCINATION RESPONSE IN OLDER ADULTS

It is important to study the psychological influences on immunity in older adults, given that they have less efficient immune systems due to immune ageing or immunosenescence, which contributes to increased infectious disease susceptibility (Ginaldi, Loreto, Corsi, Modesti, and De Martinis, 2001). The effects of ageing on immune function may alter individuals' susceptibility to disease in part via a less efficient antibody response. In fact, it has been shown that, for example, the influenza vaccine has poorer efficacy in older populations (Allsup, Haycox, Regan, and Gosney, 2004; Patriarca, 1994). Further, it is possible that ageing of the immune system and stress interact such that stress takes its greatest toll on immunity in those who have existing immunosenescence (Graham, Christian, and Kiecolt-Glaser, 2006; Phillips, Burns, and Lord, 2007). The vaccination response in older adults has mainly been considered in the context of care-giving for a spouse with dementia. Studies have shown that caregivers have poorer antibody responses to vaccination in comparison to matched control participants (Glaser et al., 1992; Glaser et al., 2000; Vedhara, Cox et al., 1999). However, care-giving studies in younger populations are less conclusive (Vedhara et al., 2002) and suggest that factors other than chronic stress, such as the disease/condition of the care recipient and the burden of care, may also be important. Caregiving is a very specific stressor, and care-givers are likely to differ from the general population in ways other than the stress of care-giving, for example, in the amount of social support they receive. Research examining the impact of more general psychological stress on antibody levels following vaccination is sparse. However, it is important to study older adults in this context as they are likely to have different stress exposure histories than younger samples (Carroll, Phillips, Ring, Der, and Hunt, 2005). One study found that older adults reporting higher perceived stress had lower antibody levels following influenza vaccination (Kohut, Cooper, Nickolaus, Russell, and Cunnick, 2002). As baseline antibody level prior to vaccination was not known, however, the impact on the actual response to the vaccine could not be assessed. More recently, we observed that the stress of bereavement in the year prior to influenza vaccination was associated with a poorer antibody response in a community sample of adults aged 65 and over (Phillips et al., 2006). Although overall negative life events exposure was not associated with vaccine response in this study, the effect found for bereavement suggests that stress is related to pervasive immune effects throughout the life course, although what constitutes stress will vary depending on the age of the sample studied.

OTHER PSYCHOLOGICAL FACTORS AND VACCINATION

The support of friends and loved ones may also be an important determinant of immune health. Studies have assessed both functional social support, a measure of the quality and availability of social resources a person has, and structural social support, the number of friends a person can call on. First, students who reported greater social support demonstrated a stronger combined immune response to the booster third inoculation of the three-dose hepatitis B vaccination (Glaser et al., 1992). Second, in a study of college freshmen, loneliness and smaller social network size were associated with a poorer antibody response to the A/New Caledonian strain of the influenza vaccination (Pressman et al., 2005). Third, students with greater functional social support showed higher titres to the A/Panama influenza strain at both five weeks and five months following vaccination (Phillips, Burns et al., 2005). Interestingly, in a study described above, elderly caregivers, who showed greater deterioration in antibody protection against the thymus-independent pneumococcal vaccination than non-caregivers, also reported poorer social support (Glaser et al., 2000). Social support was also negatively correlated with pre- and post-vaccination titres against the A/Panama influenza strain yet positively with pre-vaccination antibody titres against the A/New Caledonia strain in elderly nursing home residents (Moynihan et al., 2004), a finding which even the authors were unable to explain. Further, older adults who were married, and particularly those who were happily married, showed a better antibody response to the influenza vaccination than those who were unmarried or less happily married (Phillips et al.,

2006). However, more general functional social support and social network size was not associated with antibody response in this older population (Phillips et al., 2006). These findings perhaps lend weight to the suggestion above that different factors become important, in terms of the influence on immunity, across the life course.

Personality factors, although often examined in the context of health outcomes (see e.g., Smith, Glazer, Ruiz, and Gallo, 2004) have scarcely been investigated relative to the vaccination response. First, among a group of 12-year old girls who had not sero-converted prior to a live-attenuated rubella virus vaccination and were thus exhibiting a primary vaccine response, those characterized by higher internalizing scores, a concept linked to neuroticism, and lower self-esteem at baseline exhibited lower antibody titres following vaccination (Morag, Morag, Reichenberg, Lerer, and Yirmiya, 1999). Similarly, in a study of female graduates and hepatitis, trait negative affect was negatively associated with the secondary antibody response to the second hepatitis B injection (Marsland et al., 2001). A related trait, neuroticism, was measured in undergraduate students, and was negatively associated with both the peak antibody response to the A/Panama strain of an influenza vaccination, and the maintenance of antibody titres to this strain; those with higher neuroticism scores had a poorer antibody response (Phillips, Carroll, Burns, and Drayson, 2005). In contrast, dispositional optimism was measured in exercising and sedentary elderly individuals, but was not found to be associated with antibody titres following influenza vaccination (Kohut et al., 2002). Inconsistencies in results could be attributable to the different populations and the different measures of personality studied.

ACUTE STRESS AND VACCINATION RESPONSE

In contrast to the immunosuppressive effects of chronic stress discussed so far, it has also been suggested that acute stress may be immune enhancing when experienced close to the immune challenge. It has been argued that immune enhancement by acute stress would be an adaptive mechanism, and might be regarded as an integral component of the fight or flight response (Dhabhar and McEwen, 1996). From this perspective, circumstances that elicit a fight or flight response are likely to also involve exposure to antigens and, therefore, a robust immune response would be adaptive for survival. There is now convincing evidence from animal studies of acute stressors in close temporal proximity to vaccination that provide support for an immune enhancing effect of stress on the antibody response (Dhabhar and Viswanathan, 2005). Only one study has examined the effect of acute psychological stress on antibody response to vaccination in humans. Participants completed a 45 min time pressured, socially evaluated mental arithmetic task, or a resting control period, immediately prior to influenza vaccination. An enhancement of the antibody response to one of the influenza viral strains was found in women in the psychological stress group compared to control (Edwards et al., 2006).

IMPLICATIONS FOR INTERVENTIONS

The clinical implications arising from a better understanding of the varied relationships between psychological factors and the vaccination response are important, particularly in the context of older adults who already display increased susceptibility to disease. Psychological interventions to improve vaccination response in these populations could include techniques such as stress management, relaxation, cognitive behavioural therapy, and emotional disclosure. One study showed an improvement in the ability of older caregivers for a spouse with dementia to mount a four-fold increase in antibody titre following influenza vaccination relative to matched controls, although the mechanisms of effect were unclear (Vedhara et al., 2003). Similarly, participants taking part in a written emotional disclosure intervention, where they wrote about their emotions about a previously undisclosed stressful event, showed significantly higher antibody titres at four and six months following vaccination with hepatitis B compared to a control non-intervention group (Petrie et al., 1995). However, Black individuals who wrote about their feelings and experience about racism in an emotional disclosure study showed poorer antibody titres to two out of three strains of an influenza vaccine relative to those writing about a neutral topic, although this may have been due to ambiguity about attributions of whether experience was due to racism or other factors (Stetler, Chen, and Miller, 2006). Consequently, at this stage, the results are mixed, and much more work is required to establish what types of intervention are likely to be the most beneficial for psychological, and hence immunological, health.

Another potential clinical application of the vaccination model has arisen from the positive immune effects demonstrated in response to acute stress (Edwards et al., 2006). In students, an acute eccentric arm exercise protocol was applied six hours before giving an influenza vaccination in the exercised arm. The antibody response was assessed at six and 20 weeks post-vaccination, and interferon-gamma production in response to in vitro stimulation by the whole vaccine, an index of the cell-mediated response to vaccination, was assessed at 8 weeks post-vaccination. Eccentric exercise enhanced the antibody response in women, and the cell-mediated response in men (Edwards et al., 2007). This suggests that the development of such a behavioural challenge that could be applied in GP settings could be a way forward for improving the vaccination response. This would be particularly important for groups at risk of infectious disease such as older adults, the bereaved, and care-givers.

CONCLUSION

In conclusion, vaccination has had a substantial impact on public health, although not everyone mounts a satisfactory and protective antibody response to vaccination. This increasingly appears to be the case with progressing age. Studying antibody responses to vaccination is now contributing to the understanding of how psychosocial exposures can influence immunity and, consequently, resistance to disease. The current challenges are to unravel the underlying mechanisms and to develop and apply feasible behavioural interventions to boost the response to vaccination and, thus, optimize our resistance against infectious disease.

REFERENCES

Ader, R., and Cohen, N. (1993). Psychoneuroimmunology: conditioning and stress. *Annual Review of Psychology, 44*, 53-85.

Allsup, S., Haycox, A., Regan, M., and Gosney, M. (2004). Is influenza vaccination cost effective for healthy people between ages 65 and 74 years? A randomised controlled trial. *Vaccine, 23*, 639-645.

Boyce, W. T., Adams, S., Tschann, J. M., Cohen, F., Wara, D., and Gunnar, M. R. (1995). Adrenocortical and behavioral predictors of immune response to starting school. *Pediatric Research, 38*, 1009-1017.

Burns, V. E., Carroll, D., Drayson, M., Whitham, M., and Ring, C. (2003). Life events, perceived stress and antibody response to influenza vaccination in young healthy adults. *Journal of Psychosomatic Research, 55*, 569-572.

Burns, V. E., Carroll, D., Ring, C., and Drayson, M. (2003). Antibody response to vaccination and psychosocial stress in humans: relationship and mechanisms. *Vaccine, 21*, 2523-2534.

Burns, V. E., Carroll, D., Ring, C., Harrison, L. K., and Drayson, M. (2002). Stress, coping and hepatitis B antibody status. *Psychosomatic Medicine, 64*, 287-293.

Burns, V. E., Drayson, M., Ring, C., and Carroll, D. (2002). Perceived stress and psychological well-being are associated with antibody status following meningitis C conjugate vaccination. *Psychosomatic Medicine, 64*, 963-970.

Carroll, D., Phillips, A. C., Ring, C., Der, G., and Hunt, K. (2005). Life events and hemodynamic stress reactivity in the middle-aged and elderly. *Psychophysiology, 42*, 269-276.

Cohen, N., Ader, R., Green, N., and Bovbjerg, D. (1979). Conditioned suppression of a thymus-independent antibody response. *Psychosomatic Medicine, 41*, 487-491.

Cohen, S., Miller, G. E., and Rabin, B. S. (2001). Psychological Stress and Antibody Response to Immunization: A Critical Review of the Human Literature. *Psychosomatic Medicine, 63*, 7-18.

De Gucht, V., Fischler, B., and Demanet, C. (1999). Immune dysfunction associated with chronic professional stress in nurses. *Psychiatry Research, 85*, 105-111.

Deinzer, R., Kleineidam, C., Stiller-Winkler, R., Idel, H., and Bachg, D. (2000). Prolonged reduction of salivary immunoglobulin A (sIgA) after a major academic exam. *Int Journal of Psychophysiology, 37*, 219-232.

Dhabhar, F. S., and McEwen, B. S. (1996). Stress-induced enhancement of antigen-specific cell-mediated immunity. *Journal of Immunology, 156*, 2608-2615.

Dhabhar, F. S., and Viswanathan, K. (2005). Short-term stress experienced at time of immunization induces a long-lasting increase in immunologic memory. *American Journal of Physiology, 289*, R738-744.

Edwards, K. M., Burns, V. E., Allen, L. M., McPhee, J. S., Bosch, J. A., Carroll, D., et al. (2007). Eccentric exercise as an adjuvant to influenza vaccination in humans. *Brain, Behavior and Immunity, 21*, 209-217.

Edwards, K. M., Burns, V. E., Reynolds, T., Carroll, D., Drayson, M., and Ring, C. (2006). Acute stress exposure prior to influenza vaccination enhances antibody response in women. *Brain, Behavior and Immunity, 20*, 159-168.

Futterman, A. D., Wellisch, D. K., Zighelboim, J., Luna-Raines, M., and Weiner, H. (1996). Psychological and immunological reactions of family members to patients undergoing bone marrow transplantation. *Psychosomatic Medicine, 58*, 472-480.

Ginaldi, L., Loreto, M. F., Corsi, M. P., Modesti, M., and De Martinis, M. (2001). Immunosenescence and infectious diseases. *Microbes and Infection, 3*, 851-857.

Glaser, R., Kiecolt-Glaser, J. K., Bonneau, R. H., Malarkey, W., Kennedy, S., and Hughes, J. (1992). Stress-induced modulation of the immune response to recombinant hepatitis B vaccine. *Psychosomatic Medicine, 54*, 22-29.

Glaser, R., Sheridan, J. F., Malarkey, W., MacCallum, R. C., and Kiecolt-Glaser, J. K. (2000). Chronic stress modulates the immune response to a pneumococcal pneumonia vaccine. *Psychosomatic Medicine, 62*, 804-807.

Graham, J. E., Christian, L. M., and Kiecolt-Glaser, J. K. (2006). Stress, age, and immune function: toward a lifespan approach. *Journal of Behavioral Medicine, 29*, 389-400.

Jabaaij, L., Grosheide, P. M., Heijtink, R. A., Duivenvoorden, H. J., Ballieux, R. E., and Vingerhoets, A. J. J. M. (1993). Influence of perceived psychological stress and distress on antibody response to low dose rDNA hepatitis B vaccine. *Journal of Psychosomatic Research, 37*, 361-369.

Jabaaij, L., Van Hattum, J., Vingerhoets, A. J. J. M., Oostveen, F. G., Duivenvoorden, H. J., and Ballieux, R. E. (1996). Modulation of immune response to rDNA hepatitis B vaccination by psychological stress. *Journal of Psychosomatic Research, 41*, 129-137.

Jemmott, J. B., 3rd, Borysenko, J. Z., Borysenko, M., McClelland, D. C., Chapman, R., Meyer, D., et al. (1983). Academic stress, power motivation, and decrease in secretion rate of salivary secretory immunoglobulin A. *Lancet, 1*, 1400-1402.

Jemmott, J. B., 3rd, and Magloire, K. (1988). Academic stress, social support, and secretory immunoglobulin A. *Journal of Personality and Social Psychology, 55*, 803-810.

Kiecolt-Glaser, J. K., Fisher, L. D., Ogrocki, P., Stout, J. C., Speicher, C. E., and Glaser, R. (1987). Marital quality, marital disruption, and immune function. *Psychosomatic Medicine, 49*, 13-34.

Kiecolt-Glaser, J. K., Glaser, R., Cacioppo, J. T., MacCallum, R. C., Snydersmith, M., Kim, C., et al. (1997). Marital conflict in older adults: endocrinological and immunological correlates. *Psychosomatic Medicine, 59*, 339-349.

Kiecolt-Glaser, J. K., Glaser, R., Shuttleworth, E. C., Dyer, C. S., Ogrocki, P., and Speicher, C. E. (1987). Chronic stress and immunity in family caregivers of Alzheimer's disease victims. *Psychosomatic Medicine, 49*, 523-535.

Kiecolt-Glaser, J. K., Malarkey, W., Chee, M., Newton, T., Cacioppo, J. T., Mao, H. Y., et al. (1993). Negative behavior during marital conflict is associated with immunological down-regulation. *Psychosomatic Medicine, 55*, 395-409.

Kohut, M. L., Cooper, M. M., Nickolaus, M. S., Russell, D. R., and Cunnick, J. E. (2002). Exercise and psychosocial factors modulate immunity to influenza vaccine in elderly individuals. *Journal of Gerontology, 57*, 557-562.

Maier, S. F., and Watkins, L. R. (1998). Cytokines for psychologists: implications of bidirectional immune-to-brain communication for understanding behaviour, mood and cognition. *Psychological Review, 105*, 83-107.

Marsland, A. L., Cohen, S., Rabin, B. S., and Manuck, S. B. (2001). Associations between stress, trait negative affect, acute immune reactivity, and antibody response to hepatitis B injection in healthy young adults. *Health Psychology, 20*, 4-11.

McClelland, D. C., Alexander, C., and Marks, E. (1982). The need for power, stress, immune function, and illness among male prisoners. *Journal of Abnormal Psychology, 91*, 61-70.

McKinnon, W., Weisse, C. S., Reynolds, C. P., Bowles, C. A., and Baum, A. (1989). Chronic stress, leukocyte subpopulations, and humoral response to latent viruses. *Health Psychology, 8*, 389-402.

Miller, G. E., Cohen, S., Pressman, S., Barkin, A., Rabin, B. S., and Treanor, J. J. (2004). Psychological stress and antibody response to influenza vaccination: when is the critical period for stress, and how does it get inside the body? *Psychosomatic Medicine, 66*, 215-223.

Morag, M., Morag, A., Reichenberg, M. A., Lerer, B., and Yirmiya, R. (1999). Psychological variables as predictors of rubella antibody titers and fatigue - a prospective double blind study. *Journal of Psychiatric Research, 33*, 389-395.

Moynihan, J. A., Larson, M. R., Treanor, J., Duberstein, P. R., Power, A., Shore, B., et al. (2004). Psychosocial factors and the response to influenza vaccination in older adults. *Psychosomatic Medicine, 66*, 950-953.

Patriarca, P. A. (1994). Editorial: A randomized controlled trial of influenza vaccine in the elderly: Scientific scrutiny and ethical responsibility. *Journal of the American Medical Association, 272*, 1700-1701.

Petrie, K. J., Booth, R. J., Pennebaker, J. W., Davison, K. P., and Thomas, M. G. (1995). Disclosure of trauma and immune response to a hepatitis B vaccination program. *Journal of Consulting and Clinical Psychology, 63*, 787-792.

Petrovsky, N. (2001). Towards a unified model of neuroendocrine-immune interaction. *Immunology and Cell Biology, 79*, 350-357.

Petry, J., Weems, L. B., and Livingstone, J. N. I. (1991). Relationship of stress, distress, and the immunologic response to a recombinant hepatitis B vaccine. *Journal of Family Practice, 32*, 481-486.

Phillips, A. C., Burns, V. E., Carroll, D., Ring, C., and Drayson, M. (2005). The Association between Life Events, Social Support and Antibody Status Following Thymus-Dependent and Thymus-Independent Vaccinations in Healthy Young Adults. *Brain, Behaviour and Immunity, 19*, 325-333.

Phillips, A. C., Burns, V. E., and Lord, J. M. (2007). Stress and exercise: getting the balance right for an ageing immune system. *Exercise and Sports Sciences Reviews, 35*, 35-39.

Phillips, A. C., Carroll, D., Burns, V. E., and Drayson, M. (2005). Neuroticism, cortisol reactivity, and antibody response to vaccination. *Psychophysiology, 42*, 232-238.

Phillips, A. C., Carroll, D., Burns, V. E., Ring, C., Macleod, J., and Drayson, M. (2006). Bereavement and marriage are associated with antibody response to influenza vaccination in the elderly. *Brain, Behavior and Immunity, 20*, 279-289.

Pressman, S. D., Cohen, S., Miller, G. E., Barkin, A., Rabin, B. S., and Treanor, J. J. (2005). Loneliness, social network size, and immune response to influenza vaccination in college freshmen. *Health Psychology, 24*, 297-306.

Schaeffer, M. A., Baum, A., Reynolds, C. F., Rikli, P., Davidson, L. M., and Fleming, I. (1985). Immune status as a function of chronic stress at Three Mile Island. *Psychosomatic Medicine, 47*, 85.

Smith, A. P., Vollmer-Conna, U., Bennett, B., Wakefield, D., Hickie, I., and Lloyd, A. (2004). The relationshp between distress and the development of a primary immune response to a novel antigen. *Brain, Behaviour and Immunity, 18*, 65-75.

Smith, T. W., Glazer, K., Ruiz, J. M., and Gallo, L. C. (2004). Hostility, anger, aggressiveness, and coronary heart disease: an interpersonal perspective on personality, emotion, and health. *Journal of Personality, 72*, 1217-1270.

Snyder, B. K., Roghmann, K. J., and Sigal, L. H. (1990). Effect of stress and other biopsychosocial factors on primary antibody response. *Journal of Adolescent Health Care, 11*, 472-479.

Stetler, C., Chen, E., and Miller, G. E. (2006). Written disclosure of experiences with racial discrimination and antibody response to an influenza vaccine. *International Journal of Behavioral Medicine, 13*, 60-68.

Stone, A. A., Cox, D. S., Valdimarsdottir, H., Jandorf, L., and Neale, J. M. (1987). Evidence that secretory IgA antibody is associated with daily mood. *Journal of Personality and Social Psychology, 52*, 988-993.

Stone, A. A., Neale, J. M., Cox, D. S., Napoli, A., Valdimarsdottir, H., and Kennedy-Moore, E. (1994). Daily events are associated with a secretory immune response to an oral antigen in men. *Health Psychology, 13*, 440-446.

Vedhara, K., Bennett, P. D., Clark, S., Lightman, S. L., Shaw, S., Perks, P., et al. (2003). Enhancement of antibody responses to influenza vaccination in the elderly following a cognitive-behavioural stress management intervention. *Psychotherapy and Psychosomatics, 72*, 245-252.

Vedhara, K., Cox, N. K. M., Wilcock, G. K., Perks, P., Hunt, M., Anderson, S., et al. (1999). Chronic stress in elderly carers of dementia patients and antibody response to influenza vaccination. *Lancet, 20*, 627-631.

Vedhara, K., Fox, J. D., and Wang, E. C. Y. (1999). The measurement of stress-related immune dysfunction in psychoneuroimmunology. *Neuroscience and Biobehavioural Reviews, 23*, 699-715.

Vedhara, K., McDermott, M. P., Evans, T. G., Treanor, J. J., Plummer, S., Tallon, D., et al. (2002). Chronic stress in non-elderly caregivers: psychological, endocrine and immune implications. *Journal of Psychosomatic Research, 53*, 1153-1161.

In: Life Style and Health Research Progress
Editors: A. B. Turley, G. C. Hofmann

ISBN: 978-1-60456-427-3
© 2008 Nova Science Publishers, Inc.

Chapter VI

Losing Weight through Lifestyle Modification: A Focus on Young Women

Siew S. Lim[*1,2], **Robert J. Norman**[*3],
Peter M. Clifton[1,2] **and Manny Noakes**[2]

[1] Discipline of Physiology, School of Molecular and Biomedical Science,
Adelaide University, Adelaide SA 5000, Australia
[2] CSIRO Human Nutrition, Kintore Avenue, Adelaide, SA 5000, Australia
[3] Resesarch Centre for Reproductive Health, Discipline of Obstetrics and
Gynaecology, Adelaide University, Adelaide, SA 5000, Australia

ABSTRACT

Women, especially those who enter adulthood with a higher BMI, have a greater risk of age-related weight gain. Weight gain from early adulthood has been associated with an increased risk of heart disease, ischemic stroke, cancer, diabetes, kidney stones, asthma, and even premature death in mid-adulthood. Carrying excess weight poses an additional burden on young women as it increases the risk of infertility, reduces the success of assisted reproductive techniques and increases the risk of complications during pregnancy and delivery. Data from national surveys, population studies and intervention studies suggests a number of reasons for weight gain in young women. The main reason for weight gain is likely to be due to changes in lifestyle that occur in young adulthood, resulting in higher levels of energy intake and lower levels of physical activity. Further investigations reveal that life events such as getting married, having children, or starting work coincides with weight gain and undesirable changes in lifestyles of young women. Social roles acquired at these milestones may affect the priorities and time availability of young women, which in turn influence their ability to maintain a healthy lifestyle. On the other hand, individual psychological characteristics such as the sense of control over one's health mediate the impact of these life events on

---

[*] Tel: +618-83038901; Fax: +618-83038899; Email: siew.lim@csiro.au, peter.clifton@csiro.au,
manny.noakes@csiro.au
[*] Tel: +618-83038166; Fax: +618-83034099; Email: robert.norman@adelaide.edu.au

the lifestyles of young women. We have noted the high prevalence of weight loss attempts and costly investments on weight management strategies in this group which indicated their strong desire to lose weight. Current research in weight loss suggest that lifestyle modification involving a combination of energy-restricted diets, exercise and behavioural therapy are effective for short term weight loss and metabolic improvements in young women. However, weight loss interventions consistently report a higher dropout rate among young women, suggesting that current weight loss approaches do not meet the needs of this group. From what we have learned about the causes of weight gain in young women, future interventions may need to address the underlying broader issues which shape the lifestyles of young women in order to produce sustainable behavioural change in this group.

INTRODUCTION

An average adult in the western world puts on weight until around 60 years old before stabilising and then losing weight [1, 2]. The greatest rate of weight gain occurs in early adulthood [3, 4]. The National Longitudinal Survey of Youth in the United States reported that more than 80% of those who were obese by mid-thirties had became obese in early adulthood [5]. Young women are at greater risk of weight gain compared to men and older women [3, 6]. The first section of this chapter will discuss the implications and causes of weight gain in young women while the second section reviews what we know about weight loss in young women.

A) YOUNG WOMEN AND WEIGHT GAIN

Women are twice as likely to develop obesity during adulthood compared to men [3, 5]. Currently the average weight gain for US white women aged 25-35 years old is 0.39kg/year [2]. The average weight gain for younger women in Australia aged 18-23 years old is even higher, at about 0.67kg/year [7]. If young women continue to gain weight at this rate until 60 years old, they would gain 28kg during adulthood. This magnitude of weight gain has serious health implications.

Not only do young women gain more weight than young men, each generation of young women also supersedes the previous generation in weight gain. A study by Allman-Farinelli et al (2006) have shown that the average body weight of women in each age group increased with time [1]. In the US, women born in 1964 were gaining weight at 28% more rapidly than women born in 1957 [5]. An Australian study in women similarly found that Generation X (born in 1966-1970) gained weight more rapidly than the baby boomers (born 1951-55), whose weight gain was in turn greater than the pre-war generations (born 1936-40) [1]. While data is not yet available for the Generation Y women (born 1976-1985), greater exposure to the obesogenic environment is likely to sustain if not worsen weight gain trends in this generation.

Weight gain affects a large proportion of young women, with 40% of them gaining more than 5% BMI in 4 years [8]. Those with a higher body weight at baseline were at greater risk of significant weight gain [5, 8]. Even moderately excess weight (eg 25-27 kg/m^2) at the age of 20-22 years old could increase the risk of obesity by mid-thirties by 60% [5]. Considering that more than 50% of young women are currently overweight or obese in the US, the weight trajectory of this group is of concern.

Long Term Consequences of Excess Weight or Weight Gain in Young Women

Being overweight or obese in young adulthood has been linked to a number of chronic diseases in mid-adulthood (Table 1.), as reported in a number of large prospective cohort studies. The Nurses Health Study, which is one of the largest prospective cohort study conducted in women, found that those with higher body mass index (BMI) at 18 years old (above 23.3 kg/m^2) had twice the risk of having coronary heart disease (CHD) by mid-age (RR=1.99) compared to women with BMI of less than 19.1 kg/m^2 at 18 years old [9]. As even the highest quintile of BMI of this cohort is within the normal range, we can only speculate that those who were overweight or obese at 18 years may be at even higher risk of developing CHD in later life.

Being overweight or obese in young adulthood could also increase the risk of certain cancers and overall mortality in later life. Women who were overweight at 18 years old had a two-fold increased risk for premenopausal ovarian cancer after adjustment for smoking, age, and oral contraceptive use [10]. Other hormone-related cancers (of breast, uterus and ovary) were also associated with obesity in early adulthood [11]. Body weight in early adulthood also predicted overall mortality. Women who were overweight at 18 years old were 1.66 times more likely to suffer premature death while those who were obese were nearly 3 times more likely to face premature death compared to the women with BMI between 18.5 kg/m^2 and 21.5 kg/m^2 [12]. These data suggest that overweight and obesity in young women could be a progressive health condition with debilitating and even fatal outcomes if left untreated.

Weight gain since early adulthood itself is also emerging to be a risk factor for a number of diseases (Table 1). Women who gained a significant amount of weight throughout adulthood (more than 20kg) were found to be 2.7 times more likely to develop heart disease compared to those who more or less maintained their weight (within 5 kg of 18 years old body weight) [13]. However, even smaller weight gain was associated with increased risk. For example, those who gained 5 kg to 7.9 kg since 18 years old had a 25% increased risk of CHD independent of other risk factors such as age, menopausal status, parental history of CHD, smoking and postmenopausal hormone use [9]. Similar relationships between weight gain and disease risks were also reported for other cardiovascular-related events such as the thickening of carotid artery wall, high blood pressure, heart attack and ischemic stroke [14-16]. Thus, weight gain since adulthood could be quite a strong predictor of cardiovascular health in mid-age.

Adulthood weight gain was also associated with increased risks of other lifestyle diseases such as diabetes, cancer, kidney stone formation, and adult-onset asthma [16-19]. Overweight young women who gained weight throughout adulthood were 20 times more likely to develop diabetes compared to normal weight, weight stable young women [16]. Significant weight gain (25 kg or more) since 18 years old also increased the risk of breast cancer by 45% [19]. No relationship was observed between adulthood weight gain and colon cancer or premenopausal ovarian cancer [10, 13]. Finally, weight gain (more than 20kg) since 18 years old increased the risk of all-cause mortality by 60% [20]. Thus, weight maintenance may be a worthwhile goal for young women.

The adverse effect of weight gain also applies to those whose weight changes were within the normal weight range. Previous weight gain increased the risk of CHD even among those with normal weight [9]. However, the effect of weight gain was far more detrimental for those who were already overweight or obese. Results from the Iowa Women's Health Study showed that normal weight young women who gained weight consistently till mid-age were 6.6 times as likely to develop diabetes as normal weight, weight stable women. In comparison, overweight young women with similar weight gain were 20 times as likely to develop diabetes compared to the same reference group [16]. Similar effects were also seen in shorter-term changes in the Coronary Artery Risk Development in Young Adults (CARDIA) study, in which overweight young adults who gained weight had more adverse changes in glucose, blood pressure, HDL-cholesterol and triglycerides than normal weight young adults with similar weight gain [21]. The greater impact of weight gain in overweight and obese young adults is of concern, as those who were already overweight or obese were more likely to gain weight.

Several studies have found a stronger association between health outcomes with young adult body weights than with older adult body weights, even though the latter were measured closer to the actual diagnoses [11]. For example, a study in men found that BMI at age 22 years old was more strongly associated with cardiovascular disease than BMI at age 38 years old [22]. Cancer and mortality was also significantly related to early adulthood body weight, but not to later body weights [10, 11]. This observation is consistent with the known pathogenesis of these chronic diseases which involve gradual cumulative change over a period time. It is possible that physiological stress caused by excess weight or weight gain in early adulthood initiated the processes of disease development which subsequently progress into disease states that are detectable only in later years. If so, active prevention of chronic diseases may have to begin as early as young adulthood.

Shorter Term Consequences of Excess Weight or Weight Gain in Young Women

In addition to the increased long term risks of chronic diseases, overweight and obesity has immediate impact on young women's lives. Obese young women had poorer health, as seen in greater rates of asthma, headaches, back pain, sleeping difficulties and more visits to their medical practitioners [23]. Weight gain also increases arterial stiffness and worsen the metabolic profile of young women through adverse changes in LDL-cholesterol, HDL-cholesterol, triglycerides, fasting insulin, fasting glucose and blood pressure [24-26]. These changes in early adulthood may culminate in cardiovascular or other metabolically-related chronic diseases in mid-age. However, some of these classic 'mid-age lifestyle diseases' are starting to appear in young adulthood, as seen in a more recent and younger cohort study.

This study found a 23% increased risk of metabolic syndrome in young adults with each 4.5 kg weight gain [27].

Table 1. The long term consequences of excess weight or weight gain in early adulthood: a summary of results from prospective studies in women

Study	n	Consequences of excess weight [RR, 95%CI]	Consequences of weight gain [RR unless specified, 95%CI]
Nurses Health Study [9, 10, 13, 15, 18-20]	121 700 women	• Coronary heart disease [1.99, 1.64-2.40] • Premenopausal ovarian cancer [2.05, 0.73-1.51]	• Coronary heart disease [2.65, 2.17-3.22] • Ischemic stroke [1.69, 1.26-2.29] • All cancers [1.5, 1.1-1.9] • Breast cancer [1.45, 1.27-1.66] • Kidney stone formation [1.70, 1.4-2.05] • Type 2 diabetes [2.4, 2.0-2.9] • All cause mortality [1.6, 1.3-1.9]
Nurses Health Study II [12, 17]	102400 women	• Premature death [2.79, 2.04-3.81]	• Adult-onset asthma [2.5, 2.0-3.1]
Iowa Women's Health Study [16]	17252 women		• Diabetes [OR 19.14, 13.38-27.40] • Blood pressure [OR 7.63, 5.69-10.24] • Heart attack [OR 3.47, 1.94-6.20] • Other heart diseases [OR 2.94, 2.01-4.32]
Atherosclerosis Risk in Communities (ARIC) Study [14]	13282 men and women		• Increase in carotid artery wall thickness [change in white women: 0.013mm, 0.009-0.017]
United Kingdom's Royal College of General Practitioners Oral Contraception Study [11]	9918 women	• Cancer [1.48, 0.98-2.24]	

In the short term, overweight and obesity can affect the quality of life in young women by impairing their reproductive health. Obese young women are at greater risk of irregular periods, infertility, and polycystic ovaries syndrome (PCOS) [23, 28, 29]. PCOS is the most common cause of anovulatory infertility and is characterised by hyperandrogenism, irregular menses and anovulation [30]. Post-adolescence weight gain, especially in the abdominal area, was associated with greater self-reported symptoms of PCOS [31]. Not only does obesity affect natural fertility, it may also decrease the efficacy of assisted reproductive technology. Women with higher BMI generally require higher doses of gonadotropin and longer periods of stimulation during *in vitro* fertilisation treatments [32-35]. When conception is successfully achieved, there are concerns about greater obstetrics and neonatal risks associated maternal obesity. Higher maternal BMI is associated with increased risks of gestational diabetes, pregnancy-related hypertensive disorders, caesarean delivery, and prolonged hospital stay [36]. In addition, there were also greater risks of neonatal complications such as birth defect, hypoglycaemia, jaundice and prematurity associated with higher maternal BMI [36]. Weight gain is also a risk factor in this area. An increase of 5 to 10 kg from 18 years old to pregnancy was associated with a two-fold increase in the risk of gestational diabetes after adjusted for age, baseline BMI, ethnicity, parity and education [37]. Thus, obesity and weight gain in young women is not just a metabolic issue, but also a gynaecologic and paediatric issue as well.

The effect of obesity on mental health of young women also deserves attention. In Australia, anxiety and depression was the leading burden of disease and injury among young adults (aged 15-24 years), accounting for 32% of total burden in females and 17% in males [38]. Women were 1.5 times more likely to report anxiety and affective disorders compared to men [39]. Overweight or obesity exacerbates the mental health of young women. The prevalence of mental disorders increases with body weight, with 57% of obese young women having had mental disorders at some point in their life, compared to 43% in overweight young women and 38% in normal weight young women [40]. Overweight women were also more vulnerable to depression or low self-esteem compared to overweight men [41, 42]. In view of the prevalence of mental disorders in young women especially among those who are overweight and obese, improving mental health should be one of the treatment goals of weight loss interventions in young women.

Struggling with overweight or obesity in early adulthood can have significant social implications for young women. Overweight or obese young women were less likely to report satisfaction with work or study, family relationships or social activities. They were also less likely to aspire to further education and more likely to have low perceived work ability [43, 44]. These may affect their vocational success and eventually, their socioeconomic status. The impact of obesity on career aspiration and satisfaction may be one of the causes for the observed relationship between obesity and socioeconomic status. In addition to jeopardising their own future, overweight and obese young women could also pass on their obesity-related problems to their offspring, not just through genetic predisposition, but also through physiological processes such as fetal programming and environmental processes such as modelling of lifestyle attitudes and patterns [45]. In this sense, addressing the issue of obesity in young women before they enter motherhood is a pivotal point in reversing the trends of obesity in future generations.

In summary, obesity and weight gain affects the metabolic, reproductive and mental health of young women. Further, it also increases the long term risk of chronic diseases. The risk of obesity could also be passed on to their offspring, thus perpetuating the epidemic into future generations. There is an urgent need to promote weight loss or prevent weight gain in young women.

Table 2. The short-term consequences of excess weight or weight gain in early adulthood: a summary of results in young women

Health domains	Consequences (Change, CI)
Metabolic [21, 24-27]	• Increase in LDL cholesterol (+0.17 mmol/L, 0.06-0.20) • Decrease in HDL-cholesterol (-0.09 mmol/L, -0.10- -0.08) • Increase in triglyceride (+1.13 mmol/L, 1.10-1.15) • Increase in fasting insulin (+1.23, 1.20-1.26) • Increase in blood pressure (+1.7, 1.2-2-2) • Increase arterial stiffness (+18.2 cm/s per year) • Increased risk of metabolic syndrome (23%, 20-27%)
Reproductive [29, 31, 36, 46]	• Increased risk of PCOS (RR 1.71, 1.30-2.24) • Reduced fecundity (OR 0.66, 0.49-0.89) • Increased risk of gestational diabetes (OR 2.95, 2.05-4.25) • Increased risk of pregnancy-related hypertensive disorders (OR 3.00, 2.40-3.74) • Increased risk of caesarean section (OR 2.02, 1.79-2.29) • Increased risk of neonates admission to intensive care (OR 2.77, 1.81-4.25)
Psychological [41, 42, 47]	• Depression (OR 1.4, 1.06-3.68) • External locus of control (OR 1.86, 1.24-2.78)
Social [43, 44]	• Low perceived work ability (χ^2=26.81) • Less satisfaction with work or studies (χ^2=37.5) • Less satisfaction with family relationships (χ^2=32.55) • Less satisfaction with social activities (χ^2=40.81) • Less likely to aspire for further education (χ^2=14.4)
General physical health [23]	• Back pain (OR 1.26, 1.08-1.48) • Sleeping difficulties (OR 1.35, 1.15-1.59) • Asthma (OR 1.30, 1.09-1.54) • Headaches (OR 1.47, 1.25-1.73) • More visits to medical practitioners (OR 1.28, 1.09-1.51)

Why Young Women Gain Weight: Biological Factors

A number of factors could contribute to weight gain in young women. The widespread phenomenon of age-related weight gain suggests that the biological changes with aging may play a role. It is well-known that metabolic rate decreases as one ages, as reflected by the estimation of total energy expenditure by Schofield equations. Recent study suggests that basal metabolic rate (BMR), which is the single largest component of total energy expenditure, decreases by 2% per decade among normal weight women aged between 20 and 96 years [48]. Given that Australian young women aged 18 to 23 years were gaining weight at the rate of about 10% per decade, decreasing BMR with aging is unlikely to account for all the weight gain. Moreover, the BMR-lowering effect of aging could be counteracted by the increase in BMR resulted from body mass gain. Accordingly, the same database reported that the BMR of those who had gained weight until 40-50 years old remained stable for that period before decreasing rapidly. The thermic effect of feeding, which is another biological component of the total energy expenditure also did not appear to be affected by age [48]. Therefore, 'age-related' weight gain as we observed may not be due to the biological process of aging, but a result of other concurrent changes that take place as one ages.

Why Young Women Gain Weight: Behavioral Factors

When asked about the reasons for their weight gain, more women cited changes in physical activity and changes in the amount of food and drink consumed than for any other reasons [49]. This was supported by objective data obtained from research studies and national surveys. The last National Nutrition Survey in Australia conducted in 1995 found that the proportion of purchased food and beverages peaked in the age group of 19 to 24 years old among females [50]. Greater consumption of fast food and take-away foods has been associated with weight gain in young women [8, 51, 52]. National data has also shown that about half of all young Australian women had inadequate fruit consumption while nearly 90% of them had inadequate vegetable consumption [39]. The picture emerging from these data suggest that young women were having poor quality diets dominated by convenience food while lacking in foods from the main food groups. This dietary pattern is high in energy but low in nutrients. Dietary patterns which are high in refined foods and low in fruits and vegetables have been associated with weight gain in women [53]. On the contrary, higher intakes of fruits, vegetables and wholegrains were associated with greater weight loss in women, with a greater effect in obese women [54].

Excessive alcohol consumption is also a growing issue in young women. Australian young women who were drinking alcohol at levels linked to long term risk (15 standard drinks or more per week) and short term risk (5 standard drinks or more per occasion) peaked in the age group of 18 to 24 years old, with 20% at long term risk and 45% at short term risk [55]. Women are also drinking more. The proportion of women drinking at excessive levels has nearly doubled from 1995 to 2004-2005 [39]. In a recent analysis on the lifestyle behaviours of overweight or obese young women registered for weight loss trial, we found that 46% of these young women were drinking at levels exceeding the recommendation of no more than 2 standard drinks in a day. High alcohol consumption could contribute to excessive energy intake. In addition to the significant health and social risks, high alcohol intakes could also be one of the factors of overweight and obesity in young women.

Low levels of physical activity could be another possible cause of weight gain in young women. About one-third of young women in Australia between the ages of 18 and 44 were physically inactive [39]. Among overweight and obese young women registered for a weight loss trial, 72% did not meet the physical activity guidelines of at least 30 minutes of activity most days per week, suggesting a higher prevalence of physical inactivity among overweight and obese young women compared to the young women in general. The CARDIA study, which involved young adults from 18 to 30 years old at baseline, found a significant decrease in self-reported physical activity among young women during the 7-years follow-up period [56]. Those in the study who increased their physical activity had an attenuated age-related weight gain, with a more pronounced effect among overweight and obese women [57]. Thus a decrease in physical activity may contribute to weight gain in young women, especially in overweight and obese young women.

Besides low levels of physical activity, high levels of sedentary behaviours could also lead to weight gain. Heavy television viewing (more than 4 hours per day) was associated with greater BMI in American young women [58]. Similarly, an Australian study found that those who watched television for more than 4 hours per day were four times more likely to be overweight [59]. About 10% of young adults in Australia aged 18 to 44 years old watched 4 hours of television in a day [59]. Lower levels of television watching also increased the risks of obesity. About 1 to 2.5 hour of television watching per day could increase the risk of overweight to nearly 2 fold [59]. According to the CARDIA study, the average television viewing time for American young women aged 23 to 29 years old was 2hr/day for white women and 3 hr/day for black women [58], which is sufficient to increase their risk of becoming overweight. Interestingly, high levels of physical activity did not eliminate the obesogenic effects of television viewing. The relationship between television viewing time and obesity existed even among those who were physically active [59]. This is possibly due to the inevitable compensatory decrease in incidental physical activities during television viewing. It is probably for the same reason that young women who spent more time sitting were more likely to gain weight [8]. Increase in energy intake among those with higher levels of television viewing may also explain greater weight gain in this group, however it is unclear if that is due to overall poorer dietary pattern or greater intake of energy dense food while watching television [59].

One of the lifestyle changes that occur during young adulthood is the decrease in sleep duration. The Zurich Cohort Study started in 1978 with 4547 men and women aged 19 found that sleep duration decreases with age [60]. A significant association between short sleep duration and obesity was found in younger adults (at age 27, 29, and 34) but not in older adults (age 40) [60]. This remained significant after adjusted for sex, education level, physical activity level, smoking, binge eating, childhood depression and family history of obesity [60]. Dietary intake was not adjusted for in the analyses, and thus could account for the relationship between sleep duration and obesity. Recent opinion on this topic suggests that short sleep duration could lead to increases in appetite, alterations in glucose metabolism and decreases in energy expenditure [61], all of which are potential mechanisms linking short sleep duration to obesity. Further research should be conducted to explore this relationship in young adults.

All the causes discussed up to this point suggest that weight gain in young women are unlikely to be due to biological reasons, but due to a range of 'modifiable' health behaviours such as dietary intake, physical activity, alcohol consumption, sedentary behaviours and sleep deprivation. However, decades of research in lifestyle modification alongside with the ever growing problem of obesity suggests that these factors are more difficult to modify than it seems. To change the health behaviour of young women, it may be helpful to understand the underlying factors driving these behaviours.

Why Young Women Gain Weight: Psychosocial Factors and Life Events

Young adulthood is a life-stage characterised by change. Many of these changes occur as part of the process of taking up adult responsibilities, such as being financially independent, caring for significant others, nurturing the next generation, or finding one's niche in society. This section will explore the effect of these events on the body weight and lifestyles of young women.

Marriage

Marriage predicts weight gain in young women. The NHANES cohort in the US found that those who married had a 50% increase in risk for major weight gain (ie more than 13 kg weight gain during 10 years of follow-up) [62]. Similar trends were noted in young women in other countries such as Finland and Australia [8, 63]. Changes in lifestyle since marriage have been noted in young women. Marriage was associated with decreased physical activity in young women while living with a partner has been shown to increase energy intake [64, 65]. A study on cohabitation found that couples living together had greater motivation to prepare meals and increased alcohol intake during meals [65]. There were also feelings of shared guilt over temptations and shared motivation over dietary restriction which may affect restraint [65]. This evidence supports marriage as one of the correlates of weight gain in young women.

Pregnancy and Child-Rearing

Women who have had children were more likely to gain weight [8, 66]. Pregnancy could also change body shape by increasing waist-to-hip ratio independent of weight gain at 12 months postpartum [66]. On average women retain 0.5 to 3kg from pregnancy, although this can vary greatly between individuals [67]. Gestational weight gain has increased over time across all BMI categories [68]. While some women are able to return to their pre-pregnancy weight at 6-12 months postpartum, majority (~73%) remained at higher BMI [67]. Normal weight women who became overweight after pregnancy had slightly higher pre-pregnancy BMI, greater weight gain during pregnancy, and less weight loss after pregnancy compared to those who returned to their normal weight after pregnancy [69]. Those who did not return to normal weight at 1 year after delivery had a steeper weight trajectory over the following 14 years, so that they ended up with greater weight gain in the long term compared to their counterparts [69]. Women who retained more weight after pregnancy tended to have higher energy intake, more frequent snacking, less regular lunch and less physical activity during or after pregnancy [70]. These studies suggest that pregnancy is a vulnerable period during which some young women could experience significant permanent weight gain. In some cases, pregnancy could trigger a new pattern of body weight characterised by greater long term weight gain.

As having children involves more than the biological process of pregnancy and childbirth, the child-rearing responsibilities that follow could also affect the lifestyles of young women. Women with children were more than twice as likely to be physically inactive compared to those who did not have any children after controlling for age, BMI and baseline physical activity level [64]. Women with children also perceived leisure time physical activity, incidental physical activity and transport physical activity as less feasible, but perceived work or domestic physical activity as more feasible [71]. Anecdotally, certain tasks associated with childcare such as 'running after the kids the whole day' seem to imply a high level of domestic physical activity. However, its contribution to energy expenditure has not been investigated. Caring for children may also affect dietary intake of young women but this has alsp not been investigated. A greater understanding on the impact of child-rearing on young women's lifestyle pattern may help to determine appropriate strategies to improve the lifestyle of young women with children.

Employment

Starting work is also a risk factor for weight gain. Young women who were still studying were less likely to gain weight [8]. This too could be due to changes in lifestyle associated with beginning employment. Starting paid work is associated with increased risk of physical inactivity while returning to study is associated with decreased risk of inactivity in young women [64]. Among overweight and obese women registered for a weight loss trial, young women who were working consumed significantly greater number of meals away from home compared to women who were not working (unpublished data). Although this may not be synonymous with greater frequency of consuming purchased meals, it is plausible that employment increases the incidence of eating out or takeaways among young women. One study suggested that working women expressed greater dislike for food shopping, greater time concerns with cooking, and had less tendency to value family's health and preference in food preparation compared to housewives [72]. Less time availability coupled with greater financial ability provided the option for women to pay for services that were traditionally women's responsibilities, such as child-caring, cleaning and cooking [73]. Further research is required to explore the effect of employment on the health of young women.

Social Environment

Social influence seems to be an important determinant of young women's health behaviour, to a greater extent than it is for young men. Young women were more likely to perceive social situations as barriers to healthy eating or being physically active [74]. Support or sabotage by friends and family predicted the success of weight maintenance in young women [75]. Women with children perceived the lack of support from partner, children or friends as barriers to physical activity and healthy eating [76]. Dietary habits such as fruits, vegetables and wholegrains intakes were also predicted by perceived social norm (eg how important healthy eating was to their parent's) and subjective norm (eg whether their parents think you should eat healthier) [77]. Thus, friends and family may have a significant influence on the lifestyle choices of young women.

Psychological Characteristics

Life events or social environment do not have the same effect on all young women. Personal characteristics such as perceived behavioural control, self-efficacy (i.e. a person's belief on his/her ability to attain a particular goal), and internal weight locus of control (i.e. more likely to perceive weight as a result to own control than to external circumstances) could determine the responses of young women to these life challenges [77]. Young women who did not gain weight had greater self-efficacy in avoiding weight gain [75]. Self-efficacy has also been found to predict physical activity levels in obese females [78]. Higher exercise self-efficacy predicted long term (16 months) success in weight management in young women [79]. Having a sense of confidence or control could help young women to overcome barriers to healthy living. For example, a study found that certain young women were able to engage in regular physical activity despite facing barriers such as having young children, low partner support in physical activity, and low socioeconomic status [80]. However, overweight women also had lower self-efficacy in weight loss compared to overweight men [42]. Women with excess weight also tend to have lower internal locus of control compared to normal weight women [47]. Among overweight and obese women, those with lower internal locus of control had higher BMI and poorer diets with lower levels of micronutrient intakes (unpublished data). Thus, low sense of control could play a role in overweight and obesity in young women.

Why Young Women Gain Weight: Social Roles and Priorities

An interesting point to note is that even though young men also go through these life events (except for pregnancy and childbirth), their body weight were somewhat less affected by these events [81]. Perhaps the reason young women gained weight at these time points were not just due to a change in the physical circumstance, which equally affects young men, but also due to changes in the social circumstance (eg living with a partner versus being a wife). At each of these life events mentioned above, young women gained an additional social role, such as mother, partner, or family caregiver. At times this occurs in addition to their existing roles of employee or student. Being involved in more than one of these social roles was associated with worse overall health in young women, while the reverse is true in older women [82]. It is possible that pressing responsibilities accompanying these roles compete for priorities in young women's lives such that health was no longer the main focus. This may explain why nutrition and physical education alone, even if delivered with behavioural therapy, may have short-lived effects in this group.

Time Pressure

Social roles may affect young women's lifestyle choices through their time availability. Fulfilment of these roles places a high demand on young women's time. 'Time poverty' may be an important cause of poor lifestyle habits and poor health in this group. Young women cited lack of time and lack of motivation as the most important barriers to physical activity and healthy eating [76]. Lack of motivation for healthy eating and exercise could be a reflection of lower priority for these agenda compared to other life responsibilities. Data from the Australian Bureau of Statistics revealed that the percentage of individuals who were chronically time pressured increases with age (measured from 15 years old) and peak in age 35 to 39 years old before decreasing. More women than men felt that they were chronically time pressured [83]. In support of our discussion on social roles, marital status and the number of children were also positively associated with time pressure [83]. Thus, time pressure could be the mediating factor through which life events affect the lifestyle patterns of young women.

Ideologies and Beliefs

As social role is an artefact of ideologies and beliefs held by the individual and her society, some of these beliefs may have generated the challenges related to these roles. For example, young women with children felt guilty for taking time out for themselves and leaving their children in other's care because to them this constitutes failure in fulfilling their role as a 'good mother'[80]. On the other hand, those who made a commitment to take care of their own health operated from a different set of ideology. For the latter group, being a good mother does not involve only caring for their children but also include being a good role model in health for their children [80]. Thus motherhood, instead of being a barrier, became a compelling reason for them to engage in physical activity. In the same way, certain beliefs and ideologies defining the roles of a 'good wife', 'good employee', 'good mother' and 'good friend' may affect the choices of young women either positively or negatively. Perhaps some of these ideologies need to be challenged. For example, despite a greater proportion of women engaged in paid occupations, gender inequalities still exist in childcare and household responsibilities within the household [80]. Inequalities also exist in the entitlement for personal leisure time within the household, whereby men were more likely to prioritise personal leisure time over household chores whereas the opposite is probably true for women [80]. This may explain why women in general are more time-pressured than men [83]. Re-adjustment of some of these beliefs by the individual and the society may be necessary to improve the lifestyles of young women.

Lifestyle behaviours are shaped by powerful influences in young women's life, such as the perceived responsibilities associated with being a wife, mother, employee, or a part of a social network. These perceived roles could impact on young women's lifestyle, possibly through their time availability. On the other hand, low self-efficacy especially among those who are overweight or obese undermines their ability to respond positively to these challenges.

B) YOUNG WOMEN AND WEIGHT LOSS

At first glance, targeting young women for weight loss may seem unnecessary as it is generally assumed that young women were probably one of the most motivated demographic sectors for weight loss. On average, 30-50% of young women across all BMI attempted to lose weight [84]. The prevalence of young women who attempted weight loss increases with BMI [84]. A study in female college students (age 18 to 24 years) in the United States reported that as many as 91% of overweight young women and 86% of obese young women tried to lose weight [85]. Primary sources of pressure to lose weight were self (54%), followed by media (37%) and friends (32%) [85]. The most common methods of losing weight were restricting the amount of food eaten, eating low fat versions of food and drinks, and exercising [85], suggesting the lifestyle modification is quite a common method to lose weight among young women. Young women were also willing to spend money on losing weight. In 2001, Australian young women spent $414 million in weight management strategies which included commercial weight loss programs, gym memberships, or exercise equipment [86].

Unfortunately, weight loss attempts do not often equate to weight loss success. Women were more than twice as likely (OR 2.4, CI 2.2-2.7) than men to attempt weight loss, but men were 40% more likely to succeed in these attempts (OR 1.4, CI 1.0-2.1) [87]. In a large clinic-based weight loss program involving meal replacements and group sessions (n=866), females were found to be 30% more likely to drop out of the study, while those who were under the age of 40 were 66% more likely to drop out of the study [88], making age and gender the most important predictors of attrition. Findings from other large-scale weight loss studies similarly found that young, female participants tended to drop out of weight loss interventions [89, 90]. Despite the lack of effectiveness of conventional approaches in retaining young women in weight loss treatments, there has been very limited research in this group.

Efficacy of Lifestyle Modification on Weight Loss and General Health

A small number of studies have looked at the effect of lifestyle modification on young women's health. This section will review the efficacy of various components of lifestyle modification on body weight and metabolic health in young women. Due to limited studies conducted in young women, findings from the general population will also be discussed.

Diet

Lifestyle intervention typically encourages participants to reduce their energy intake by 500-1000 kcal/day to achieve a gradual weight loss of 0.5kg/week.[91] Traditionally, energy restriction is achieved by having a low-fat, high carbohydrate diet. However, increasingly studies suggest that diets with reduced glycemic loads such as high protein diets, low glycemic index diets or even very low carbohydrate diets were associated with greater metabolic benefit compared to the conventional low-fat high (mostly refined) carbohydrate diet [92-95]. In particular, diets with higher protein recommendations were beneficial in preserving muscle mass during weight loss [96]. *Ad libitum* studies reported a spontaneously lower energy intake with higher protein diet compared to high carbohydrate diet [97, 98] possibly due to the satiating properties of protein [99]. On the contrary, *ad libitum* low carbohydrate high fat diets tended to result in greater energy intake than the high carbohydrate-low fat diets possibly owing to the increased intake of energy-dense foods. Nevertheless, long term studies (1-year) are usually marked by high attrition rate and poor adherence to diet regardless of the prescribed dietary pattern [100-102], suggesting that manipulation of macronutrient composition alone is insufficient to maintain long term adherence.

In young women, energy restricted high carbohydrate or high protein diets were found to be equally effective in producing weight loss of around 8kg in 16 weeks [103]. Other energy restricted dietary strategies such as very low calorie diet (4200KJ per day), very low carbohydrate diet (<20g carbohydrate per day) and meal replacements for 16 to 24 weeks have also been shown to be effective in weight loss in young women [104-106]. Weight loss from lifestyle interventions improved metabolic parameters in young women, such as fasting insulin, LDL cholesterol and triglyceride levels [103-105]. Reproductive outcomes such as ovulation rates, menstrual cyclicity, testosterone and sex-hormone binding globulin levels, hirsutism, and pregnancy rates were also improved following weight loss through lifestyle modification [103, 107, 108]. These findings suggest that energy restriction is efficacious in producing weight loss and its associated benefits in metabolic and reproductive health but insufficient studies were conducted in young women to determine if certain dietary strategies were associated with greater metabolic or reproductive benefit beyond weight loss.

Physical Activity

It is commonly assumed that physical activity assists in weight management by contributing to the increase in energy expenditure. The International Association for the Study of Obesity consensus statement stated that 60 to 90 minutes of moderate intensity activity per day is required for the secondary prevention of obesity [109]. This statement was based mainly on prospective studies conducted at the population level [109]. The National Weight Control Registry similarly found an important role for physical activity on long term weight loss maintenance [110]. Although these observational studies support the role of physical activity in weight management, these results have not been consistently reproduced in randomised controlled trials (RCT). In a recent review on physical activity and weight management, only 2 out of 17 RCT reported a significant benefit of adding physical activity to dietary intervention for weight loss [111]. Physical activities ranging from 60 to 240 minutes per week resulted in a 1.5kg weight loss advantage compared to diet-only interventions, but this do not always reach statistical significance [111]. Despite the increasingly acknowledged role of physical activity in weight maintenance, only 3 out of 8 RCT confirmed the additional benefit of physical activity to diet-only interventions in weight maintenance [111]. It could be that the physical activity levels in these interventions were not sufficient to have an effect on body weight. However, a greater physical activity requirement may not be a sustainable behavioural goal for many overweight or obese individuals. Moreover, it is also unclear if incidental activities were accounted for in these studies. Individuals who compensated the increase in leisure-time physical activity with a decrease in incidental activity may have attenuated the potential weight loss benefits of the intervention.

In women, a prospective cohort study found that those who had more than 5 hours of vigorous activity per week gained 0.5 kg less than their inactive peers in 6 years, suggesting a small effect for the effort involved [112]. Intervention studies similarly reported negligible effects of exercise alone in weight loss in young women. An exercise-only intervention in overweight young women consisting of aerobic exercise (mainly treadmill, target intensity of 55%-70% of maximum oxygen capacity, 45 minutes per session, 5 sessions per week for 16 months) did not result in significant weight or fat loss [113]. In the absence of weight or fat loss, aerobic exercise produced improvement in insulin sensitivity in normal weight young women but not in overweight young women [114, 115]. In overweight and obese young women with PCOS, exercise decreased waist-hip-ratio, body mass index and homocysteine levels [116, 117]. Physical activity was also found to be beneficial in producing weight loss in men [113, 118]. As the studies conducted in young women were exercise-only interventions, the combined effects of diet and exercise in this group remain to be investigated.

Comprehensive Lifestyle Programs

Expert panels such as the National Health Institutes recommended a combination of diet, exercise and behavioural therapy for long term obesity treatment [119]. Self-monitoring, which is an important aspect of behavioural modification, was found to be an important correlate of long term weight maintenance in the US National Weight Control Registry. Findings from the Registry reported that those who frequently monitored their food intake lost significantly more weight than those who monitor their intake less frequently (18 kg vs 5 kg) [110]. Self-monitoring of body weight by frequent weighing was also associated with better weight maintenance [120]. In support of this observational evidence, intervention studies found that the addition of behavioural therapy which included self-monitoring and other self-regulatory aspects improved the efficacy of diet and exercise interventions on weight loss [121-124].

Very few combined interventions (ie including diet, exercise and behavioural therapy) were conducted in young women. The Health Hunters from Sweden is the only weight management lifestyle program developed specifically for this group [125]. This one-year program was developed for young women at high risk of weight gain, between the ages of 18 to 28 years with at least one obese parent. The aim of the program was to prevent weight gain through diet, exercise and behavioural therapy. The program provided information and self-help materials in three main areas: diet, physical activity and weight control. All participants in the intervention group received some core materials from all three areas, but they could choose when and which area they wish to focus on at any time. The program consisted of one face-to-face visit at baseline followed by regular contact through telephone, email, occasional group sessions and visits with dietitians. Thirty out of the 40 young women completed the program. Intention-to-treat analysis found that the intervention group lost 1.9 kg while control group gained 2.6 kg (P<0.05). Completers analysis found that the intervention group had significantly greater improvement in BMI, waist circumference and waist-hip-ratio compared to the control group.

The Fertility Fitness program in South Australia was a lifestyle program developed for obese infertile women with the aim of improving reproductive health. Most of their participants were young women with an average age of around 30 years old [126, 127]. The program consisted of 2-hour sessions per week for 24 weeks. Each session consisted of an hour of exercise led by a coach, followed by an hour information session led by various health professionals such as psychiatrist, dietitian, and gynaecologist. The program resulted in a mean weight loss of 6.2kg [126]. The young women had a decrease in insulin and testosterone levels as well as improvement in psychological measures such as self-esteem, anxiety and depression [126, 128]. Those who completed the program also had greater rates of spontaneous ovulation, pregnancy, and live births [127]. Despite these successes, the program is no longer running due to lack of interest from young women seeking fertility treatment through lifestyle modification. Other treatments such as assisted reproductive techniques were preferred, probably due to lower time commitment.

Hoeger et al. (2004) conducted a pilot trial in young women with PCOS using a study design adapted from the Diabetes Prevention Trial. Subjects randomised to the lifestyle plus placebo arm participated in a combined lifestyle modification program [129]. This included energy restriction of 500-1000 calorie deficit per day, individualised exercise program of 150 minutes per week and behavioural therapy. The program consisted of 24 weeks weight loss phase followed by 24 weeks weight maintenance phase. Group meetings and progress monitoring took place regularly throughout the entire study period. Six out of the 11 young women randomised to the lifestyle plus placebo arm completed the program. Those who completed the program lost 6.8 kg by the end of the program. Changes in androgen levels, insulin measures, and ovulation did not reach statistical significance, probably owing to the small sample size.

In summary, energy restriction was found to be efficacious in producing weight loss and its associated metabolic and reproductive benefits in young women. The benefit of adding exercise to dietary interventions remains to be investigated in this group. Interventions which involved a combination of diet, exercise and behavioural therapy resulted in improvements in physical and mental health but the contribution of behavioural therapy per se to these outcomes have not been ascertained in this group. In addition, none of these studies went beyond 1 year, thus the long term efficacy and effectiveness is not known. Attrition is also a considerable concern in this group, as evident from nearly 40% drop out rate in Hoeger et al's study and the cessation of the Fertility Fitness program. Further research is required to address these questions.

CONCLUSION

Population studies suggest that young women are at high risk of weight gain and that weight gain in young women could be detrimental in both the short and long term. Changes in lifestyles such as an increase in energy intake through poor quality diet and a decrease in physical activity during early adulthood could account for weight gain in this group. However, lifestyle patterns seldom occur in isolation. These changes in diet and physical activity have been found to be associated with other significant changes in young women's lives, such as getting married, having children and starting work. As young women acquire the additional responsibilities at these milestones in life, growing time pressure could sap their energy and motivation to maintain a healthy lifestyle. Perhaps a screaming child, an unhappy boss, or a disgruntled spouse poses a greater threat to their wellbeing than increasing clothes size and the prospect of heart disease or even premature death in a few decades.

Causes of weight gain   **Weight loss interventions**

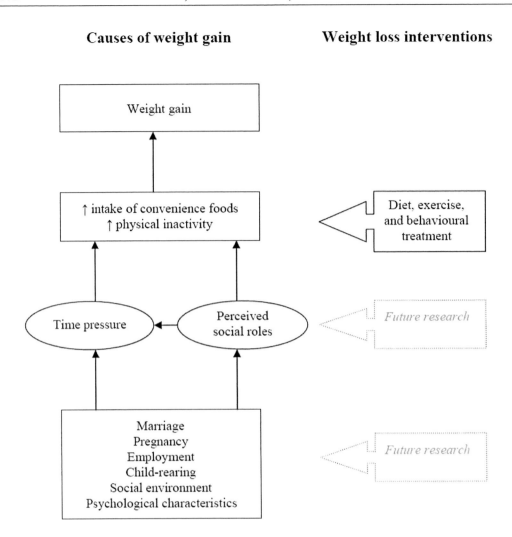

Figure 1. Causes of weight gain and weight loss interventions in young women.

On the other hand, obesity research has developed a number of efficacy-proven lifestyle modification strategies including a variety of energy-restricted diets, exercise regimes and behavioural therapies. However, these interventions depend on the costly investments of time and energy by its participants, which are both sought-after resources in young women's life. Without addressing the underlying issues which powerfully shaped the lifestyles of young women (Figure 1), behavioural change from current models of lifestyle modification is unlikely to be sustainable. A high attrition rate which follows the high attempt rate in weight loss by young women attests to this. A persistent hunger for new and novel weight loss strategies by lay and scientific communities similarly reflects the incompetency of existing approaches in producing the desired result, which is long term weight loss.

The complexity of obesity in young women highlights the importance of a multidisciplinary, multi-sectorial approach to manage obesity. Interventions targeting young women need to address not only the behavioural aspects such as food intake and energy expenditure, but also the cognitive aspects such as self-efficacy, self-esteem and perceived ideologies on social roles. Additionally, changes in the society needs to take place in order to sustain these efforts, such as the production of affordable and nutritious convenient foods and takeaways, the promotion of gender equality in the household, and a shift in workplace culture towards health. When a healthy lifestyle is valued not just by certain individuals but by every sector in the society, the healthy choice will be the easy choice.

REFERENCES

[1]   Allman-Farinelli M, King L, Bonfiglioli C, Bauman A. *The weight of time:time influences on overweight and obesity in women.* Sydney: NSW Centre for Overweight and Obesity; 2006.

[2]   Sheehan TJ, DuBrava S, DeChello LM, Fang Z. Rates of weight change for black and white Americans over a twenty year period. *Int. J. Obes. Relat. Metab. Disord.* 2003;27(4):498-504.

[3]   Kuczmarski RJ. Prevalence of overweight and weight gain in the United States. *Am. J. Clin. Nutr.* 1992;55(2 Suppl):495S-502S.

[4]   Lewis CE, Jacobs DR, Jr., McCreath H, Kiefe CI, Schreiner PJ, Smith DE, et al. Weight gain continues in the 1990s: 10-year trends in weight and overweight from the CARDIA study. Coronary Artery Risk Development in Young Adults. *Am. J. Epidemiol.* 2000;151(12):1172-81.

[5]   McTigue KM, Garrett JM, Popkin BM. The natural history of the development of obesity in a cohort of young U.S. adults between 1981 and 1998. *Ann. Intern. Med.* 2002;136(12):857-64.

[6]   Ball K, Crawford D, Ireland P, Hodge A. Patterns and demographic predictors of 5-year weight change in a multi-ethnic cohort of men and women in Australia. *Public Health Nutr.* 2003;6(3):269-81.

[7]   Brown W, Byles J, Carrigan G, Dobson A, Dolja-Gore X, Gibson R, et al. *Trends in women's health: Results from the Australian Longitudinal Study on Women's Health - priority conditions, risk factors and health behaviours*: The University of Newcastle The University of Queensland; 2006 October 2006.

[8]   Ball K, Brown W, Crawford D. Who does not gain weight? Prevalence and predictors of weight maintenance in young women. *Int. J. Obes. Relat. Metab. Disord.* 2002;26(12):1570-8.

[9]   Willett WC, Manson JE, Stampfer MJ, Colditz GA, Rosner B, Speizer FE, et al. Weight, weight change, and coronary heart disease in women. Risk within the 'normal' weight range. *Jama.* 1995;273(6):461-5.

[10] Fairfield KM, Willett WC, Rosner BA, Manson JE, Speizer FE, Hankinson SE. Obesity, weight gain, and ovarian cancer. *Obstet. Gynecol.* 2002;100(2):288-96.

[11] Elliott AM, Aucott LS, Hannaford PC, Smith WC. Weight change in adult life and health outcomes. *Obes. Res.* 2005;13(10):1784-92.

[12] van Dam RM, Willett WC, Manson JE, Hu FB. The relationship between overweight in adolescence and premature death in women. *Ann. Intern. Med.* 2006;145(2):91-7.

[13] Colditz GA, Coakley E. Weight, weight gain, activity, and major illnesses: the Nurses' Health Study. *Int. J. Sports Med.* 1997;18 Suppl 3:S162-70.

[14] Stevens J, Tyroler HA, Cai J, Paton CC, Folsom AR, Tell GS, et al. Body weight change and carotid artery wall thickness. The Atherosclerosis Risk in Communities (ARIC) Study. *Am. J. Epidemiol.* 1998;147(6):563-73.

[15] Rexrode KM, Hennekens CH, Willett WC, Colditz GA, Stampfer MJ, Rich-Edwards JW, et al. A prospective study of body mass index, weight change, and risk of stroke in women. *Jama.* 1997;277(19):1539-45.

[16] French SA, Jeffery RW, Folsom AR, McGovern P, Williamson DF. Weight loss maintenance in young adulthood: prevalence and correlations with health behavior and disease in a population-based sample of women aged 55-69 years. *Int. J. Obes. Relat. Metab. Disord.* 1996;20(4):303-10.

[17] Camargo CA, Jr., Weiss ST, Zhang S, Willett WC, Speizer FE. Prospective study of body mass index, weight change, and risk of adult-onset asthma in women. *Arch. Intern. Med.* 1999;159(21):2582-8.

[18] Taylor EN, Stampfer MJ, Curhan GC. Obesity, weight gain, and the risk of kidney stones. *Jama.* 2005;293(4):455-62.

[19] Eliassen AH, Colditz GA, Rosner B, Willett WC, Hankinson SE. Adult weight change and risk of postmenopausal breast cancer. *Jama.* 2006;296(2):193-201.

[20] Manson JE, Willett WC, Stampfer MJ, Colditz GA, Hunter DJ, Hankinson SE, et al. Body weight and mortality among women. *N. Engl. J. Med.* 1995;333(11):677-85.

[21] Truesdale KP, Stevens J, Lewis CE, Schreiner PJ, Loria CM, Cai J. Changes in risk factors for cardiovascular disease by baseline weight status in young adults who maintain or gain weight over 15 years: the CARDIA study. *Int. J. Obes. (Lond)* 2006.

[22] Jeffreys M, McCarron P, Gunnell D, McEwen J, Smith GD. Body mass index in early and mid-adulthood, and subsequent mortality: a historical cohort study. *Int. J. Obes. Relat. Metab. Disord.* 2003;27(11):1391-7.

[23] Brown WJ, Mishra G, Kenardy J, Dobson A. Relationships between body mass index and well-being in young Australian women. *Int. J. Obes. Relat. Metab. Disord.* 2000;24(10):1360-8.

[24] Folsom AR, Jacobs DR, Jr., Wagenknecht LE, Winkhart SP, Yunis C, Hilner JE, et al. Increase in fasting insulin and glucose over seven years with increasing weight and inactivity of young adults. The CARDIA Study. Coronary Artery Risk Development in Young Adults. *Am. J. Epidemiol.* 1996;144(3):235-46.

[25] Norman JE, Bild D, Lewis CE, Liu K, West DS. The impact of weight change on cardiovascular disease risk factors in young black and white adults: the CARDIA study. *Int. J. Obes. Relat. Metab. Disord.* 2003;27(3):369-76.

[26] Wildman RP, Farhat GN, Patel AS, Mackey RH, Brockwell S, Thompson T, et al. Weight change is associated with change in arterial stiffness among healthy young adults. *Hypertension.* 2005;45(2):187-92.

[27] Carnethon MR, Loria CM, Hill JO, Sidney S, Savage PJ, Liu K. Risk factors for the metabolic syndrome: the Coronary Artery Risk Development in Young Adults (CARDIA) study, 1985-2001. *Diabetes Care.* 2004;27(11):2707-15.

[28] Gambineri A, Pelusi C, Vicennati V, Pagotto U, Pasquali R. Obesity and the polycystic ovary syndrome. *Int. J. Obes. Relat. Metab. Disord.* 2002;26(7):883-96.

[29] Pasquali R, Pelusi C, Genghini S, Cacciari M, Gambineri A. Obesity and reproductive disorders in women. *Hum. Reprod. Update.* 2003;9(4):359-72.

[30] Broekmans FJ, Knauff EAH, Valkenburg O, Laven JS, Eijkemans MJ, Fauser BCJM. PCOS according to the Rotterdam consensus criteria:change in prevalence among WHO-II anovulation and association with metabolic factors. *BJOG: An International Journal of Obstetrics and Gynaecology.* 2006;Online early issue.

[31] Laitinen J, Taponen S, Martikainen H, Pouta A, Millwood I, Hartikainen AL, et al. Body size from birth to adulthood as a predictor of self-reported polycystic ovary syndrome symptoms. *Int. J. Obes. Relat. Metab. Disord.* 2003;27(6):710-5.

[32] Dokras A, Baredziak L, Blaine J, Syrop C, VanVoorhis BJ, Sparks A. Obstetric outcomes after in vitro fertilization in obese and morbidly obese women. *Obstet. Gynecol.* 2006;108(1):61-9.

[33] Balen AH, Platteau P, Andersen AN, Devroey P, Sorensen P, Helmgaard L, et al. The influence of body weight on response to ovulation induction with gonadotrophins in 335 women with World Health Organization group II anovulatory infertility. *Bjog.* 2006;113(10):1195-202.

[34] Dodson WC, Kunselman AR, Legro RS. Association of obesity with treatment outcomes in ovulatory infertile women undergoing superovulation and intrauterine insemination. *Fertil. Steril.* 2006;86(3):642-6.

[35] Dechaud H, Anahory T, Reyftmann L, Loup V, Hamamah S, Hedon B. Obesity does not adversely affect results in patients who are undergoing in vitro fertilization and embryo transfer. *Eur. J. Obstet. Gynecol. Reprod. Biol.* 2006;127(1):88-93.

[36] Callaway LK, Prins JB, Chang AM, McIntyre HD. The prevalence and impact of overweight and obesity in an Australian obstetric population. *Med. J. Aust.* 2006;184(2):56-9.

[37] Rudra CB, Sorensen TK, Leisenring WM, Dashow E, Williams MA. Weight characteristics and height in relation to risk of gestational diabetes mellitus. *Am. J. Epidemiol.* 2007;165(3):302-8.

[38] Australian Institute of Health and Welfare A. *Young Australians: Their health and wellbeing. 2007.* Canberra: AIHW; 2007.

[39] TAGOfW. *Women in Australia 2007.* Canberra: Commonwealth of Australia; 2007.

[40] Becker ES, Margraf J, Turke V, Soeder U, Neumer S. Obesity and mental illness in a representative sample of young women. *Int. J. Obes. Relat. Metab. Disord.* 2001;25 Suppl 1:S5-9.

[41] Herva A, Laitinen J, Miettunen J, Veijola J, Karvonen JT, Laksy K, et al. Obesity and depression: results from the longitudinal Northern Finland 1966 Birth Cohort Study. *Int. J. Obes. (Lond)* 2006;30(3):520-7.

[42] Forster JL, Jeffery RW. Gender differences related to weight history, eating patterns, efficacy expectations, self-esteem, and weight loss among participants in a weight reduction program. *Addict. Behav.* 1986;11(2):141-7.

[43] Ball K, Crawford D, Kenardy J. Longitudinal relationships among overweight, life satisfaction, and aspirations in young women. *Obes. Res.* 2004;12(6):1019-30.

[44] Laitinen J, Nayha S, Kujala V. Body mass index and weight change from adolescence into adulthood, waist-to-hip ratio and perceived work ability among young adults. *Int. J. Obes. (Lond)* 2005;29(6):697-702.

[45] Kral JG. Preventing and treating obesity in girls and young women to curb the epidemic. *Obes. Res.* 2004;12(10):1539-46.

[46] Gesink Law DC, Maclehose RF, Longnecker MP. Obesity and time to pregnancy. *Hum. Reprod.* 2007;22(2):414-20.

[47] Ali SM, Lindstrom M. Socioeconomic, psychosocial, behavioural, and psychological determinants of BMI among young women: differing patterns for underweight and overweight/obesity. *Eur. J. Public Health.* 2006;16(3):325-31.

[48] Roberts SB, Dallal GE. Energy requirements and aging. *Public Health Nutr.* 2005;8(7A):1028-36.

[49] Jackson M, Ball K, Crawford D. Beliefs about the causes of weight change in the Australian population. *Int. J. Obes. Relat. Metab. Disord.* 2001;25(10):1512-6.

[50] Australian Bureau of Statistics A. *National Nutrition Survey: Selected Highlights of Australia.* Canberra: Australia Bureau of Statistics; 1995.

[51] Crawford D, Jeffery RW, French SA. Can anyone successfully control their weight? Findings of a three year community-based study of men and women. *Int. J. Obes. Relat. Metab. Disord.* 2000;24(9):1107-10.

[52] Pereira MA, Kartashov AI, Ebbeling CB, Van Horn L, Slattery ML, Jacobs DR, Jr., et al. Fast-food habits, weight gain, and insulin resistance (the CARDIA study): 15-year prospective analysis. *Lancet.* 2005;365(9453):36-42.

[53] Schulze MB, Fung TT, Manson JE, Willett WC, Hu FB. Dietary patterns and changes in body weight in women. *Obesity. (Silver Spring)* 2006;14(8):1444-53.

[54] Newby PK, Weismayer C, Akesson A, Tucker KL, Wolk A. Longitudinal changes in food patterns predict changes in weight and body mass index and the effects are greatest in obese women. *J. Nutr.* 2006;136(10):2580-7.

[55] Australian Institute of Health and Welfare A. AIHW analysis of the 1998 and 2001 National Drug Strategy Household Surveys.

[56] Sternfeld B, Sidney S, Jacobs DR, Jr., Sadler MC, Haskell WL, Schreiner PJ. Seven-year changes in physical fitness, physical activity, and lipid profile in the CARDIA study. Coronary Artery Risk Development in Young Adults. *Ann. Epidemiol.* 1999;9(1):25-33.

[57] Schmitz KH, Jacobs DR, Jr., Leon AS, Schreiner PJ, Sternfeld B. Physical activity and body weight: associations over ten years in the CARDIA study. Coronary Artery Risk Development in Young Adults. *Int. J. Obes. Relat. Metab. Disord.* 2000;24(11):1475-87.

[58] Sidney S, Sternfeld B, Haskell WL, Jacobs DR, Jr., Chesney MA, Hulley SB. Television viewing and cardiovascular risk factors in young adults: the CARDIA study. *Ann. Epidemiol.* 1996;6(2):154-9.

[59] Salmon J, Bauman A, Crawford D, Timperio A, Owen N. The association between television viewing and overweight among Australian adults participating in varying levels of leisure-time physical activity. *Int. J. Obes. Relat. Metab. Disord.* 2000;24(5):600-6.

[60]   Hasler G, Buysse DJ, Klaghofer R, Gamma A, Ajdacic V, Eich D, et al. The association between short sleep duration and obesity in young adults: a 13-year prospective study. *Sleep.* 2004;27(4):661-6.

[61]   Knutson KL, Spiegel K, Penev P, Van Cauter E. The metabolic consequences of sleep deprivation. *Sleep Med. Rev.* 2007;11(3):163-78.

[62]   Kahn HS, Williamson DF, Stevens JA. Race and weight change in US women: the roles of socioeconomic and marital status. *Am. J. Public Health.* 1991;81(3):319-23.

[63]   Rissanen AM, Heliovaara M, Knekt P, Reunanen A, Aromaa A. Determinants of weight gain and overweight in adult Finns. *Eur. J. Clin. Nutr.* 1991;45(9):419-30.

[64]   Brown WJ, Trost SG. Life transitions and changing physical activity patterns in young women. *Am. J. Prev. Med.* 2003;25(2):140-3.

[65]   Anderson AS, Marshall DW, Lea EJ. Shared lives-an opportunity for obesity prevention? *Appetite.* 2004;43(3):327-9.

[66]   Smith DE, Lewis CE, Caveny JL, Perkins LL, Burke GL, Bild DE. Longitudinal changes in adiposity associated with pregnancy. The CARDIA Study. Coronary Artery Risk Development in Young Adults Study. *Jama.* 1994;271(22):1747-51.

[67]   Gore SA, Brown DM, West DS. The role of postpartum weight retention in obesity among women: a review of the evidence. *Ann. Behav. Med.* 2003;26(2):149-59.

[68]   Kinnunen TI, Luoto R, Gissler M, Hemminki E. Pregnancy weight gain from 1960s to 2000 in Finland. *Int. J. Obes. Relat. Metab. Disord.* 2003;27(12):1572-7.

[69]   Linne Y, Dye L, Barkeling B, Rossner S. Weight development over time in parous women--the SPAWN study--15 years follow-up. *Int. J. Obes. Relat. Metab. Disord.* 2003;27(12):1516-22.

[70]   Ohlin A, Rossner S. Trends in eating patterns, physical activity and socio-demographic factors in relation to postpartum body weight development. *Br. J. Nutr.* 1994;71(4):457-70.

[71]   Ball K, Crawford D, Warren N. How feasible are healthy eating and physical activity for young women? *Public Health Nutr.* 2004;7(3):433-41.

[72]   Jackson RW, McDaniel SW, Rao CP. Food shopping and preparation: psychographic differences of working wives and housewives. *The Journal of Consumer Research.* 1985;12(1):110-13.

[73]   Warde A, Martens L. *Eating out: social differentiation, consumption and pleasure.* New York: Cambridge University Press; 2000.

[74]   Milligan RA, Burke V, Beilin LJ, Richards J, Dunbar D, Spencer M, et al. Health-related behaviours and psycho-social characteristics of 18 year-old Australians. *Soc. Sci. Med.* 1997;45(10):1549-62.

[75]   Ball K, Crawford D. An investigation of psychological, social and environmental correlates of obesity and weight gain in young women. *Int. J. Obes. (Lond)* 2006.

[76]   Andajani-Sutjahjo S, Ball K, Warren N, Inglis V, Crawford D. Perceived personal, social and environmental barriers to weight maintenance among young women: A community survey. *Int. J. Behav. Nutr. Phys. Act.* 2004;1(1):15.

[77]   Kvaavik E, Lien N, Tell GS, Klepp KI. Psychosocial predictors of eating habits among adults in their mid-30s: the Oslo Youth Study follow-up 1991-1999. *Int. J. Behav. Nutr. Phys. Act.* 2005;2:9.

[78] McAuley E, Jacobson L. Self-efficacy and exercise participation in sedentary adult females. *Am. J. Health Promot.* 1991;5(3):185-91.

[79] Teixeira PJ, Going SB, Houtkooper LB, Cussler EC, Metcalfe LL, Blew RM, et al. Pretreatment predictors of attrition and successful weight management in women. *Int. J. Obes. Relat. Metab. Disord.* 2004;28(9):1124-33.

[80] Miller DY, Brown WJ. Determinants of active leisure for women with young children-- an 'ethic of care' prevails. *Leisure Sciences.* 2005;27:405-420.

[81] Sobal J, Rauschenbach B, Frongillo EA. Marital status changes and body weight changes: a US longitudinal analysis. *Soc. Sci. Med.* 2003;56(7):1543-55.

[82] Lee C, Powers JR. Number of social roles, health, and well-being in three generations of Australian women. *Int. J. Behav. Med.* 2002;9(3):195-215.

[83] Gunthorpe W, Lyons K. A predictive model of chronic time pressure in the Australian population: implications for leisure research. *Leisure Sciences.* 2004;26:201-213.

[84] Wardle J, Haase AM, Steptoe A. Body image and weight control in young adults: international comparisons in university students from 22 countries. *Int. J. Obes. (Lond)* 2006;30(4):644-51.

[85] Malinauskas BM, Raedeke TD, Aeby VG, Smith JL, Dallas MB. Dieting practices, weight perceptions, and body composition: a comparison of normal weight, overweight, and obese college females. *Nutr. J.* 2006;5:11.

[86] Ball K, Andajani-Sutjahjo S, Crawford D. The costs of weight control: what do young women pay? *Med. J. Aust.* 2003;179(11-12):586.

[87] Assaf AR, Parker D, Lapane KL, Coccio E, Evangelou E, Carleton RA. Does the Y chromosome make a difference? Gender differences in attempts to change cardiovascular disease risk factors. *J. Womens Health (Larchmt)* 2003;12(4):321-30.

[88] Honas JJ, Early JL, Frederickson DD, O'Brien MS. Predictors of attrition in a large clinic-based weight-loss program. *Obes. Res.* 2003;11(7):888-94.

[89] Bautista-Castano I, Molina-Cabrillana J, Montoya-Alonso JA, Serra-Majem L. Variables predictive of adherence to diet and physical activity recommendations in the treatment of obesity and overweight, in a group of Spanish subjects. *Int. J. Obes. Relat. Metab. Disord.* 2004;28(5):697-705.

[90] Dalle Grave R, Calugi S, Molinari E, Petroni ML, Bondi M, Compare A, et al. Weight loss expectations in obese patients and treatment attrition: an observational multicenter study. *Obes. Res.* 2005;13(11):1961-9.

[91] Wadden TA, Foster GD. Behavioral treatment of obesity. *Med. Clin. North. Am.* 2000;84(2):441-61, vii.

[92] McMillan-Price J, Petocz P, Atkinson F, O'Neill K, Samman S, Steinbeck K, et al. Comparison of 4 diets of varying glycemic load on weight loss and cardiovascular risk reduction in overweight and obese young adults: a randomized controlled trial. *Arch. Intern. Med.* 2006;166(14):1466-75.

[93] Nordmann AJ, Nordmann A, Briel M, Keller U, Yancy WS, Jr., Brehm BJ, et al. Effects of low-carbohydrate vs low-fat diets on weight loss and cardiovascular risk factors: a meta-analysis of randomized controlled trials. *Arch. Intern. Med.* 2006;166(3):285-93.

[94] Farnsworth E, Luscombe ND, Noakes M, Wittert G, Argyiou E, Clifton PM. Effect of a high-protein, energy-restricted diet on body composition, glycemic control, and lipid

concentrations in overweight and obese hyperinsulinemic men and women. *Am. J. Clin. Nutr.* 2003;78(1):31-9.

[95] Appel LJ, Sacks FM, Carey VJ, Obarzanek E, Swain JF, Miller ER, 3rd, et al. Effects of protein, monounsaturated fat, and carbohydrate intake on blood pressure and serum lipids: results of the OmniHeart randomized trial. *Jama.* 2005;294(19):2455-64.

[96] Krieger JW, Sitren HS, Daniels MJ, Langkamp-Henken B. Effects of variation in protein and carbohydrate intake on body mass and composition during energy restriction: a meta-regression 1. *Am. J. Clin. Nutr.* 2006;83(2):260-74.

[97] Due A, Toubro S, Skov AR, Astrup A. Effect of normal-fat diets, either medium or high in protein, on body weight in overweight subjects: a randomised 1-year trial. *Int. J. Obes. Relat. Metab. Disord.* 2004;28(10):1283-90.

[98] Skov AR, Toubro S, Ronn B, Holm L, Astrup A. Randomized trial on protein vs carbohydrate in ad libitum fat reduced diet for the treatment of obesity. *Int. J. Obes. Relat. Metab. Disord.* 1999;23(5):528-36.

[99] Gerstein DE, Woodward-Lopez G, Evans AE, Kelsey K, Drewnowski A. Clarifying concepts about macronutrients' effects on satiation and satiety. *J. Am. Diet. Assoc.* 2004;104(7):1151-3.

[100] Brinkworth GD, Noakes M, Keogh JB, Luscombe ND, Wittert GA, Clifton PM. Long-term effects of a high-protein, low-carbohydrate diet on weight control and cardiovascular risk markers in obese hyperinsulinemic subjects. *Int. J. Obes. Relat. Metab. Disord.* 2004;28(5):661-70.

[101] Foster GD, Wyatt HR, Hill JO, McGuckin BG, Brill C, Mohammed BS, et al. A randomized trial of a low-carbohydrate diet for obesity. *N. Engl. J. Med.* 2003;348(21):2082-90.

[102] Stern L, Iqbal N, Seshadri P, Chicano KL, Daily DA, McGrory J, et al. The effects of low-carbohydrate versus conventional weight loss diets in severely obese adults: one-year follow-up of a randomized trial. *Ann. Intern. Med.* 2004;140(10):778-85.

[103] Moran LJ, Noakes M, Clifton PM, Tomlinson L, Galletly C, Norman RJ. Dietary composition in restoring reproductive and metabolic physiology in overweight women with polycystic ovary syndrome. *J. Clin. Endocrinol. Metab.* 2003;88(2):812-9.

[104] Andersen P, Seljeflot I, Abdelnoor M, Arnesen H, Dale PO, Lovik A, et al. Increased insulin sensitivity and fibrinolytic capacity after dietary intervention in obese women with polycystic ovary syndrome. *Metabolism.* 1995;44(5):611-6.

[105] Mavropoulos JC, Yancy WS, Hepburn J, Westman EC. The effects of a low-carbohydrate, ketogenic diet on the polycystic ovary syndrome: A pilot study. *Nutr. Metab. (Lond)* 2005;2:35.

[106] Moran LJ, Noakes M, Clifton PM, Wittert GA, Williams G, Norman RJ. Short-term meal replacements followed by dietary macronutrient restriction enhance weight loss in polycystic ovary syndrome. *Am. J. Clin. Nutr.* 2006;84(1):77-87.

[107] Kiddy DS, Hamilton-Fairley D, Bush A, Short F, Anyaoku V, Reed MJ, et al. Improvement in endocrine and ovarian function during dietary treatment of obese women with polycystic ovary syndrome. *Clin. Endocrinol. (Oxf)* 1992;36(1):105-11.

[108] Tolino A, Gambardella V, Caccavale C, D'Ettore A, Giannotti F, D'Anto V, et al. Evaluation of ovarian functionality after a dietary treatment in obese women with polycystic ovary syndrome. *Eur. J. Obstet. Gynecol. Reprod. Biol.* 2005;119(1):87-93.

[109] Saris WH, Blair SN, van Baak MA, Eaton SB, Davies PS, Di Pietro L, et al. How much physical activity is enough to prevent unhealthy weight gain? Outcome of the IASO 1st Stock Conference and consensus statement. *Obes. Rev.* 2003;4(2):101-14.

[110] Wing RR, Hill JO. Successful weight loss maintenance. *Annu. Rev. Nutr.* 2001;21:323-41.

[111] Catenacci VA, Wyatt HR. The role of physical activity in producing and maintaining weight loss. *Nat. Clin. Pract. Endocrinol. Metab.* 2007;3(7):518-29.

[112] Field AE, Wing RR, Manson JE, Spiegelman DL, Willett WC. Relationship of a large weight loss to long-term weight change among young and middle-aged US women. *Int. J. Obes. Relat. Metab. Disord.* 2001;25(8):1113-21.

[113] Donnelly JE, Hill JO, Jacobsen DJ, Potteiger J, Sullivan DK, Johnson SL, et al. Effects of a 16-month randomized controlled exercise trial on body weight and composition in young, overweight men and women: the Midwest Exercise Trial. *Arch. Intern. Med.* 2003;163(11):1343-50.

[114] Potteiger JA, Jacobsen DJ, Donnelly JE, Hill JO. Glucose and insulin responses following 16 months of exercise training in overweight adults: the Midwest Exercise Trial. *Metabolism.* 2003;52(9):1175-81.

[115] Poehlman ET, Dvorak RV, DeNino WF, Brochu M, Ades PA. Effects of resistance training and endurance training on insulin sensitivity in nonobese, young women: a controlled randomized trial. *J. Clin. Endocrinol. Metab.* 2000;85(7):2463-8.

[116] Vigorito C, Giallauria F, Palomba S, Cascella T, Manguso F, Lucci R, et al. Beneficial effects of a three-month structured exercise training program on cardiopulmonary functional capacity in young women with polycystic ovary syndrome. *J. Clin. Endocrinol. Metab.* 2007;92(4):1379-84.

[117] Randeva HS, Lewandowski KC, Drzewoski J, Brooke-Wavell K, O'Callaghan C, Czupryniak L, et al. Exercise decreases plasma total homocysteine in overweight young women with polycystic ovary syndrome. *J. Clin. Endocrinol. Metab.* 2002;87(10):4496-501.

[118] Dunn CL, Hannan PJ, Jeffery RW, Sherwood NE, Pronk NP, Boyle R. The comparative and cumulative effects of a dietary restriction and exercise on weight loss. *Int. J. Obes. (Lond)* 2006;30(1):112-21.

[119] National Heart L, and Blood Institute, NHLBI, NIH. Clinical guidelines on the identification, evaluation, and treatment of overweight and obesity in adults: The evidence report. *NIH Publications.* 1998;No. 98-4083:1-262.

[120] Wing RR, Phelan S. Long-term weight loss maintenance. *Am. J. Clin. Nutr.* 2005;82(1 Suppl):222S-225S.

[121] Tate DF, Wing RR, Winett RA. Using Internet technology to deliver a behavioral weight loss program. *Jama.* 2001;285(9):1172-7.

[122] Williamson DA, Martin PD, White MA, Newton R, Walden H, York-Crowe E, et al. Efficacy of an internet-based behavioral weight loss program for overweight adolescent African-American girls. *Eat. Weight Disord.* 2005;10(3):193-203.

[123] Tate DF, Jackvony EH, Wing RR. Effects of Internet behavioral counseling on weight loss in adults at risk for type 2 diabetes: a randomized trial. *Jama.* 2003;289(14):1833-6.

[124] Perri MG, McAllister DA, Gange JJ, Jordan RC, McAdoo G, Nezu AM. Effects of four maintenance programs on the long-term management of obesity. *J. Consult. Clin. Psychol.* 1988;56(4):529-34.

[125] Eiben G, Lissner L. Health Hunters-an intervention to prevent overweight and obesity in young high-risk women. *Int. J. Obes. (Lond)* 2006;30(4):691-6.

[126] Galletly C, Clark A, Tomlinson L, Blaney F. Improved pregnancy rates for obese, infertile women following a group treatment program. An open pilot study. *Gen. Hosp. Psychiatry.* 1996;18(3):192-5.

[127] Clark AM, Thornley B, Tomlinson L, Galletley C, Norman RJ. Weight loss in obese infertile women results in improvement in reproductive outcome for all forms of fertility treatment. *Hum. Reprod.* 1998;13(6):1502-5.

[128] Clark AM, Ledger W, Galletly C, Tomlinson L, Blaney F, Wang X, et al. Weight loss results in significant improvement in pregnancy and ovulation rates in anovulatory obese women. *Hum. Reprod.* 1995;10(10):2705-12.

[129] Hoeger KM, Kochman L, Wixom N, Craig K, Miller RK, Guzick DS. A randomized, 48-week, placebo-controlled trial of intensive lifestyle modification and/or metformin therapy in overweight women with polycystic ovary syndrome: a pilot study. *Fertil. Steril.* 2004;82(2):421-9.

In: Life Style and Health Research Progress
Editors: A. B. Turley, G. C. Hofmann

ISBN: 978-1-60456-427-3
© 2008 Nova Science Publishers, Inc.

Chapter VII

Diet Is a Four-Letter Word: What Can Be Done about America's Unhealthy Obsession with Weight?

Mary E. Pritchard

Department of Psychology, Boise State University

ABSTRACT

Although diagnostic rates of eating disorders (e.g., anorexia, bulimia) are relatively small in the United States (Ogden, 2003), disordered eating behaviors (including weight control behaviors through excessive exercise and restrictive eating, as well as body dissatisfaction are much more common (Anorexia Nervosa and Related Eating Disorders, Inc., 2005a, sub clinical eating disorders section). Fifty-one percent of U.S. adults did something to control their weight in 2001-2002 (Weiss, Galuska, Khan, and Serdula, 2006). However, it is difficult for many to keep the weight off, in large part because a post-diet binge occurs in nearly half of people who end a diet (successfully or not; Tribole and Resch, 1995). The 'dieting lifestyle' is beginning at younger and younger ages. Half of 3rd to 6th graders want to weigh less (Schur, Sanders, and Steiner, 2000) and half of 8- to 10-year-olds have done something to try to alter their weight (Thomas, Ricciardelli, and Williams, 2000). Although disordered eating behaviors are not considered serious enough to be diagnosed as eating disorders, these behaviors do need attention as they can have damaging mental, social, and physical effects (O'Dea and Yager, 2006). With over half of children, adolescents, and adults currently engaging in some type of disordered eating or exercise behavior, these cultural trends can no longer be ignored. The purpose of this chapter will be to discuss factors influencing disordered eating and exercise behaviors in children, adolescents, and adults. In addition, possible solutions at the familial and societal levels will be proposed. This chapter should be informative for parents, school officials, and those who are either suffering from disordered eating behaviors or know someone who is.

INTRODUCTION

In American society today – in the land of plenty – an interesting paradox is occurring. On the one hand, obesity rates are skyrocketing in all age groups. A recent study found that over the past three decades, the prevalence of obesity and overweight has increased at an average annual rate of 0.3%–0.9%; depending on the demographic and socioeconomic group in question (Wang and Beydoun, 2007). In 2003-2004 data, 66% of U.S. adults and 16% of children and adolescents were overweight. If obesity rates continue to grow unchecked, it is estimated that by 2015, 75% of U.S. adults and 24% of U.S. children and adolescents will be overweight or obese (Wang and Beydoun). This data is perhaps not surprising given that while obesity rates have increased, physical activity has decreased, especially among adults. In 2002, 77% of children aged 9-13 participated in some type of physical activity during their free time during the week preceding the survey, whereas 23% did not participate in any physical activity during their free time (Centers for Disease Control, 2003). Yet, in 2005, only 36% of high school students met the physical activity standards set forth by the federal government, with 10% engaging in no physical activity in the seven days prior to survey administration (Eaton et al., 2006). Finally, in 2005, only 24% of U.S. adults engage in physical activity three or more times per week, with 62% of U.S. adults engaging in no regular physical activity (Pleis and Lethbridge-Çejku, 2006; see also Weiss et al., 2006).

What is interesting is that while as a nation rates of obesity and overweight are growing (no pun intended); rates of eating disorders, body dissatisfaction and other disordered eating behaviors are also on the rise. As a culture, Americans are very unhappy with their appearance and increasing numbers of individuals are doing something about it. Researchers estimate that eating disorders (anorexia nervosa, bulimia nervosa, binge eating disorder) affect 3% to 10% of females and 2.4% of males (Espina, Ortego, Ochoa de Alda, Aleman, and Juaniz, 2002; Polivy and Herman, 2002). Perhaps more alarming are the increasing rates of disordered eating behaviors (including weight control behaviors through excessive exercise, restrictive eating, and binge/purge behaviors as well as body dissatisfaction). Estimates are hard to pin down because these disorders are typically not diagnosed and prevalence estimates vary based on what criteria are used, but disordered eating behaviors are much more common than are eating disorders (Anorexia Nervosa and Related Eating Disorders, Inc, 2005). In 2005, 17% of high school females and 8% of high school males went without eating for more than 24 hours in order to either lose weight or keep from gaining weight. In addition, 8% of high school females and 5% of high school males took diet pills/powders/liquids to either lose weight or keep from gaining weight. 6% of high school females and 3% of high school males vomited or took laxatives to lose weight or keep from gaining weight (Eaton et al., 2006). Estimates of disordered eating behaviors among college students range from 13% in female non-athletes (Reinking and Alexander, 2005) to 58% among female athletes (Johnson, Powers and Dick, 1999). In a community-based sample of adults, 22% of females and 17% of males reported that in the past year, they had engaged in an 'unhealthy' weight control behavior (Neumark-Sztainer et al., 1999).

When considering only the two disordered eating behaviors of body dissatisfaction and dieting, researchers now claim that these behaviors are considered normative in adolescents (Cook-Cottone and Phelps, 2006; Polivy and Herman, 1987) and adults (French, Jeffrey, and

Murray, 1999; Neumark-Sztainer et al., 1999; Polivy and Herman). For example, 50% of 3rd through 6th graders want to weigh less (Schur et al., 2000), half of 8- to 10-year-olds diet at least some of the time, and two-thirds of girls and nearly half of boys this age are concerned about becoming overweight (Thomas et al., 2000). Similar numbers have been reported in adult populations. Over 70% of adults have used some sort of diet strategy in the past few years, including increasing exercise (82% of those responding), decreasing fat intake (79%), reducing food intake (78%), and reducing caloric intake (73%; French et al., 1999). In 2002 alone, 51% of U.S. adults did something to control their weight (Weiss et al., 2006).

The sad fact is that over 90% of dieters ultimately fail. Furthermore, a post-diet binge occurs in nearly half of people who end a diet (successfully or not; Tribole and Resch, 1995). Thus, many of us have lost touch with what 'healthy' actually means. Now that we realize that there is a problem, the next question that needs to be addressed is: Why? How did we get to be this way? There are a number of theories and factors accounting for Americans' obsession with food and weight loss. Each will be addressed in turn.

FACTORS INFLUENCING DISORDERED EATING AND EXERCISE BEHAVIORS

Gender

Traditionally, disordered eating has been viewed as a problem primary facing women. Research certainly supports the notion that women may be more vulnerable to certain aspects of disordered eating behaviors. For example, Smolak and Levine (1994) reported that girls in elementary school reported no more body dissatisfaction than did boys, but they report more weight loss attempts (see also Sands, Tricker, Sherman, Armatas, and Maschette, 1997). In a survey of high school students, nearly twice as many female adolescents were found to engage in disordered eating than their male counterparts (Croll, Neumark-Sztainer, Story, and Ireland, 2002). In addition, one study of high school students found that females were three times more likely than their male counterparts to practice weight reduction techniques, and were four times more likely than males to express drive for thinness (Brook and Tepper, 1997). Muth and Cash (1997) found that female undergraduates express higher levels of body dissatisfaction, body image dysphoria, and are more invested in their appearance than their male counterparts (see also Anderson and Bulik, 2004). Milligan and Pritchard (2006) found that among Division I collegiate athletes, more female than male athletes displayed disordered eating behaviors (see also Johnson et al., 2004). Similarly, female undergraduates report lower levels of satisfaction with several specific body parts and are more likely to utilize a variety of weight-loss strategies than are their male counterparts (Kashubeck-West et al., 2005; see also Mintz and Kashubeck, 1999). Similarly, adult women report higher levels of body dissatisfaction and dieting than do adult men (Brunner et al., 1994; Kiefer, Rathmanner, and Kunze, 2005), as well as more restrained eating and disordered eating behaviors (Kiefer et al., 2005). In fact, in a study of factors predicting disordered eating in college students, gender was the primary predictor of drive for thinness and body dissatisfaction, and was also a predictor of bulimic behaviors (Shea and Pritchard, 2007).

Recent research indicates that gender differences in disordered eating behaviors may be tied to differences in both prenatal exposure to testosterone as well as production of estradiol in adulthood (Klump et al., 2006). Klump et al. further suggest that when estrogen production increases during puberty, the genes contributing to disordered eating get 'turned on.' O'Dea and Abraham (1999) found support for this idea, as females become increasingly dissatisfied with their bodies following menarche and vulnerable to engaging in disordered eating behaviors (but see Hermes and Keel, 2003; and Sands et al., 1997 for conflicting findings). In addition, Thelen, Powell, Lawrence, and Kuhnert (1992) reported that whereas no gender differences existed in 2nd graders, 4th and 6th grade girls were more likely than were their male counterparts to express body dissatisfaction and concerns about becoming overweight. Finally, Phelps, Johnson, Jiminez, and Wilczenski (1993) reported that body dissatisfaction increased with age in females, and that females in high school displayed significantly higher levels of body dissatisfaction than middle school females and males.

However, research is beginning to question the gender gap in disordered eating behaviors. Furthermore, some researchers argue that the type of disordered eating behavior matters. For example, Smolak and Levine (1994) reported no gender differences in body dissatisfaction, but found that girls reported more weight loss attempts than did boys. Similarly, Wilcox (1997) found no differences in body attitudes in a sample of U.S. adults. Tata, Fox, and Cooper (2001) found that although female undergraduates exhibited higher levels of most disordered eating behaviors, males actually exhibited higher levels of excessive exercise (see also Anderson and Bulik, 2004; see Kiefer et al., 2005 for similar findings in adults). In addition, whereas adolescent females are more likely to report wanting to lose weight, adolescent males are more likely to report wanting to gain weight (O'Dea and Abraham, 1999; see also Brook and Tepper, 1997; Furnham, Badmin, and Sneade, 2002). Similar results have been found in college students, with correct weight males believing they were underweight and wishing to be heavier, and correct weight females believing they were overweight and wishing to be thinner (Raudenbush and Zellner, 1997). In addition, further research has suggested that sexual orientation matters as well, with heterosexual females and gay males engaging in more disordered eating behaviors than heterosexual males and lesbians (Schneider, O'Leary, and Jenkins, 1995). Finally, sex role orientation may also make a difference, with men and women exhibiting higher levels of masculinity also reporting more body satisfaction (Wilcox, 1997). Thus, to say that there are gender differences in patterns of disordered eating seems to be too simplistic, as it may depend on the behavior in question. In addition, gender may interact with other factors (such as age) in its influence on disordered eating patterns. Similarly, other factors related to gender, such as sex role orientation and sexual orientation cannot be ruled out as factors influencing any reported gender differences.

Race

Croll et al. (2002) found that Hispanic and American Indian adolescents reported higher levels of disordered eating behaviors than adolescents of other races. Hermes and Keel (2003) reported that White girls reported greater internalization of the thin ideal than did their non-White counterparts, but that there were no differences in eating pathologies as a result of race. However, Leon, Fulkerson, Perry, and Early-Zaid (1995) found that being Caucasian was a significant predictor of disordered eating in adolescent females. Logio (2003) found White girls and boys engaged in more disordered eating and dieting than did their Black counterparts. Parker et al. (1995) reported that White female high school students reported higher levels of body dissatisfaction than did their African-American counterparts. However, Chandarana, Helmes, and Benson (1988) found that race did not predict disordered eating attitudes in high school students. In addition, White female undergraduates are more likely to perceive themselves as being overweight than are Black female undergraduates (Perez and Joiner, 2003; see Logio, 2003 for similar results in adolescents). Johnson et al. (2004) reported that White female athletes displayed significantly more body dissatisfaction, disordered eating, and a higher drive for thinness than did their Black female counterparts (see also Chandler, Abood, Lee, Cleveland, and Daly, 1994). Similarly, Edwards-Hewitt and Gray (1993) found that White female undergraduates displayed more binge eating and bulimic behaviors than did their Black counterparts. Mintz and Kashubeck (1999) reported that whereas Caucasian female undergraduates were more likely to engage in dieting and binging behaviors, Asian American female undergraduates reported more dissatisfaction with their racially defined body and facial features. Thus, it seems unclear what role race actually plays in predicting disordered eating behavior. Although many studies seem to support the notion that being Caucasian is a risk factor in the development of certain disordered eating behaviors, other studies have found the opposite or found no racial differences. Future research may wish to examine other factors underlying the reported racial differences to better ascertain whether true racial differences exist.

Loss of the Ability to Recognize Our Bodies' Hunger Signals

Regardless of race and gender, and long before the hormonal surges of adolescence kick in, most of us begin to face food-related challenges. Young children are often very skilled at determining when they are hungry, when they are full, and what food would best satisfy their body's physiological cravings (Birch, Johnson, Andresen, Peters, and Schulte, 1991). But we tend to lose the ability to read our biological hunger cues as we age. There are a number of reasons that this may occur. According to the internal-external hypothesis, we tend to eat for either internal reasons (e.g., hunger) or external reasons (e.g., taste, smell, time of day; Schachter, 1971). As we age and become sensitive to body image 'norms', we begin to restrain our eating by ignoring internal cues and paying attention to external cues (e.g., judgments of what and how much we should be eating; Herman and Polivy, 1975). This often happens quite early in childhood as a result of parental restrictions on children's eating behaviors. If parents restrict how much or when we eat, this restriction can lead to binge behaviors when the children are left unsupervised (Fisher and Birch, 1986). In addition, as we become more motivated to eat for external reasons, we also become more vulnerable to binge eating as we learn to eat for the purposes of mood regulation (e.g., eating to make yourself feel better when you experience stress, anxiety, or depression; Arnow, Kenardy, and Agras, 1992; 1995) or as a reward (Birch, Zimmerman, and Hind, 1980). This can lead us to set up cycles of eating where we binge for a time, but then follow that binge with restrained eating in order to punish ourselves for the binge and to try to lose any weight gain that resulted from the binge (Foreyt and Goodrick, 1992; Tribole and Resch, 1995).

Self-Esteem

As we age, we tend to begin to eat (or fail to eat when hungry) for external reasons (Herman and Polivy, 1975). These external cues are influenced by a variety of factors, including our baseline level of self esteem. Self-esteem is negatively correlated with body dissatisfaction (Wiseman, Peltzman, Halmi, and Sunday, 2004), as well as disordered eating symptoms in adolescent males and females (McCabe and Vincent, 2003). In addition, Button, Loan, Davies, and Sonuga-Barke (1997) found that adolescent females who displayed lower levels of self-esteem were more likely to report eating disordered behaviors, as well as higher levels of dissatisfaction with themselves and their appearance (see also Granillo, Jones-Rodriguez, and Carvajal, 2005). Finally, Finstad (2003) reported that lower levels of self-esteem predicted internalization and personal investment in the thin-ideal, disordered eating scores, and placing a greater importance on appearance.

Similar studies with college students have shown that low self-esteem is positively correlated with disordered eating (Milligan and Pritchard, 2006; Shea and Pritchard, 2007), poorer body image (Abell and Richards, 1996; Gleason, Alexander, and Somers, 2000; Shea and Pritchard) and bulimic symptoms (Gilbert and Meyer, 2005; Mora-Giral, Raich-Escursell, Segues, Torras, Claraso, and Huon, 2004; Shea and Pritchard; Vohs, Bardone, Joiner, Abramson, and Heatherton, 1999). Finally, lower levels of self esteem have been correlated with chronic dieting and dietary restraint in adult women (Cachelin and Regan, 2006), as well as body dissatisfaction (Kashubeck-West, Mintz, and Weigold, 2005; Olivardia, Pope, Borowiecki, Cohane, 2004), and disordered eating (Ghaderi, 2003). In addition, self-esteem predicts body satisfaction in both adult men and women (Green and Pritchard, 2003).

Perfectionism

In addition to self esteem, other personal characteristics influence our eating behaviors, including personality factors such as perfectionism. Ruggiero, Levi, Ciuna, and Sassaroli (2003) found that perfectionism is associated with body dissatisfaction and drive for thinness in female high school students. In addition, Hopkinson and Lock (2004) found a correlation between disordered eating and perfectionism in both male and female collegiate recreational and varsity athletes. In fact, Hopkinson and Lock reported that the greatest risk factor for disordered eating attitudes in females was perfectionism. Similarly, Haase, Prapavessis, and Owens (2002) reported that perfectionism predicted both physique anxiety and disordered eating attitudes in male and female collegiate athletes. Forbush, Heatherton, and Keel (2007) found that perfectionism predicted fasting and purging in female undergraduates and fasting in male undergraduates. Furthermore, a study of male amateur cyclists found that other-oriented perfectionism predicted disordered eating, dieting, and bulimic behaviors, whereas socially prescribed perfectionism predicted anorexic behaviors (Ferrand and Brunet, 2004).

Attachment

Another intrinsic factor found to relate to the presence of disordered eating is attachment style. A study of high school students revealed that insecurely attached students reported more concerns about their weight than did securely attached students (Sharpe et al., 1998). Furthermore, attachment predicted disordered eating in a study of Latina adolescents (Hodson, Newcomb, Locke, and Goodyear, 2006). In a study of college students, secure attachment scores were significantly negatively correlated with body dissatisfaction, and fearful attachment scores were positively correlated with bulimia in women, whereas secure attachment was significantly negatively correlated to drive for thinness, bulimia, and body dissatisfaction in men (Elgin and Pritchard, 2006). In addition, Kiang and Harter (2006) found that female undergraduates who were insecurely attached (avoidant or anxious attachment) exhibited higher levels of disordered eating behaviors than did their securely attached counterparts (see also Broberg, Hjalmers, and Nevonen, 2001; Evans and Wertherim, 1998). Becker, Bell, and Billington (1987) found a similar relation between insecure attachment and bulimic behaviors in undergraduate women. Similarly, Salzman (1997) found that female undergraduates who exhibited anorexic and bulimic behaviors were more likely to be ambivalently attached. Cash, Thériault, and Ames (2004) found higher levels of body image dysfunction in male and female undergraduates who exhibited preoccupied and anxious attachment styles. However, Cole-Detke and Kobak (1996) found that female undergraduates who were avoidantly attached had higher levels of disordered eating, whereas those with preoccupied did not. Brennan and Shaver (1995) found secure attachment ratings were negatively correlated with eating disorder symptomatology, yet both anxious-ambivalent and avoidant attachment ratings were positively associated with disordered eating female college students. Finally, Eggert, Levendosky, and Klump (2007) found a relation between insecure attachment and disordered eating in adult female twin pairs.

Media Pressure

Although intrinsic factors (e.g., self esteem, perfectionism) can influence our eating behaviors, extrinsic factors such as media exposure often play a role as well. In a longitudinal study of preadolescent girls, baseline television viewing predicted disordered eating and having a thinner body ideal one year later (Harrison and Hefner, 2006). In fact, some studies have suggested that media pressure to be thin is one of the top two predictors of drive for thinness and disturbed eating patterns in adolescent females (Levine, Smolak, and Hayden, 1994; Wertheim, Paxton, Schutz, and Muir, 1997; Taylor et al., 2000). In fact, the more adolescents compare themselves to television characters and celebrities, the more they endorse the thinness ideal, are dissatisfied with their bodies, have a drive to be thin, and exhibit bulimic tendencies (Botta, 1999). Harrison and Cantor (1997) found a relation between how often undergraduate women viewed media that promotes thinness and their own drive for thinness, body dissatisfaction, and disordered eating behaviors. Hawkins, Richards, Granley, and Stein (2004) reported that exposure to thin-ideal magazine images increased body dissatisfaction and disordered eating in undergraduate women. Heinberg and Thompson (1995) found similar results following exposure to television commercials. Tiggerman (2003) found that different types of media may influence different aspects of disordered eating. Specifically, whereas both magazine reading and television watching correlate with body dissatisfaction, magazine reading alone correlated with the internalization of thin ideals in female undergraduates. Regardless of the type of media exposure, Twamley and Davis (1999) explain that the Western thin-ideal and the body dissatisfaction associated with it have been shown to be important risk factors for eating pathology among young women (see also Thompson and Heinberg, 1999; but see Hawkins et al., 2004). Furthermore, research has linked the increasing number of diet food and diet product commercials to the increase in disordered eating over the past few decades (Wiseman, Gunning, and Gray, 1993).

Although research has clearly linked media exposure to eating disordered behaviors and body dissatisfaction in women (Groesz, Levine, and Murmen, 2002), research is less clear about the affects of media exposure on men. Some studies report no effects of media exposure on men's body image (Green and Pritchard, 2003; Kalodner, 1997), whereas others have reported that exposure to ideal image advertisements causes higher levels of muscle dissatisfaction in men (Agliata and Tantleff-Dunn, 2004). Ogden and Mundray (1996) argue that media exposure affects both genders, but the effect is stronger for women than for men (but see Vartanian, Giant, and Passino, 2001). Stephens, Hill, and Hanson (1994) hypothesize that whereas young girls are taught to use their body to attract others, boys are taught to use their bodies to master the environment.

Family Environment

In addition to media exposure, studies have shown that family environment can play a role in the development of disordered eating. In fact, Twamley and Davis (1999) found that family pressure to control weight moderated the relation between media exposure to thinness norms and the internalization of the thin ideal in college women. Research has linked low levels of family cohesion and family pressure to diet with disordered eating in female undergraduates and in male and female adolescents (Felker and Stivers, 1994; Levine et al., 1994; Pauls and Daniels, 2000; Pike and Rodin, 1991). Weight-related teasing by family members (Fabian and Thompson, 1989; Levine et al., 1994; Neumark-Sztainer et al., 2002) and maternal body image (Attie and Brooks-Gunn, 1989) predicted disordered eating and body dissatisfaction in adolescents. Similarly, childhood weight or shape related criticism or teasing by family members or others and maternal dieting behaviors and body image was found to contribute significantly to body dissatisfaction in undergraduates (Gleason et al., 2000; Rieves and Cash, 1996) and adult women (Annus, Smith, Fischer, Hendricks, and Williams, 2007). It is perhaps not surprising, then, that many children learn dieting behaviors from family members. In fact, 77% of children reported learning about dieting from family

(Schur et al., 2000). In addition, children often learn body satisfaction from their parents (Guiney and Furlong, 1999; Pike and Rodin), and maternal disordered eating is predictive of daughters' disordered eating (Pike and Rodin).

Social Group Pressure

Although family pressure clearly influences children's eating behaviors, as children begin to interact more with their peers in adolescence, they become more susceptible to societal pressures and peer pressure. Peer pressure to be thin is one of the strongest predictors of eating behavior and body image in girls and women (Lieberman, Gauvin, Bukowski, and White, 2001; Pauls and Daniels, 2000; Taylor et al., 1998). When this pressure comes in the form of weight-related teasing by peers, it is predictive disordered eating in adolescents and adult women (Annus et al., 2007; Neumark-Sztainer et al., 2000; Shisslak et al., 1998) and body satisfaction in adolescent boys and girls (Guiney and Furlong, 1999). The pressure does not even have to be direct for it to have consequences. For example, Schutz, Paxton, and Wertheim (2002) found that girls frequently compare their bodies to those of their friends, and these comparisons can lead to drive for thinness, body dissatisfaction, and dieting (see also Wertheim et al., 1997). Friends' attitudes alone can predict body dissatisfaction and disordered eating (Paxton, Schutz, Wertheim, and Muir, 1999), and often girls will diet simply to avoid social disapproval (Wertheim et al., 1997). In addition, when social circles engage in "fat talk," it can motivate its members to engage in dieting behaviors regardless of their current weight status (Nichter and Vuckovic, 1994; see also Wertheim et al., 1997). In fact, many adolescents learn about disordered eating from their friends. Pauls and Daniels (2000) found that when a female undergraduate's friends exhibit bulimic behaviors, she is more likely engage in bulimic behaviors as well. In fact, Crandall (1988) suggests that many female social groups set norms concerning group members' eating behaviors. In order to avoid social rejection by the group, group members likely model behaviors and attitudes associated with disordered eating.

Participation in Athletics

One form of social group interaction for many children and adolescents comes in the form of athletic teams. Engel et al. (2003) found that participation in athletics was a significant predictor of food restriction, body dissatisfaction, and drive for thinness. Similarly, Picard (1999) found that athletes were more vulnerable to developing disordered eating behaviors than were non-athletes (see also Patel, Greydanus, Pratt, and Phillips, 2003; Smolak, Murnen, and Ruble, 2000; Thompson and Sherman, 1999). However, some research has found no differences between female athletes and non-athletes who engaged in regular exercise in body dissatisfaction, drive for thinness, bulimia, social physique anxiety (Krane, Stiles-Shipley, Waldron, and Michalenok, 2001), and disordered eating behaviors (Kirk, Singh, and Getz, 2001). Furthermore, some studies have found that participation in athletics can serve as a buffer to disordered eating behaviors (Powers, 1999; Smolak et al.; Warren,

Stanton, and Blessing, 1990). For example, Reinking and Alexander (2005) found that female collegiate athletes had lower levels of body dissatisfaction and disordered eating than did female non-athletes. In addition, non-athletes reported a lower ideal bodyweight than did athletes. One explanation for this apparent disparity is the type of sport in which the student athlete participates (Patel et al.; Powers; Smolak et al.; but see Kirk et al. who found no differences in type of sport). For example, Engel et al. found that wrestlers and gymnasts were more vulnerable to drive for thinness, bulimic behaviors, and food restrictions than were other athletes. Warren et al. reported that female cross country runners had a lower level of risk of body dissatisfaction than did non-athletes, but that gymnasts had higher levels of weight preoccupation. Similarly, Reinking and Alexander found that female collegiate athletes participating in sports than emphasize leanness reported significantly more body dissatisfaction and disordered eating and lower ideal and actual body weights than did athletes participating in sports that do not emphasize leanness (see also Picard, 1999; Stoutjesdyk and Jevne, 1993). Milligan and Pritchard (2006) reported that female collegiate athletes participating in non-lean sports (basketball, tennis, golf, soccer, and skiing) and males participating in lean sports (track, wrestling) displayed higher levels of disordered eating behavior and body dissatisfaction than did men in non-lean sports and women in lean sports. Furthermore, athletes participating at higher levels of competition (e.g., Division I) are more vulnerable to developing disordered eating behaviors than are athletes who participate at lower levels of competition (e.g., Division III; Picard).

SOLUTIONS: WHAT CAN PARENTS/FAMILIES DO?

As the research mentioned above demonstrates, there are a variety of factors that can influence the development of disordered eating behaviors. However, perhaps the first and most critical factors in the development of disordered eating in children involve the home environment. Things that happened in childhood can have lasting impressions on our eating patterns and behaviors well into our adult years. Thus, parents and families play a critical role in the development of our eating behaviors in multiple ways. Not only are families typically the primary caregivers that provide food for us, but also we learn eating behaviors from them. We learn when to eat, what we should eat, how much we should eat, and even, to some extent, what we like to eat from our parents (Falciglia, Pabst, Couch, and Goody, 2004; Robinson, 2000; Vereecken, Keukelier, and Maes, 2004; Weber Cullen et al., 2001). We also learn about body satisfaction and disordered eating behaviors through direct modeling of our families or indirectly as a result of teasing and criticism about our weight (Attie and Brooks-Gunn, 1989; Fabian and Thompson, 1989; Felker and Stivers, 1994; Fisher and Birch, 1986; Guiney and Furlong, 1999; Levine et al., 1994; Neumark-Sztainer et al., 2002; Pauls and Daniels, 2000; Pike and Rodin, 1991; Schur et al., 2000). So what can parents and families do to ensure their children grow up with healthy habits, a good relationship with food, and a healthy body image?

Be a Positive Role Model

Parents are the earliest influence on their children's health habits. Thus, perhaps the most important thing parents and families can do for children is to set healthy examples for their children in their words and actions. Having a parent who does not eat a healthy diet is a contributing factor to children's dieting behaviors and body dissatisfaction (Pritchard, 2004; Schur et al., 2000). Similarly, children with overweight parents are likely to be overweight as well (Johannsen, Johannsen, and Specker, 2006; Sallis, Patterson, McKenzie, and Nader, 1988). In addition, children learn exercise habits from those of their parents (Bois, Sarrazin, Brustad, Trouilloud, and Cury, 2005), and parents who support children's physical activities have more physically active children (Gustafson and Rhodes, 2006; Heitzler, Martin, Duke, and Huhman, 2006). Even parental smoking habits are related to children's body dissatisfaction (Pritchard, 2004). Finally, parents should realize the impact that their criticism of their own bodies has on their children. Children often learn body satisfaction from their parents (Guiney and Furlong, 1999; Pike and Rodin, 1991), and maternal disordered eating is predictive of daughters' disordered eating (Pike and Rodin).

Make Positive Family Meal Times a Priority

Often we live in a fast-paced, fast-food world, not taking the time to make and eat healthy meals together as a family. However, Neumark-Sztainer, Wall, Story, and Fulkerson (2004) found that adolescents who reported more frequent family meals displayed lower frequencies of disordered eating behaviors than did adolescents who ate fewer meals per week with their families (see also Mellin, Neumark-Sztainer, Patterson, and Sockalosky, 2004). The topics of discussion during mealtime are also important. Research suggests that the discussion of physical appearance in a negative way during childhood family mealtimes is predictive of disordered eating in female college students (Worobey, 2002). In addition, refusing to eat certain foods is associated with negative family mealtime management in nursery school children (Whitehouse and Harris, 1998). However, positive family meal time experiences can help prevent disordered eating behaviors in adolescents (Neumark-Sztainer et al.). Furthermore, the combination of having meals together and making them stress free is critical. Mellin et al. reported that 58% of girls who reported infrequent meals and had parents who made negative comments about weight and eating also reported disordered eating behaviors, whereas only 7% of girls who reported frequent family meals with no negative weight comments reported disordered eating behaviors.

Do Not Label Foods as Good or Bad

Forbidding children to eat certain foods can set up a binge/purge eating pattern when the child is left unsupervised (Fisher and Birch, 1996). In a study of 5-year-old girls, Fisher and Birch found that following an unsupervised snacking session, 50% of the girls reported that they ate "too much," 44% said they felt bad or guilty about some of the foods they ate, and approximately one-third of the girls reported they would feel bad if their parents found out about what they had eaten. Similarly, forcing children to eat 'good foods' in order to obtain a reward (e.g., "if you eat your Brussels sprouts, you can have dessert") is not desirable either as Birch, Marlin, and Rotter (1984) found that children learn to dislike foods eaten to obtain rewards.

Do Not Use Food as a Reward

Children learn to prefer foods that are eaten as the reward of a certain behavior (e.g., cleaning their room, Birch et al., 1980). This can ultimately lead to patterns of binge emotional eating (Arnow et al., 1992; 1995), as repeated stimulation of physiological pathways through intake of foods we enjoy can lead neurobiological adaptations that promote compulsive overeating of those foods (Adam and Epel, 2007). In fact, research indicates that overweight individuals may be even more vulnerable to these kinds of food reward patterns than normal weight individuals (Davis, Strachan, and Berkson, 2004).

Do Not Have a "Clean Plate" Policy

When children are trained to rely on external cues (e.g., cleaning their plates) instead of internal cues of satiety, they fail to respond to caloric density, which can result in overeating (Birch, McPhee, Shoba, Steinberg, and Krehbeil, 1987). Furthermore, emphasizing a "clean plate" policy can interfere with a child's ability to learn self control (Alger, 1984).

Limit Media Exposure

Because baseline television viewing predicts disordered eating (Harrison and Hefner, 2006), it is important to limit television exposure, especially when parents find their children comparing themselves to television characters and celebrities (Botta, 1999). It is not simply enough to limit television exposure, however. Other media forms need to be carefully scrutinized as well, as even exposure to thin-ideal magazine images increases body dissatisfaction and disordered eating (Hawkins et al., 2004; Tiggerman, 2003).

Never Tease or Make Disparaging Remarks about Yourself or Your Child

Weight-related teasing by family members and maternal body image predicts disordered eating and body dissatisfaction (Attie and Brooks-Gunn, 1989; Annus et al., 2007; Fabian and Thompson, 1989; Gleason et al., 2000; Levine et al., 1994; Neumark-Sztainer et al., 2002; Rieves and Cash, 1996). Thus, parents need to not only be good role models for their children, but they also need to let their children be who they are – regardless of what they weigh.

SOLUTIONS: WHAT CAN SCHOOLS DO?

As children enter school-age, some of the responsibilities for a child's care and welfare transfer from the family to the schools. In addition, as children get older, parental influence on eating patterns becomes less prevalent and peer influence becomes more important. Given this, what can school officials do to provide a safe, nurturing environment for children and adolescents to ensure the development of healthy habits and a healthy relation with food?

Provide Quality Meals in a Pleasant Environment

Research has demonstrated that frequent positive family meal times are important for the prevention of disordered eating in adolescents (Neumark-Sztainer et al., 2004). Because most children and adolescents eat at least 5 meals a week at school (and sometimes 10 or more), having a positive dining environment is important at school as well. Recently the USDA (2000; 2007) began advocating that schools do just this by: 1) giving children enough time to eat, 2) never forcing them to eat anything they do not want to eat, 3) scheduling meals at appropriate times when nothing else is scheduled, 4) making sure students do not have to wait in line too long to get their meal, 5) having attractive dining settings with appropriately sized tables and chairs, 6) scheduling recess before lunch so that children are ready to eat, 7) encouraging socializing with proper adult supervision and noise control, 8) providing hand washing equipment and drinking fountains, 9) protecting the identity of students who eat free or at a reduced rate, and 10) having children clean up after themselves. In addition, specific guidelines for foodservice staff exist regarding meal preparation according to the Food Guide Pyramid and USDA nutrition standards (USDA, 2000).

Do Not Use Food as a Reward or Withdraw Food as Punishment

As previously mentioned, studies have indicated that using foods as rewards or withdrawing foods as punishment can lead children to have an unhealthy relation with food (Birch et al., 1980). The USDA (2000) recognizes this and encourages teachers to replace rewards with non-food items and avoid withholding food as punishment.

Allow Time for Physical Activity

Research has shown that students who are more physically active also have lower levels of body dissatisfaction (Malinauskas, Cucchiara, Aeby, and Bruening, 2007), drive for thinness, and bulimia (Sands et al., 1997). Yet, students are becoming increasingly less physically active (Kann et al., 1998). Thus, the USDA (2000) recommends that physical activity be included as a daily part of the educational program from provided by schools from pre-kindergarten through grade 12.

Provide Appropriate Nutrition Education

Research has demonstrated that students who eat low-fat or fat-free diets are more likely to suffer from disordered eating (Rasnake, Laube, Lewis, and Linscheid, 2005). Unfortunately, many adolescents are not aware of what constitutes a healthy diet (Zenner and Pritchard, 2007). In fact, 16% of students believe that a fat-free diet is the healthiest diet (Rasnake et al.). Research suggests that educating students about nutrition can help prevent disordered eating (Patel et al., 2003). Unfortunately, Chapman and Toma (1997) found that most adolescents do not receive nutrition education in school. Thus, the USDA (2000) recommends that nutrition education be included as a daily part of the educational program from provided by schools from pre-kindergarten through grade 12.

Promote Weight and Size Acceptance

It is well established that peer pressure to be thin is one of the strongest predictors of eating behavior and body image in children and adolescents (Lieberman et al., 2001; Taylor et al., 1998), especially when this pressure comes in the form of weight-related teasing by peers (Guiney and Furlong, 1999; Neumark-Sztainer et al., 2000; Shisslak et al., 1998). Thus, it is imperative that schools encourage students to acceptance one another "as is." In fact, the Society for Nutrition Education (SNE, 2003) recommends that schools promote size and weight acceptance as part of their overall school policies on acceptance of diversity and have a no tolerance policy for appearance-related teasing and harassment (see also Levine, 1999).

Sensitivity in Assessment

Weighing and measuring of students in school is a common practice that can potentially have long-term negative effects (SNE, 2003). Furthermore, the use of body mass index (BMI) as the sole measure of health status can lead to inaccurate labeling of children as obese or overweight (Ellis, Abrams, and Wong, 1999). Thus, the SNE (2003) recommends that screenings involving weight, height, and body fat percentage only be conducted when necessary. In addition, any weight assessment should be conducted under private and safe conditions by someone with whom the child is comfortable. This person must understand individual differences in growth rates and body shape and size and must be careful not to convey any negative feedback to the child or label them in any way. Children should never be made to feel intimidated or humiliated about weight-related issues.

CONCLUSION

Although we can wish that society will change overnight and appearance will no longer be an issue, we must be realistic. In the end, what we do and say as parents, teachers, friends, family members, etc. will ultimately have the greatest impact on the lives of our loved ones.

Perhaps the best thing that any of us can do is to try to change ourselves – find contentment with our current size, re-learn to recognize our bodies' hunger signals, eat more healthfully and exercise. A friend of mine once told me that she could not understand why her daughter was so obsessed with her weight and why her daughter thought she had to be model-thin. My friend proudly told me that she always told her daughter that "It's what's on the inside that counts." She always encouraged her daughter to excel in school and focus on non-appearance related aspects of herself. She tried to limit media exposure and keep healthful food choices around the house. Her daughter was 17, borderline anorexic, and she was at a loss about what to do. As we talked about the different factors that influence disordered eating behaviors, she looked at me as though a light bulb had gone off in her head. She said, "So… the fact that my daughter sees me weigh myself daily and make disparaging remarks about my body probably isn't a good thing, is it?" I told her that, no, it probably was not the best thing, but that she still had the ability to be a powerful positive role model in her daughter's life. After all, what child will take us seriously when we tell them that appearance does not matter when our behaviors obviously show that it does?

The purpose of the present chapter was to shed light on some of the factors that have been found to relate to disordered eating behaviors. In addition, it offered some practical suggestions for families and schools – two of our most powerful influences on the development of a healthy relationship with our bodies. We may not be able to make sweeping changes in media or society, but every small change that we can make at the individual, familial, or local level adds up. Will you be the one to make the change?

REFERENCES

Abell, S. C., and Richards, M. H. (1996). The relationship between body shape satisfaction and self-esteem: An investigation of gender and class differences. *Journal of Youth and Adolescence, 25,* 691-703.

Adam, T. C., and Epel, E. S. (2007). Stress, eating and the reward system *Physiology and Behavior, 91,* 449-458.

Agliata, D., and Tantleff-Dunn, S. (2004). The impact of media exposure on males' body image. *Journal of Social and Clinical Psychology, 23,* 7-22.

Alger, H. A. (1984). Transitions: Alternatives to manipulative management techniques. *Young Children, 39,* 16-25.

Anderson , C. B., and Bulik, C. M. (2004) Gender differences in compensatory behaviors, weight and shape salience, and drive for thinness. *Eating Behaviors, 5,* 1-11.

Annus, A. M., Smith, G. T., Fischer, S., Hendricks, M., and Williams, S. F. (2007). Associations among family and peer food-related experiences, learning about eating and dieting, and the development of eating disorders. *The International Journal of Eating Disorders, 40,* 179-186.

Anorexia Nervosa and Related Eating Disorders, Inc. (2005). Retrieved March 7, 2007, from: http://www.anred.com/stats.html

Arnow, B., Kenardy, J., and Agras, W.S. (1992). Binge eating among the obese: A descriptive study. *Journal of Behavioral Medicine, 15,* 155–170.

Arnow, B., Kenardy, J., and Agras,W.L. (1995). The Emotional Eating Scale: A development of a measure to assess coping with negative affect by eating. *International Journal of Eating Disorders, 18,* 79–90.

Becker, B., Bell, M., and Billington, R. (1987). Object relations ego deficits in bulimic college women. *Journal of Clinical Psychology, 43,* 92-95.

Birch, L. L., Johnson, S. L., Andresen, G., Peters, J. C., and Schulte, M. C. (1991). The variability of young children's energy intake. *New England Journal of Medicine, 324,* 232-235.

Birch L. L., Marlin D. W., and Rotter J. (1984). Eating as the "means" activity in a contingency: effects on young children's food preference. *Child Development, 55,* 432-439.

Birch, L. L., McPhee, L., Shoba, B. C., Steinberg, L., and Krehbiel, R. (1987) "Clean up your plate": Effects of child feeding practices on the conditioning of meal size. *Learning and Motivation, 18,* 301-317.

Birch, L. L., Zimmerman, S., and Hind, H. (1980). The influence of social-affective context on preschoolers' food preferences. *Child Development, 51,* 856-861.

Bois, J., Sarrazin, P., Brustad, R., Trouilloud, D, and Cury, F. (2005). Elementary school children's perceived competence and physical activity involvement: The influence of parents' role modelling behaviours and perceptions of their child competence. *Psychology of Sport and Exercise, 6,* 381-414.

Botta, R. A. (1999). Television images and adolescent girls' body image disturbance. *Journal of Communication, 49,* 22 – 41.

Brennan, K. A., and Shaver, P. R. (1995). Dimensions of adult attachment, affect regulation, and relationship functioning. *Personality and Social Psychology Bulletin, 21,* 267-283.

Broberg, A. G., Hjalmers, I., and Nevonen, L. (2001). Eating disorders, attachment and interpersonal difficulties: A comparison between 18- to 24-year-old patients and normal controls. *European Eating Disorders Review, 9,* 381-396.

Brook, U., and Tepper, I. (1997). High school students' attitudes and knowledge of food consumption and body image: Implications for school based education. *Patient Education and Counseling, 30,* 283-288.

Brunner, R. L., St. Jeor, S. T., Scott, B. J., Miller, G. D., Carmody, T. P., Brownell, K. D., and Foreyt, J. (1994). Dieting and disordered eating correlates of weight fluctuation in normal and obese adults. *Eating Disorders: The Journal of Treatment and Prevention, 2,* 341-356.

Button, E. J., Loan, P., Davies, J., and Sonuga-Barke, E. J. (1997). Self-esteem, eating problems, and psychological well-being in a cohort of schoolgirls aged 15-16: a questionnaire and interview study. *International Journal of Eating Disorders, 21,* 39-47.

Cachelin, F. M., and Regan, P. C. (2006). Prevalence and correlates of chronic dieting in a multi-ethnic U.S. community sample. *Eating and Weight Disorders, 11,* 91-99.

Cash, T. F., Thériault, J., and Annis, N. M. (2004). Body image in an interpersonal context: Adult attachment, fear of intimacy, and social anxiety. *Journal of Social and Clinical, Psychology Special Issue: Body Image and Eating Disorders, 23,* 89-103.

Centers for Disease Control (2003). Physical activity levels among children aged 9-13 years – United States, 2002. *Morbidity and Mortality Weekly Report, 52 (33),* 785-788.

Chandarana, P., Helmes, E., and Benson, N. (1988). Eating attitudes as related to demographic and personality characteristics: A high school survey. *Canadian Journal of Psychiatry, 33,* 834-837.

Chandler, S. B., Abood, D. A., Lee, D. T., Cleveland, M. Z., and Daly, J. A. (1994). Pathogenic eating attitudes and behaviors and body dissatisfaction differences among black and white college Students. *Eating Disorders: The Journal of Treatment and Prevention, 2,* 319-328.

Chapman, P., and Toma, R. B. (1997). Nutrition knowledge among adolescent high school female athletes. *Adolescence, 32,* 437-446.

Cole-Detke, H., and Kobak, R. (1996). Attachment processes in eating disorder and depression. *Journal of Consulting and Clinical Psychology, 64,* 282-290.

Cook-Cottone, C. P., and Phelps, L. (2006). Adolescent eating disorders. In G. Bear, K. Minke, and A. Thomas (Eds.), *Children's needs III: Understanding and addressing The developmental needs of children* (pp. 977-988). Bethesda, MD: National Association of School Psychologists Publications.

Croll, J. K., Neumark-Sztainer, D., Story, M., and Ireland, M. (2002). Prevalence and risk and protective factors related to disordered eating behaviors among adolescents: Relationship to gender and ethnicity. *Journal of Adolescent Health, 31,* 166-175.

Davis, C., Strachan, S., and Berkson, M. (2004). Sensitivity to reward: implications for overeating and overweight. *Appetite, 42,* 131–138.

Eaton, D. K., Kann, L., Kinchen, S., Ross, J., Hawkins, J., Harris, W. A. et al. (2006). Youth risk behavior surveillance – United States, 2005. *Morbidity and Mortality Weekly Report, 55 (SS-5),* 1-108.

Edwards-Hewitt, T., and Gray, J. J. (1993). The prevalence of disordered eating attitudes and behaviors in Black-American and White-American college women: Ethnic, regional, class, and media differences. *Eating Disorders Review, 1,* 41-54.

Eggert, J., Levendosky, A., and Klump, K. (2007). Relationships among attachment styles, personality characteristics, and disordered eating. *International Journal of Eating Disorders, 40,* 149-155.

Elgin, J., and Pritchard, M. E. (2006). Adult attachment and disordered eating in undergraduate men and women. *Journal of College Student Psychotherapy, 21,* 25-40.

Ellis, K. J., Abrams, S. A., and Wong, W. W. (1999). Monitoring childhood obesity: Assessment of the weight/height^2 index. *American Journal of Epidemiology, 150,* 939-946.

Engel, S.G., Johnson, C., Powers, P. S., Crosby, R. D., Wonderlich, S. A., Wittrock, D. A., and Mitchell, J. E. (2003). Predictors of disordered eating in a sample of Elite Division I college athletes. *Eating Behaviors, 4,* 333-343.

Evans, L., and Wertheim, E. H. (1998). Intimacy patterns and relationship satisfaction of women with eating problems and the mediating effects of depression, trait anxiety and social anxiety. *Journal of Psychosomatic research, Special Issues: Current Issues in Eating Disorder Research, 44,* 355-365.

Espina A., Ortego M. A., Ochoa de Alda I., Aleman A., and Juaniz M. (2002). Body shape and eating disorders in a sample of students in the Basque country: A pilot study. *Psychology in Spain, 6,* 3-11, 2002.

Fabian, L., and Thompson, J. K. (1989). Body image and eating disturbance in young females. *International Journal of Eating Disorders, 8,* 63-74.

Falciglia, G. Pabst, S. Couch, S. and Goody, C. (2004). Impact of parental food choices on child food neophobia. *Children's Health Care, 33,* 217-225.

Felker, K. R., and Stivers, C. (1994). The relationship of gender and family environment to eating disorder risk in adolescents. *Adolescence, 29,* 821-834.

Ferrand, C., and Brunet, E. (2004). Perfectionism and risk for disordered eating among young French male cyclists of high performance. *Perceptual and Motor Skills, 99,* 958-967.

Finstad, E. (2003). Identity and disordered eating in white, Hispanic, and American Indian adolescents. *Dissertation Abstracts International: Section B: The Sciences and Engineering, 64(2-B),* 961.

Fisher, J. O., and Birch, L. L. (1996). Maternal restriction of young girls' food access is related to intake of those foods in an unrestricted setting. *FASEB Journal, 10,* A225.

Forbush, K., Heatherton, T. F., and Keel, P. K. (2007). Relationships between perfectionism and specific disordered eating behaviors. *International Journal of Eating Disorders, 40,* 37-41.

Foreyt, J. P., and Goodrick, G. K. (1992). *Living without dieting.* Houston: Harrison.

French, S. A., Jeffrey, R. W., and Murray, D. (1999). Is dieting good for you?: Prevalence, duration and associated weight and behaviour changes for specific weight loss strategies over four year in US adults. *International Journal of Obesity and Related Metabolic Disorders: Journal of the International Association for the Study of Obesity, 23,* 320-327.

Furnham, A., Badmin, N., and Sneade, I. (2002). Body image dissatisfaction: Gender differences in eating attitudes, self-esteem, and reasons for exercise. *The Journal of Psychology, 136,* 581-596.

Ghaderi, A. (2003). Structural modeling analysis of prospective risk factors for eating disorder. *Eating Behaviors, 3,* 387–396.

Gilbert, N., and Meyer, C. (2005). Fear of negative evaluation and the development of eating psychopathology: A longitudinal study among nonclinical women. *International Journal of Eating Disorders, 37,* 307-312.

Gleason, J. H., Alexander, A. M., and Somers, C. L. (2000). Later adolescents' reactions to three types of childhood teasing: Relations with self-esteem and body image. *Social Behavior and Personality, 28,* 472-480.

Granillo, T., Jones-Rodriguez, G. and Carvajal, S. C. (2005). Prevalence of eating disorders in Latina adolescents: Associations with substance use and other correlates. *Journal of Adolescent Health, 36,* 214-220.

Green, S. P., and Pritchard, M. E. (2003). Predictors of body image dissatisfaction in adult men and women. *Social Behavior and Personality, 31,* 215-222.

Groesz, L. M., Levine, M. P., and Murmen, S. K. (2002). The effect of experimental presentation of thin media images on body satisfaction: A meta-analytic review. *International Journal of Eating Disorders, 31,* 1-16.

Guiney, K M., and Furlong, N.E. (1999). Correlates of body satisfaction and self-concept in third and sixth Graders. *Current Psychology, 18,* 353-368.

Gustafson, S. L., and Rhodes, R. E. (2006). Parental correlates of physical activity in children and early adolescents. *Sports Medicine, 36*, 79-97.

Haase, A., Prapavessis, H., and Owens, R. G. (2002). Perfectionism, social physique anxiety and disordered eating: a comparison of male and female elite athletes. *Psychology of Sport and Exercise, 3*, 209-222.

Harrison, K., and Cantor, J. (1997). The relationship between media consumption and eating disorders. *Journal of Communication, 47*, 40-67.

Harrison, K., and Hefner, V. (2006). Media exposure, current and future body ideals, and disordered eating among preadolescent girls: A longitudinal panel study. *Journal of Youth and Adolescence, 35*, 153-163.

Hawkins, N., Richards, R. S., Granley, H. M., and Stein, D. M. (2004). The impact of exposure to the thin-ideal media image on women. *The Journal of Treatment and Prevention, 12*, 35-50.

Heinberg, L. J., and Thompson, J. K. (1995). Body image and televised images of thinness and attractiveness: A controlled laboratory investigation. *Journal of Social and Clinical Psychology, 14*, 325-338.

Heitzler, C. D., Martin, S. L., Duke, J., and Huhman, M. (2006). Correlates of physical activity in a national sample of children aged 9–13 years. *Preventive Medicine, 42*, 254–260.

Herman, C. P., and Polivy, J. (1975). Anxiety, restraint, and eating behavior *Journal of Abnormal Psychology, 84*, 666-672.

Hermes, S. F., and Keel, P. K. (2003). The influence of puberty and ethnicity on awareness and internalization of the thin ideal. *International Journal of Eating Disorders, 33*, 465-467.

Hodson, C., Newcomb, M., Locke, T., and Goodyear, R. (2006). Childhood adversity, poly-substance use, and disordered eating in adolescent Latinas: Mediated and indirect paths in a community sample. *Child Abuse and Neglect, 30*, 1017-1036, 2006.

Hopkinson, R. A., and Lock, J. (2004). Athletics, perfectionism, and disordered eating. *Eating and Weight Disorders, 9*, 99-106.

Johannsen, D., Johannsen, N., and Specker, B. (2006). Influence of parent's eating behaviors and child-feeding practices on children's weight status. *Obesity, 14*, 431-439.

Johnson, C., Crosby, R., Engel, S., Mitchell, J., Powers, P.S., Wittrock, D. and Wonderlich, S. (2004) Gender, ethnicity, self-esteem and disordered eating among college athletes. *Eating Behaviors, 5*, 147-156.

Johnson, C., Powers, P. S., and Dick, R. (1999). Athletes and eating disorders: The National Collegiate Athletic Association study. *International Journal of Eating Disorders, 26*, 179-188.

Kalodner, C. R. (1997). Media influence on males and female non-eating-disordered college students: A significant issue. *Eating Disorders, 5*, 47-51.

Kann, L., Kinchen, S. A., Williams, B. I., Ross, J., Lowry, R., Hill, C. V., Grunbaum, J. A., Blumson, P. S., Collins, J. L., and Kolb, L. J. (1998). Youth risk behavior surveillance-United States, 1997. *Morbidity and Mortality Weekly Report 47*, 1-89.

Kashubeck-West, S., Mintz, L. B., and Weigold, I. (2005). Separating the effects of gender and weight-loss desire on body satisfaction and disordered eating behavior. *Sex Roles, 53,* 505-518.

Kiang, L., and Harter, S. (2006). Sociocultural values of appearance and attachment processes: An integrated model of eating disorder symptomatology. *Eating Behaviors, 7,* 134-51.

Kiefer, I., Rathmanner, T., and Kunze, M. (2005) Eating and dieting differences in men and women. *The Journal of Men's Health and Gender, 2,* 194-201.

Kirk, G., Singh, K., and Getz, H. (2001). Risk of eating disorders among female college athletes and non-athletes. *Journal of College Counseling, 4,* 122-133.

Klump, K. L., Gobrogge, K. L., Perkins, P. S., Thorne, D., Sisk, C., and Breedlove, S. M. (2006). Preliminary evidence that gonadal hormones organize and activate disordered eating. *Psychological Medicine, 36, 539-46.*

Krane, V., Stiles-Shipley, J. A., Waldron, J., and Michalenok, J. (2001). Relationships among body satisfaction, social physique anxiety, and eating behaviors in female athletes and exercisers. *Journal of Sport Behavior, 24,* 247-265.

Leon, G. R., Fulkerson, J. A., Perry, C. L., and Early-Zaid, M. B. (1995). Prospective analysis of personality and behavioral vulnerabilities and gender influences in the later development of disordered eating. *Journal of Abnormal Psychology, 104,* 140-149.

Levine, M. P. (1999). Prevention of eating disorders, eating problems and negative body image. In R. Lemberg (Ed.), *Controlling Eating Disorders with Facts, Advice and Resources (2nd ed., pp. 64-72).* Phoenix: Oryx Press.

Levine, M. P., Smolak, L., and Hayden, H. (1994). The relation of sociocultural factors to eating attitudes and behaviors among middle school girls. *Journal of Early Adolescence, 14,* 471-490.

Lieberman, M., Gauvin, L., Bukowski, W. M., and White, D. R. (2001). Interpersonal influence and disordered eating behaviors in adolescent girls: The role of peer modeling, social reinforcement and body-related teasing. *Eating Behaviors, 2,* 215–236.

Logio, K. A. (2003). Gender, race, childhood abuse, and body image among adolescents. *Violence Against Women, 9,* 931-954.

Malinauskas, B. M ., Cucchiara, A. J ., Aeby, V. G ., and Bruening, C. C. (2007). Physical activity, disordered eating risk, and anthropometric measurement: A comparison of college female athletes and non athletes. *College Student Journal, 41,* 217-222.

McCabe, M. P., and Vincent, M. A. (2003). The role of biodevelopmental and psychological factors in disordered eating among adolescent males and females. *European Eating Disorder Review, 11,* 315-328.

Mellin, A., Neumark-Sztainer, D., Patterson, J., and Sockalosky, J. (2004). Unhealthy weight management behaviors among adolescent girls with type 1 diabetes mellitus: The role of familial eating patterns and weight-related concerns. *Journal of Adolescent Health, 35,* 278-289.

Milligan, B., and Pritchard, M. E. (2006). The relationship between gender, sport, self-esteem and eating disordered behaviors in Division I athletes. *Athletic Insight, 8,* 9-43.

Mintz, L. B., and Kashubeck, S. (1999). Body image and disordered eating among Asian American and Caucasian college students: An examination of race and gender differences. *Psychology of Women Quarterly, 23,* 781-796.

Mora-Giral, M., Raich-Escursell, R. M., Segues, V. C., Torras-Claraso, J. and Huon, G. 2004). Bulimia symptoms and risk factors in university students. *Eating and Weight Disorders, 9,* 163-169.

Muth, J. L., and Cash, T. F. (1997). Body–image attitudes: What difference does gender make? *Journal of Applied Social Psychology, 27,* 1438-1452.

Neumark-Sztainer, D., Falkner, N., Story, M., Perry, C., Hannan, P., and Mulert, S. (2002). Weight-teasing among adolescents: Correlations with weight status and disordered eating behaviors. *International Journal of Obesity, 1,* 123-131.

Neumark-Sztainer, D., Sherwood, N. E., French, S. A., and Jeffrey, R. W. (1999). Weight control behaviors among adult men and women: Cause for concern? *Obesity Research, 7,* 179-188.

Neumark-Sztainer, D., Wall, M., Story, M., and Fulkerson, J. A. (2004). Are family meal patterns associated with disordered eating behaviors among adolescents? *Journal of Adolescent Health, 35,* 350-359.

Nichter, M., and Vuckovic, N. (1994). Fat talk: Body image among adolescent females. In N. Sault (Ed.), *Many mirrors: Body image and social relations* (pp. 109-131).

New Brunswick, N.J.: Rutgers University Press.

O'Dea, J. A., and Abraham, S. (1999). Onset of disordered eating attitudes and behaviors in early adolescence: Interplay of pubertal status, gender, weight and age. *Adolescence, 34,* 671-679.

O'Dea, J. A., and Yager, Z. (2006). Body image and eating disorders in male adolescents and young men. In P. I. Swain (Ed.), *New developments in eating disorders research (pp. 1-36).* Hauppauge, NY: Nova Science Publishers.

Ogden, J. (2003). *The psychology of eating.* United Kingdom: MPG Books.

Ogden, J., and Mundray, K. (1996). The effect of media on body satisfaction: The role of gender and size. *European Eating Disorders Review, 4,* 171-182.

Olivardia, R., Pope, H. G., Borowieki, J. J., and Cohane, G. H. (2004). Biceps and body image: The relationship between muscularity and self-esteem, depression, and eating disorder symptoms. *Men and Masculinity, 5,* 112-120.

Parker, S., Nichter, M., Nichter, M., Vuckovic, N., Sims, C., and Ritenbaugh, C. (1995). Body image and weight concerns among African American and white adolescent females: differences that make a difference. *Human Organization, 54,* 103-113.

Patel, D. R., Greydanus, D. E., Pratt, H. D., and Phillips, E. L. (2003). Eating disorders in adolescent athletes. *Journal of Adolescent Research, 18,* 280-296.

Pauls, B. S., and Daniels, T. (2000). Relationship among family, peer networks, and bulimic symptomatology in college women. *Canadian Journal of Counseling, 34,* 260-272.

Paxton, S. J., Schutz, H. K., Wertheim, E. H., and Muir, S. L. (1999). Friendship clique and peer influences on body image attitudes, dietary restraint, extreme weight loss behaviors and binge eating in adolescent girls. *Journal of Abnormal Psychology, 108,* 255-266.

Perez, M., and Joiner, Jr., T. E. (2003). Body image dissatisfaction and disordered eating in black and white females. *International Journal of Eating Disorders, 33,* 342-350.

Phelps, L., Johnston, L. S., Jimenez, D. P., and Wilczenski, F L. (1993). Figure preference, body dissatisfaction, and body distortion in adolescence. *Journal of Adolescent Research, 8,* 297-310.

Picard, C. L. (1999). The level of competition as a factor for the development of eating disorders in female collegiate athletes. *Journal of Youth and Adolescence, 28(5),* 583-594.

Pike, K. M., and Rodin, J. (1991). Mothers, daughters, and disordered eating. *Journal of Abnormal Psychology, 100,* 198-204.

Pleis, J. R., and Lethbridge-Çejku, M., (2005). Summary health statistics for U.S. adults: National health interview survey, 2005. National Center for Health Statistics. *Vital Health Stat 10(232).*

Polivy, J., and Herman, C. P. (1987). Diagnosis and treatment of normal eating. *Journal of Consulting and Clinical Psychology, 55,* 635-644.

Polivy J., and Herman P. C. (2002). Causes of eating disorders. *Annual Review of Psychology, 53,* 187-213.

Powers, P. S. (1999). The last word: Athletes and eating disorders. *Eating Disorders: The Journal of Treatment and Prevention, 7,* 249-255.

Pritchard, M. E. (2004). Body satisfaction in male and female adolescents: Associations with parental behavior. *Perceptual and Motor Skills, 99,* 257-258.

Rasnake, L. K., Laube, E., Lewis, M., and Linscheid, T. R. (2005). Children's nutritional judgments: Relation to eating attitudes and body image. *Health Communication, 18,* 275-289.

Raudenbush, B., and Zellner, D. A. (1997). Nobody's satisfied: Effects of abnormal eating behaviors and actual and perceived weight status on body image satisfaction in males and females. *Journal of Social and Clinical Psychology, 16,* 95-110.

Reinking, M. F., and Alexander, L. E. (2005). Prevalence of disordered-eating behaviors in undergraduate female collegiate athletes and non-athletes. *Journal of Athletic Training, 40,* 47-51.

Rieves, L., and Cash, T. (1996). Social developmental factors and women's body-image attitudes. *Journal of Social Behavior and Personality, 11,* 63-78.

Robinson, S. (2000). Children's perceptions of who controls their food. *Journal of Human Nutrition and Dietetics, 13,* 163-171.

Sallis, J. F., Patterson, R. L., McKenzie, T. L., and Nader, P. R. (1988). Family variables and physical activity in preschool children. *Journal of Developmental and Behavioral Pediatrics, 9,* 57-61.

Salzman, J. P. (1997). Ambivalent attachment in female adolescents: Association with affective instability and eating disorders. *International Journal of Eating Disorders, 21,* 251-259.

Sands, R., Tricker, J., Sherman, C., Armatas, C., and Maschette, W. (1997). Disordered eating patterns, body image, self esteem, and physical activity in preadolescent school children. *International Journal of Eating Disorders, 21,* 159-166.

Schachter, S. (1971). Some extraordinary facts about obese humans and rats. *American Psychologist, 26,* 129-144.

Schneider, J. A., O'Leary, A., and Jenkins, S. R. (1995). Gender, sexual orientation, and disordered eating. *Psychology and Health, 10,* 113-128.

Schutz, H. K., Paxton, S. J., and Wertheim, E. H. (2002). Investigation of body comparison among adolescent girls. *Journal of Applied Psychology, 32,* 1906-1937.

Schur, E. A., Sanders, M., and Steiner, H. (2000). Body dissatisfaction and dieting in young children. *International Journal of Eating Disorders, 27,* 339-343.

Sharpe, T. M., Killen, J. D., Bryson, S. W., Shisslak, C. M., Estes, L. S., Gray, N., Crago, M., and Taylor, C. B. (1998). Attachment style and weight concerns in preadolescent and adolescent girls. *International Journal of Eating Disorders, 23,* 39-44.

Shea, M., and Pritchard, M. E. (2007). Is self-esteem the primary predictor of disordered eating? *Personality and Individual Differences, 42,* 1527-1537.

Shisslak C. M., Crago, M., McKnight, K. M., Estes, L. S., Gray, N., and Parnaby, O. G. (1998). Potential risk factors associated with weight control behaviors in elementary and middle school girls. *Journal of Psychosomatic Research, 44,* 301-313.

Smolak, L., and Levine, M. P. (1994). Toward an empirical basis for primary prevention of eating problems with elementary school-children. *Eating Disorders: The Journal of Treatment and Prevention, 2,* 293-307.

Smolak, L., Murnen, S. K., and Ruble, A. E. (2000). Female athletes and eating problems: a meta-analysis. *International Journal of Eating Disorders, 27,* 371-380.

Society for Nutrition Education. (2003). Guidelines for childhood obesity prevention programs: Promoting healthy weight in children. *Journal of Nutrition Education and Behavior, 35,* 1-4.

Stevens, D. L., Hill, R. P., and Hanson, C. (1994). The beauty myth and female consumers: The controversial role of advertising. *The Journal of Consumer Affairs, 28,* 137-153.

Stoutjesdyk, D., and Jevne, R. (1993). Eating disorders among high performance athletes. *Journal of Youth and Adolescence, 22,* 272-282.

Striegel-Moore, R. H., Silberstein, L. R., Frensch, P., and Rodin, J. (1989). A prospective study of disordered eating among college students. *International Journal of Eating Disorders, 8,* 499-509.

Tata, P., Fox., J., and Cooper, J. (2001). An investigation into the influence of gender and parenting styles on excessive exercise and disordered eating. *European Eating Disorders Review, 9,* 194-206.

Taylor, C. B., Sharpe, T., Shisslak, C., Bryson, S., Estes, L. S., Gray, N., McKnight, K. M., Crago, M., Kraemer, H. C., and Killen, J. D. (1998). Factors associated with weight concerns in adolescent girls. *International Journal of Eating Disorders, 24,* 31-42.

Thelen, M. H., Powell, A. L., Lawrence, C., and Kuhnert, M. E. (1992). Eating and body image concerns among children. *Journal of Clinical Child Psychology, 21,* 41-46.

Thomas, K., Ricciardelli, L. A., and Williams, R. J. (2000). Gender traits and self-concept as indicators of problem eating and body dissatisfaction among children. *Sex Roles, 43,* 441-458.

Thompson, J. K., and Heinberg, L. J. (1999). The media's influence on body image disturbance and eating disorders: We've reviled them, now can we rehabilitate them? *Journal of Social Issues, 55,* 339-353.

Thompson, R. A., and Sherman, R. T. (1999). Athletes, athletic performance, and eating disorders: Healthier alternatives. *Journal of Social Issues, 55*, 317-337.

Tiggerman, M. (2003). Media exposure, body dissatisfaction and disordered eating: Television and magazines are not the same! *European Eating Disorders Review, 11*, 418-430.

Tribole, E. T., and Resch, E. (1995). *Intuitive eating.* New York: St. Martin's Press.

Twamley, E. W., and Davis, M. C. (1999). The sociocultural model of eating disturbance in young women: The effects of personal attributes and family environment. *Journal of Social and Clinical Psychology, 18*, 467-489.

United States Department of Agriculture: Food and Nutrition Service. (2000). *Changing the Scene.* Retrieved November 1, 2007 from http://www.fns.usda.gov/tn/Healthy/support.pdf.

United States Department of Agriculture: Food and Nutrition Service. (2007). *Summer Food Service Program for Children.* Retrieved November 1, 2007 from http://www.fns.usda.gov/...7/Nutrition_Guidance_2007_Ref.doc.

Vartanian, L. R., Giant, C. L., and Passino, R. M. (2001). "Ally McBeal vs. Arnold Schwarzenegger": Comparing mass media, interpersonal feedback and gender as predictors of satisfaction with body thinness and muscularity. *Social Behavior and Personality, 29*, 711-723.

Vereecken, C. A., Keukelier, E., and Maes, L. (2004). Influence of mother's educational level on food parenting practices and food habits of young children. *Appetite, 43*, 93-103.

Vohs, K. D., Bardone, A. M., Joiner, T. E., Jr., Abramson, L. Y., and Heatherton, T. F.(1999). Perfectionism, perceived weight status, and self-esteem interact to predict bulimic symptoms: A model of bulimic symptom development. *Journal of Abnormal Psychology, 4, 695-700.*

Wang, Y., and Beydoun, M. A. (2007). The obesity epidemic in the United States – Gender, age, socioeconomic, racial/ethnic, and geographic characteristics: A systematic review and meta-regression analysis. *Epidemiologic Reivews, 29*, 6-28.

Warren, B., Stanton, A., and Blessing, D. (1990). Disordered eating patterns in competitive female athletes. *International Journal of Eating Disorders, 9*, 565- 569.

Weber Cullen, K., Baranowski, T., Rittenberry, L., Cosart, C., Hebert, D., and de Moor, C. (2001). Child-reported family and peer influences on fruit, juice and vegetable consumption: Reliability and validity of measures. *Health Education Research, 16*, 187-200.

Weiss, E. C., Galuska, D. A., Khan, L. K., and Serdula, M. K. (2006). Weight-control practices among U.S. adults, 2001-2002. *American Journal of Preventive Medicine, 31*, 18-24.

Wertheim, E. H., Paxton, S. J., Schutz, H. K., and Muir, S. (1997). Why do adolescent girls watch their weight? An interview study examining sociocultural pressures to be thin. *Journal of Psychosomatic Research, 42*, 345-355.

Whitehouse, P. J., and Harris, G. (1998). The intergenerational transmission of eating disorders. *European Eating Disorders Review, 6*, 238-254.

Wilcox, S. (1997). Age and gender in relation to body attitudes: Is there a double standard of aging? *Psychology of Women Quarterly, 21*, 549-565.

Wiseman, C. V., Gunning, F. M., and Gray, J. J. (1993). Increasing pressure to be thin: 19 years of diet products in television commercials. *Eating Disorders: The Journal of Treatment and Prevention, 1,* 52-61.

Wiseman, C. V., Peltzman, B., Halmi, K. A., and Sunday, S. R. (2004). Risk factors for eating disorders: Surprising similarities between middle school boys and girls. Eating Disorders: *The Journal of Treatment and Prevention, 12,* 315-320.

Worobey, J. (2002). Interpersonal versus intrafamilial predictors of maladaptive eating attitudes in young women. *Social Behavior and Personality, 30,* 423-434.

Zenner, C., and Pritchard, M. E. (2007). What do adolescents know about health? *Academic Exchange Quarterly, 68-72.*

In: Life Style and Health Research Progress
Editors: A. B. Turley, G. C. Hofmann

ISBN: 978-1-60456-427-3
© 2008 Nova Science Publishers, Inc.

Chapter VIII

Imaginary or Real?:
The Body Image in Obese People

Monika Bąk-Sosnowska

Department of Psychology, Medical University of Silesia, Poland

ABSTRACT

Body image is the picture of one's own body in the mind. Body image contains the body mass estimation and the emotional attitude towards body. For the purpose of the research study, four aspects of body image were separated: declarative (the way of thinking about body), sensory (feeling body), imaginable (imaginary body) and perceptive (a picture of body in a mirror). The research study included 150 overweight women who participated in an outpatient complex obesity treatment. The average age of the examined was 42.97 ± 13.55. The average body mass before the treatment was 97.93 ± 16.47 kg, and the average Body Mass Index (BMI) was 37.17 ± 6.42 kg/m^2. Two research methods were used for body mass estimating: Silhouette Test (Craig, Caterson, 1990) and the Assessment Scale of a Body Mass (own method, 2005). The Scale of Satisfaction with One's Own Body (own method, 2005) was used to assess an emotional attitude towards body. The following aspects of body were analyzed with respect to the level of satisfaction: attractiveness, charm, agility, shapeliness, proportionality and firmness. All research methods were used separately for each aspect of body image at each stage out of four research stages: at the beginning of the treatment, and after weight reduction by 5%, 10% and 15% of initial body mass. The research results confirmed that at following stages of the research study an objective weight of participants was reducing considerably ($F(3.144)=987.038$; $p<0.001$). As far as a subjective assessment of body mass is concerned, the participants estimated their weight as decreasing in relation to the following aspects: declarative (Assessment Scale: $\chi^2=78.775$; $p<0.001$; Silhouette Test: $\chi^2=87.123$; $p<0,001$), sensory (Assessment Scale: $\chi^2=39.963$; $p<0.001$; Silhouette Test: $\chi^2=60.269$; $p<0.01$), and perceptive (Assessment Scale: $\chi^2=67.728$; $p<0.001$; Silhouette Test: $\chi^2=88.182$; $p<0.001$). A subjective estimation of body mass in an imaginable aspect was not changing, and it was defined as an average weight (The Assessment Scale: $\chi^2=2.727$; $p=0.436$; Silhouette Test: $\chi^2=4.211$; $p=0.240$). The adequacy of a subjective body mass estimation was decreasing at following stages of the research study with respect to a declarative aspect (Assessment Scale: $Q=21.578$; $p<0.001$; Silhouette Test:

Q=43.108; p<0.001), a sensory aspect (Silhouette Test: Q=25.114; p<0.001), and a perceptive one (Assessment Scale: Q=18.677; p<0.01; Silhouette Test: Q=51.283; p<0.01). As far as an imaginable aspect is concerned, the adequacy of the assessment was at a constant level (inadequate assessments outnumbered the adequate ones). At next research stages the increase in satisfaction with one's own body was examined, with respect to all the following aspects: declarative (Q=31.299; p<0.001), sensory (Q=22.444; p<0.001), imaginable (Q=8.250; p<0.05), and perceptive (Q=40.880; p<0.001). The conducted research shows that from the beginning of the treatment to its end, imaginable aspect of body image differed from declarative, sensory and perceptive aspects. Imagined body was younger (t(149)=13,234; p<0.001), slimmer (t (149)=17.774; p<0.001), and more attractive in respect to the appearance than the body that was declared (Z=9.460; p<0.001), felt (Z=9.345; p<0.001), and seen in a mirror (Z=9.455; p<0.001).

INTRODUCTION

"Before words appeared, there had been images …
The creation of images is not an empty concept;
It is the half of our consciousness;
It is the way of our thinking,
Perhaps, more important than other ways."

Samuels and Samuels

The body image is a complex issue which includes observations, thoughts, feelings, and actions which are connected with one's own body (Waxler, Liska, 1975 by Cohen, 1984; Lacey, Birtchnell, 1986). The body percept is an inside and visual image of body shape and size. The body percept develops during childhood. The body percept is a neural representation which determines body experience (Lacey, Birtchnell 1986; Offman, Bradley, 1992). The body concept is an attitude, i.e., beliefs, feelings and actions towards body as a whole, and its particular parts. The body concept expresses the level of satisfaction with body and its appearance. The development of the body concept is the most at puberty (Lacey, Birtchnell 1986; Waller, Barnes, 2002).

The body image influences a person's psychological and social functioning significantly. Above all, the body image influences an attitude towards oneself, an assessment of a state of health, i.e., the body image influences relations with the others (Butters, Cash, 1987; Jestes, 1997; Mandal, 2000; Cohen, 2001; Harwas – Napierala, Trempala, 2002; Thompson, 2002; Etcoff, 2002). In the case of females, the determinants of a successful life are the following aspects of the body image: sexual attractiveness, physical condition and weight acceptance (Stoke, Recascino, 2003).

Lots of factors influence the body image. That is why, some authors think that the body image is not stable and it changes under the influence of a mood, an assessment context and the others' advice (Stunkard, Mendelson, 1967; Adami et al., 1998; Glebocka, Kulbat, 2005). On the other hand, lots of researches (also with overweight people's participation) suggest that while describing and assessing ones own appearance people often follow rather an inside image than an image in the mirror. Moreover, the researches suggest that the body image is relatively stable. This confirms a hypothesis that sensory experiences and patterns belong to the foundation of a perceptive and postural model of the body, and visual perception is of secondary importance (Lacey, Birtchnell, 1986; Mandal, 2000).

The studies concerning the assessment of the body mass indicate that all people, irrespective of the body mass, show a tendency to overestimating their body mass (Cash, Hicks, 1990; Gardner et al., 1991). However, some studies suggest that obese people overestimate their body mass as a whole and its particular parts (especially tights) much more than slim people. Moreover, obese people reply faster, which may suggest that they follow rather their inside body image that their reflection in the mirror. However, other studies show that obese people perceive their body less adequately than slim people. Indeed, obese people underestimate their body weight, but they overestimate their height (Bell, Kirpatrick, Rinn, 1986; Nawaz et al., 2001; Sanchez-Villegas et al., 2001).

The studies concerning an emotional attitude towards ones own body indicate that most obese people have a negative attitude towards their body (Stunkard, Wadden, 1992; Sanchez-Villegas et al., 2001; Friedman et al., 2002). Some significant predictors of dissatisfaction with the body are: the female sex, compulsive overeating, low self-esteem (Grilo et al., 2005). However, some part of obese people may express an ambivalent or even a positive attitude toward their body. It is manifested throughout, for example, the attribution of positive physical and psychological features to obese people, the aversion to weight loss campaigns, the propagation of negative effects of losing weight (for example: irritation, the skin's elasticity decrease, the signs of aging) (Molinari, Riva, 1995; Basdevant, Le Barzic, Guy – Grand, 1993).

The inspiration for the research which is presented below was the ambiguity relating to scientific reports on the body image in obese people. The theoretical foundation of the researches included: Seymour Epstein's Cognitive-experiential Self-theory (1990) and Anthony Greenwald's concept of mental representations (1986).

Epstein claimed that Self sphere includes two systems of information processing: a rational system (which is connected with the consciousness and functions in accordance with conclusion rules; its products are words) and an experiential system (which interprets, decodes and organizes experiences automatically, and directs behaviors; the system is connected with the subconscious and it prevails over the rational system; the system's products are metaphors and representations).

Greenwald's multilevel concept of mental representations assumes that information are processed by mind at several stages. The first stage is an analysis of sensory features. The process is automatic, unconscious and it does not leave marks in memory. The second stage is a perceptive system which helps identify objects and comprehend words. The next stage is a linguistic system which decodes verbal information which becomes representations of statements which are connected with a conceptual knowledge. The fourth stage of processing information is connected with using an accumulated conceptual knowledge to conclude from observable events. According to the concept, the systems of processing information are relatively independent from each other due to different ways of coding. Thus, there is a possibility of avoiding knowledge about contents which are somehow threatening.

There are four aspects of the body image which can be distinguished on the basis of the above mentioned theories and author's professional clinical experiences. The aspects are as follows (own analysis):

- declarative – represents the sphere: I know, when for example I provide the size I wear or my body weight; it is an opinion, so according to Reber's dictionary definition (2000, p.452), i.e.: a temporary and expressible point of view; it is of intellectual character and it is based on (at least to some degree) facts or data
- sensory – represents the sphere: I feel, when I experience stimuli coming from my own body; a sensation, following Reber's dictionary definition (2000, p.834), is not subject to a secondary analysis, it is an elementary feeling or consciousness of conditions inside or outside the body, it results from a stimulation of a receptor or the receptor system; apart from unitary stimuli, a general body feeling depends on, for example: a state of health, ongoing physical and physiological processes, a feeling of hunger/satiety, physical fitness;
- imaginable – represents the sphere: I imagine, when I close my eyes and imagine my figure; an image results from bringing up or processing a content of a memory mark (a long-term memory); an image refers only to pictures (Mlodkowski, 1998); based on Reber's dictionary definition (2000, p. 847) in a narrow meaning, an image is a copy of an earlier sensory experience, in a broad meaning, an image means imagining something – it includes an imagination and a creation of mental images
- perceptive – represents the sphere: I can see, when for example I am looking in the mirror; following Reber's dictionary definition (2000, p. 835) a perception results from the operation of an attention and a random-access memory, a perception is the result of an interpretation and an analysis of sensations – in this case – visual sensations; the quality of a perception depends on cognitive skills and an attitude.

It was assumed that a separate analysis of each body image will enable to understand its general diversity and dynamics during the weight loss therapy. Two dependent variables were assumed: a subjective body mass and an emotional attitude towards the body. BMI was an independent variable. The basic aim of the research was to study, whether:

1. The following body image aspects: declarative, sensory, imaginable and perceptive, are different from each other in respect of a body mass estimation and an emotional attitude towards the body,
2. The body image aspects are changing upon the reduction in body mass in respect of a body mass estimation and an emotional attitude towards the body.

MATERIAL AND METHODS

The research group consisted of 150 overweight women who participated in the outpatient and complex weight loss therapy, organized by Ambulatory Clinic for Obesity and Metabolic Disorders (the Head of the Clinic: Prof. Barbara Zahorska-Markiewicz). The average age of the examined females was 42.97 ± 13.55. The average body mass at the beginning of the treatment was 97.93 ± 16.47 kg, and the average Body Mass Index (BMI) was 37.17± 6.42. Most of the examined females had a secondary education and during the weight loss therapy were unemployed. Most of them had a permanent partner and two children. The period of participating in the therapy was not limited. The aim of the therapy was the reduction in body mass by min 15 %. The participants attended group and individual meetings in accordance with their own desire. On the average, they saw a physician, a dietician and a psychologist once or twice a month. At the first meeting there was also a physiotherapist. The professional help provided to the patients included educating and giving emotional and instrumental support (for example, helping with calculating the calorific value of foodstuffs, prescribing medicines – under justified circumstances). The psychological work with the patients did not include detailed issues concerning body image which are significant for the conducted research. The participation in the research was voluntary. To qualify to the next research step the patients had to obtain the specified reduction in body mass by 5%, 10% and 15%. The exclusion of the research was when a participant resigned or when the reduction in body mass was less than 1 kg during the last 2 months.

The following four research methods were used: an objective check of body mass using an electronic weighing scales, the Silhouette Test (P. Craig and I. Caterson, 1990), the Assessment Scale of a Body Mass (own instrument, 2005), and the Scale of Satisfaction with Ones Own Body (own instrument, 2005). The Silhouette Test and the Assessment Scale of a Body Mass were used to study a subjective estimation of body mass. And, the Scale of Satisfaction with Ones Own Body was used to study an emotional attitude towards ones own body. Moreover, in the case of an imaginable aspect of body image, an additional research method was included – the description of an imaginary figure.

The Silhouette Test is a pictorial test. It consists of drawings of female and male figures which are arranged side by side according to increasing body mass – starting with the slimmest figures, through figures with average BMI, and ending up with overweight figures. The test was published for the first time by Furhnam and Alibhai (1983). The tests including 3, 5, 7 or 9 human silhouettes are used. The tests including 9 female silhouettes (Craig, Caterson, 1990) were used for the purpose of the presented research.

For the purpose of the presented research, using the competent judges method, 9 female silhouettes were divided into 4 categories: 1) slim (pictures 1 and 2); 2) average (pictures 3 and 4); 3) overweight (pictures 5 and 6); 4) obese (pictures 7, 8, 9). Then, pictures were assigned to an increasing BMI as follows: 1 <18 BMI; 2 = 18 – 19 BMI; 3 = 20 – 21 BMI; 4 = 22 – 24 BMI; 5 = 25 – 26 BMI; 6 = 27 – 29 BMI; 7 = 30 – 34 BMI; 8 = 35 – 40 BMI; 9 >40 BMI.

In the case of each participant, the test was conducted separately for each aspect of body image at each stage out of four research stages. Instructions for the test suggested that each female participant should point out a silhouette which is the best illustration of her body according to: the knowledge of her body (a declarative aspect), the actual feeling of her body (a sensory aspect), the image of her body (an imaginable aspect), and the reflection of her body in the mirror (a perceptive aspect).

The Assessment Scale of a Body Mass (own method, 2005) is a four-point scale that includes the following categories: 1) slim; 2) average; 3) overweight; 4) obese. The instruction for the scale suggested that a female participant should point out a term that is the best description of her body according to: the knowledge of her body (a declarative aspect), the actual feeling of her body (a sensory aspect), the image of her body (an imaginable aspect), and the reflection of her body in the mirror (a perceptive aspect). The choice of a particular term from the scale was based on a participant's subjective understanding of a term's meaning. In the case of each participant the Assessment Scale of a Body Mass was used separately for each aspect of body image at each stage out of four research stages.

The Scale of Satisfaction with Ones Own Body (own instrument, 2005) is in the form of 6 linear scales that consist of 5 points. It determines the level of satisfaction with particular aspects of ones own body. Number 1 means a very positive evaluation, number 3 means an ambivalent evaluation, and number 5 means a very negative evaluation. Particular, detailed scales related to the following, adjectival dimensions: attractiveness, charm, agility, shapeliness, proportionality, and firmness. An examined person pointed to a term that characterized her body in an analyzed aspect. The following dimensions were based on clinical experience, as something important for estimation of one's own body in obese women during weight loss. The instruction of this method suggested to point a number which best represent an actual characteristics of examined person's body, according to: knowledge about own body (declarative aspect), actual expirience of own body (sensory aspect), imaginary picture of own body (imaginable aspect) and mirror of own body (perceptive aspect). The Scale of Satisfaction with Ones Own Body was used separately for each aspects of body image, at each stage out of four research stages.

SPSS, a statistical and data management package, was used to perform a statistical analysis of the gathered data. The data from the methods studying a subjective estimation of body mass (the Silhouette Test and the Assessment Scale of a Body Mass) were contained in four categories so that the obtained in both cases results were included in the range from 1 to 4. At the same time, an objective BMI of an examined female was assigned to one out of four categories – by way of analogy, as in the Silhouette Test. As far as the Scale of Satisfaction with Ones Own Body is concerned, the variable of general satisfaction with body was divided into two categories for the purpose of some analyses. The division was as follows: a positive emotional attitude towards ones own body (assessment: 1, 2, 3) versus a negative emotional attitude towards ones own body (assessment: 4, 5).

The following statistical methods were used: descriptive statistics, R-Pearson's correlation coefficient (R), t-Student Test (t), the analysis of variance – the ANOVA Test (F), Chi-square goodness of fit Test (χ^2), Friedman Test (χ^2), Cochran Test (Q) and The Wilcoxon signed-rank Test (Z).

RESULTS

1. Objective Body Mass

At each research stage an objective BMI was calculated on the base of an objective body mass measurement.

Among 150 females who started the therapy, 37 of them was ruled out at the first stage. It means that the reduction in their weight was less than 5%. 33 females entered the second stage. 31 of them entered the third stage, and 49 of them completed the research study. Only those examined females obtained the reduction in weight by 15%.

The one-factorial analysis of variance (ANOVA) was used to study whether the reduction in body mass during therapy was significant (table 1).

Table 1. Changes in Body Mass Index (BMI) during the weight loss therapy

Stage of cure	M	SD	ANOVA Test *			
			F	df	df	p
①	38.306	6.778				
②	36.356	6.420				
③	34.444	6.106	987.038	3	144	<0.001
④	32.443	5.790				

*N = 49.

The results proved that in fact the variable (an objective body mass, here: BMI) was changing considerably during the weight loss therapy: F (3.144)= 987.038; p<0.001.

2. Subjective Body Mass Estimation

Friedman's Chi-Square Test was used in the case of each aspect of body image to study the changes of a subjective body mass estimation in time.

As far as a declarative aspect is concerned, a statistically significant variability was observed both in the Assessment Scale of a Body Mass (χ^2=78.775; p<0.001), and in the Silhouette Test (χ^2=87.123; p<0.001) (table 2).

Table 2. Changes in subjective estimation of body mass during the weight loss therapy, in declarative aspect

Method	Stage of cure	Average rank	FriedmanTest *		
			χ^2	df	p
The Assessment Scale	①	3.36			
	②	2.71	78.775	3	<0.001
	③	2.19			
	④	1.73			
Silhouette Test	①	3.29			
	②	2.93	87.123	3	<0.001
	③	2.23			
	④	1.55			

* N = 49.

As far as a sensory aspect is concerned, a subjective body mass estimation was also changing significantly during the therapy, both in the Assessment Scale of a Body Mass (χ^2=39,963; p<0,001), and in the Silhouette Test (χ^2=60,269; p<0,01) (table 3).

Table 3. Changes in subjective estimation of body mass during the weight loss therapy, in sensory aspect

Method	Stage of cure	Average rank	Friedman Test *		
			χ^2	df	p
The Assessment Scale	①	2.98	39. 963	3	<0.001
	②	2.77			
	③	2.35			
	④	1.91			
Silhouette Test	①	3.12	60.269	3	< 0.001
	②	2.99			
	③	2.17			
	④	1.71			

* N = 49.

As far as an imaginable aspect of body image is concerned, any variability of a subjective body mass estimation was not detected, either in the Assessment Scale of a Body Mass or in the Silhouette Test (table 4).

Table 4. Changes in subjective estimation of body mass during the weight loss therapy, in imaginable aspect

Method	Stage of cure	Average rank	Friedman Test *		
			χ^2	df	p
The Assessment Scale	①	2.51	2.727	3	0.436
	②	2.63			
	③	2.37			
	④	2.49			
Silhouette Test	①	2.42	4.211	3	0.240
	②	2.66			
	③	2.58			
	④	2.34			

* N = 49.

As far as a perceptive aspect is concerned, a significant variability of body mass estimation was proved during the therapy, both in the Assessment Scale of a Body Mass (χ^2=67,728; p<0,001), and in the Silhouette Test (χ^2=88,182; df=3; p<0,001) (table 5).

Table 5. Changes in subjective estimation of body mass during the weight loss therapy, in perceptive aspect

Method	Stage of cure	Average rank	Friedman Test *		
			χ^2	df	p
The Assessment Scale	①	3.34	67.728	3	<0.001
	②	2.72			
	③	2.06			
	④	1.88			
Silhouette Test	①	3.38	88.182	3	<0.001
	②	2.99			
	③	2.01			
	④	1.62			

* N = 49.

3. Consistency of Body Image Aspects in Respect to a Subjective Body Mass Estimation

R-Spearman's correlation coefficient was calculated to analyze a mutual relation of particular body image aspects in respect to a subjective body mass estimation (table 6).

As far as the Assessment Scale of a Body Mass is concerned, when participants started the weight loss therapy, some statistically significant correlations were observed. The above mentioned correlations appeared between the following aspects: a declarative aspect and a sensory one (R=0.241; p<0.01), a declarative aspect and a perceptive one (R=0.417; p<0.01), a sensory aspect and an imaginable one (R=0.313; p<0.01), a sensory aspect and a perceptive one (R=0.229; p<0.01). During the next stages of the therapy statistically significant correlations appeared between all body image aspects: a declarative aspect and a sensory one (II:R=0.484; p<0.01; III: R =0.570; p<0.01; IV: R=0.532; p<0.01), a declarative aspect and an imaginable one (II:R=0.276; p<0.01; III: R=0.372; p<0.01; IV: R=0.357; p<0.05), a declarative aspect and a perceptive one II:R=0.492; p<0.01; III: R=0.553; p<0.01; IV: R=0.526; p<0.01), a sensory aspect and an imaginable one (II:R=0.405; p<0.01; III: R=0.335; p<0.01; IV: R=0.399; p<0.01), a sensory aspect and a perceptive one (II:R=0.470; p<0.01; III: R=0.487; p<0.01; IV: R=0.624; p<0.01), an imaginable aspect and a perceptive one (II:R=0.321; p<0.01; III: R=0.461; p<0.01; IV: R=0.454; p<0.01).

Table 6. Correlations in the case of subjective estimation of body mass, during the weight loss therapy (the Assessment Scale)

Stage of cure	Aspects	① declarative	② sensory	③ imaginable	④ perceptive
I (N = 150)	①	-	0.241**	0.090	0.417**
	②	0.241**	-	0.313**	0.229**
	③	0.090	0.313**	-	0.119
	④	0.417**	0.229**	0.119	-
II (N = 113)	①	-	0.484**	0.276**	0.492**
	②	0.484**	-	0.405**	0.470**
	③	0.276**	0.405**	-	0.321**
	④	0.492**	0.470**	0.321**	-
III (N = 80)	①	-	0.570**	0.372**	0.553**
	②	0.570**	-	0.335**	0.487**
	③	0.372**	0.335**	-	0.461**
	④	0.553**	0.487**	0.461**	-
IV (N = 49)	①	-	0.532**	0.357*	0.526**
	②	0.532**	-	0.399**	0.624**
	③	0.357*	0.399**	-	0.454**
	④	0.526**	0.624**	0.454**	-

* Correlation is statistically important at the level of 0,05 (bilateral).
** Correlation is statistically important at the level of 0,01 (bilateral).

Some additional analyses were conducted due to the probable non-linear character of the relation between the variables. The consistency between particular aspects of body image in respect of a subjective body mass estimation was studied with the use of the Chi-square goodness of fit Test.

As it is shown in table 7, at the first stage of the therapy the following aspects were significantly consistent in respect of a subjective body mass estimation: a declarative aspect and a perceptive one (χ^2=15.360; p<0.001), and a sensory aspect and a perceptive one (χ^2=4.507; p<0.05). On the other hand, the following aspects were significantly inconsistent: a declarative aspect and an imaginable one (χ^2=56.427; p<0.001), a sensory aspect and an imaginable one (χ^2=20.907; p<0.001), and a perceptive aspect and an imaginable one (χ^2=49.307; p<0.001).

As far as the second stage of the therapy is concerned, the following aspects appeared to be significantly consistent: a declarative aspect and a sensory one (χ^2=3.903; p<0.05), a declarative aspect and an imaginable one (χ^2=10.841; p<0.01), and a sensory aspect and an imaginable one (χ^2= 5.531; p<0.05). On the other hand, the following aspects appeared to be significantly inconsistent: a declarative aspect and an imaginable one (χ^2= 35.124; p<0.001), a sensory aspect and an imaginable one (χ^2=16.363; p<0.001), a sensory aspect and an imaginable one (χ^2=37.389; p<0.001).

As far as the third stage of the therapy is concerned, the following aspects proved to be significantly consistent: a declarative aspect and a sensory one (χ^2=12.800; p<0.001), a declarative aspect and a perceptive one (χ^2=11.250; p<0.01), and a sensory aspect and a perceptive one (χ^2=11.250; p<0.05). On the other hand, the following aspects were significantly inconsistent: a declarative aspect and an imaginable one (χ^2= 8.050; p<0.001), a sensory aspect and an imaginable one (χ^2=6.050; p<0.05), and a perceptive aspect and an imaginable one (χ^2=8.450; p<0.01).

At the fourth stage the following aspects were significantly consistent: a declarative aspect and a sensory one (χ^2=9.000; p<0.01), a declarative aspect and an imaginable one (χ^2=10.796; p<0.01), and a sensory aspect and a perceptive one (χ^2=9.000; p<0.05). An imaginable aspect was inconsistent with other aspects, however the inconsistency was not significant statistically.

Table 7. The consistency of the aspects of a body image in the case of a subjective estimation of body mass (the Assessment Scale)

Stage	Aspects	N	Number of consistent			Test*		
			O	E	O - E	χ^2	df	p
①	declarative vs.	150	85	75.0	10.0	2.667	1	0.102
	declarative vs. imaginable	150	29	75.0	-46.0	56.427	1	< 0.001
	declarative vs. perceptive	150	99	75.0	24.0	15.360	1	< 0.001
	sensory vs. imaginable	150	47	75.0	-28.0	20.907	1	< 0.001
	sensory vs. perceptive	150	88	75.0	13.0	4.507	1	0.034
	imaginable vs. perceptive	150	32	75.0	-43.0	49.307	1	< 0,001
②	declarative vs. sensory	113	67	56.5	10.5	3.903	1	0.048
	declarative vs. imaginable	113	25	56.5	-31.5	35.124	1	< 0.001
	declarative vs. perceptive	113	74	56.5	17.5	10.841	1	0.001
	sensory vs. imaginable	113	35	56.5	-21.5	16.363	1	< 0.001
	sensory vs. perceptive	113	69	56.5	12,5	5.531	1	0.019
	imaginable vs. perceptive	113	24	56.5	-32.5	37.389	1	< 0.001

Table 7. (Continued)

| Stage | Aspects | N | Number of consistent | | | Test* | | |
			O	E	O - E	χ^2	df	p
③	declarative vs. sensory	80	56	40.0	16.0	12.800	1	< 0.001
	declarative vs. imaginable	80	21	40.0	-19.0	18.050	1	< 0.001
	declarative vs. perceptive	80	55	40.0	15,0	11.250	1	0.001
	sensory vs. imaginable	80	29	40.0	-11.0	6.050	1	0.014
	sensory vs. perceptive	80	55	40.0	15.0	11.250	1	0.001
	imaginable vs. perceptive	80	27	40.0	-13.0	8.450	1	0.004
④	declarative vs. sensory	49	35	24.5	10.5	9.000	1	0.003
	declarative vs. imaginable	49	20	24.5	-4.5	1.653	1	0.199
	declarative vs. perceptive	49	36	24.5	11.5	10.796	1	0.001
	sensory vs. imaginable	49	28	24.5	3.5	1.000	1	0.317
	sensory vs. perceptive	49	35	24.5	10.5	9.000	1	0.003
	imaginable vs. perceptive	49	21	24.5	-3.5	1.000	1	0.317

* O - value observed
  E - value expected.

As it is seen in the above table, the same tendency was present at all stages of the therapy. The tendency was connected with the consistency of the following aspects in respect of a subjective body mass estimation: a declarative aspect, a sensory aspect and a perceptive aspect. An imaginable aspect was inconsistent with other aspects.

The same analyses as the analyses above were conducted with the use of data from the Silhouette Test. R-Spearman's correlation coefficient was calculated between particular body image aspects in respect of a subjective body mass estimation (table 8).

At each stage of the research statistically significant correlations appeared between all aspects of body image: a declarative aspect and a sensory one (I: R=0.403; p<0,01; II: R=0.643; p<0.01; III: R=0.768; p<0.01; IV: R=0.778; p<0.01), a declarative aspect and an imaginable one (I: R=0.179; p<0.05; II: R=0.282; p<0.01; III: R=0.480; p<0.01; IV:

R=0.540; p<0.01), a declarative aspect and a perceptive one (I: R=0.666; p<0.01; II: R=0.664; p<0.01; III: R=0.755; p<0.01; IV: R=0.672; p<0.01), a sensory aspect and an imaginable one (I: R=0.364; p<0.01; II: R=0.377; p<0.01; III: R=0.499; p<0.01; IV: R=0.567; p<0.01), a sensory aspect and a perceptive one (I: R=0.389; p<0.01; II: R=0.646; p<0.01; III: R=0.682; p<0.01; IV: R=0.724; p<0.01), and an imaginable aspect and a perceptive one (I: R=0.232; p<0.01; II: R=0.315; p<0.01; III: R=0.584; p<0.01; IV: R=0.532; p<0.01).

Table 8. Correlations in the case of subjective estimation of body mass, during the weight loss therapy (Silhouette Test)

Stage of cure	Aspects	① declarative	② sensory	③ imaginable	④ perceptive
I (N = 150)	①	-	0.403**	0.179*	0.666**
	②	0.403**	-	0.364**	0.389**
	③	0.179*	0.364**	-	0.232**
	④	0.666**	0.389**	0.232**	-
II (N = 113)	①	-	0.643**	0.282**	0.664**
	②	0.643**	-	0.377**	0.646**
	③	0.282**	0.377**	-	0.315**
	④	0.664**	0.646**	0.315**	-
III (N = 80)	①	-	0.768**	0.480**	0.755**
	②	0.768**	-	0.499**	0.682**
	③	0.480**	0.499**	-	0.584**
	④	0.755**	0.682**	0.584**	-
IV (N = 49)	①	-	0.778**	0.540**	0.672**
	②	0.778**	-	0.567**	0.724**
	③	0.540**	0.567**	-	0.532**
	④	0.672**	0.724**	0.532**	-

* Correlation is statistically important at the level of 0,05 (bilateral).
** Correlation is statistically important at the level of 0,01 (bilateral).

As is the case of the data from the Assessment Scale of a Body Mass, the Chi-square goodness of fit Test was conducted in respect of the Silhouette Test. The table below (Table 9) presents the results of consistency concerning particular body image aspects in respect of a subjective body mass estimation at all stages of the weight loss therapy.

As far as the first stage of the therapy is concerned, the following aspects were significantly consistent in respect of a subjective body mass estimation: a declarative aspect and a sensory one ($\chi^2=32.667$; p<0.001), a declarative aspect and a perceptive one ($\chi^2=96.000$; p<0.001), and a sensory aspect and a perceptive one ($\chi^2=34.560$; p<0.01). On the other hand, the following aspects were significantly inconsistent: a declarative aspect and an imaginable one ($\chi^2=54.000$; p<0.001), a sensory aspect and an imaginable one ($\chi^2=29.040$; p<0.001), and a perceptive aspect and an imaginable one ($\chi^2=44.827$; p<0.001).

Table 9. The consistency of the aspects of a body image in the case of a subjective estimation of body mass (Silhouette Test)

Stage	Aspects	N	Number of consistent estimates			Test*		
			O	E	O - E	χ^2	df	p
①	declarative vs.	150	110	75.0	35.0	32.667	1	< 0.001
	declarative vs. imaginable	150	30	75.0	-45.0	54.000	1	< 0.001
	declarative vs. perceptive	150	135	75.0	60.0	96.000	1	< 0.001
	sensory vs. imaginable	150	42	75.0	-33.0	29.040	1	< 0.001
	sensory vs. perceptive	150	111	75.0	36.0	34.560	1	< 0.001
	imaginable vs. perceptive	150	34	75.0	-41.0	44.827	1	< 0.001
②	declarative vs. sensory	113	80	56.5	23.5	19.549	1	< 0.001
	declarative vs. imaginable	113	27	56.5	-29.5	30.805	1	< 0.001
	declarative vs. perceptive	113	88	56.5	31.5	35.124	1	< 0.001
	sensory vs. imaginable	113	37	56.5	-19.5	13.460	1	< 0.001
	sensory vs. perceptive	113	80	56.5	23.5	19.549	1	< 0.001
	imaginable vs. perceptive	113	25	56.5	-31.5	35.124	1	< 0.001
③	declarative vs. sensory	80	56	40.0	16.0	12.800	1	< 0.001
	declarative vs. imaginable	80	21	40.0	-19.0	18.050	1	< 0.001
	declarative vs. perceptive	80	60	40.0	20.0	20.000	1	< 0.001
	sensory vs. imaginable	80	24	40.0	-16.0	12.800	1	< 0.001
	sensory vs. perceptive	80	60	40.0	20.0	20.000	1	< 0.001
	imaginable vs. perceptive	80	22	40.0	-18.0	16.200	1	< 0.001

Table 9. (Continued).

Stage	Aspects	N	Number of consistent estimates			Test*		
			O	E	O - E	χ^2	df	p
④	declarative vs. sensory	49	35	24.5	10.5	9.000	1	0.003
	declarative vs. imaginable	49	21	24.5	-3.5	1.000	1	0.317
	declarative vs. perceptive	49	32	24.5	7.5	4.592	1	0.032
	sensory vs. imaginable	49	24	24.5	-0.5	0.020	1	0.886
	sensory vs. perceptive	49	36	24.5	11.5	10.796	1	0.001
	imaginable vs. perceptive	49	20	24.5	-4.5	1.653	1	0.199

* O - value observed
E - value expected.

As far as the second stage of the therapy is concerned, the following aspects appeared to be significantly consistent: a declarative aspect and a sensory one (χ^2=19.549; p<0.001), a declarative aspect and a perceptive one (χ^2=35.124; p<0.001), and a sensory aspect and a perceptive one (χ^2=19.549; p<0.001). The following aspects were significantly inconsistent: a declarative aspect and an imaginable one (χ^2=30.805; p<0.001), a sensory aspect and an imaginable one (χ^2=13.460; p<0.001), and a perceptive aspect and an imaginable one (χ^2=35.124; p<0.001).

At the third stage of the therapy the following aspects proved to be significantly consistent: a declarative aspect and a sensory one (χ^2=12.800; p<0.001), a declarative aspect and a perceptive one (χ^2=20.000; p<0.001), and a sensory aspect and a perceptive one (χ^2=20.000; p<0.001). The following aspects were significantly inconsistent: a declarative aspect and an imaginable one (χ^2=18.050; p<0.001), a sensory aspect and an imaginable one (χ^2=12.800; p<0.001), and a perceptive aspect and an imaginable one (χ^2=16.200; p<0.001).

As far as the fourth stage of the therapy is concerned, a significant consistency was observed between the following aspects: a declarative aspect and a sensory one (χ^2=9.000; p<0.01), a declarative aspect and a perceptive one (χ^2=4.592; p<0.05), and a sensory aspect and a perceptive one (χ^2= 10.796; p<0.01). An imaginable aspect was not consistent with other aspects, however the inconsistency was not significant statistically.

As it is seen in the above table, the following aspects: a declarative aspect, a sensory aspect and a perceptive aspect, were significantly consistent in respect of a subjective body mass estimation at all stages of the therapy. An imaginable aspect was inconsistent with other aspects, however the inconsistency was statistically significant at the first three stages.

4. The Adequacy of a Subjective Body Mass Estimation

The adequacy of a subjective body mass estimation with respect to the examined females was analyzed. The adequacy of a subjective body mass estimation means the consistency of a subjective body mass estimation with an objective body mass. The adequacy was examined with the use of the Chi-square goodness of fit Test.

As far as a declarative aspect is concerned (table 10), using the Assessment Scale of a Body Mass most of the examined females estimated their body mass adequately to reality only at the beginning of the therapy. However, the consistency was not significant. At the next stages of the research the participants declared their body mass significantly inadequate to an objective body mass. The situation appeared after reduction in body weight by 5% (χ^2=7.442; p<0.01), by 10% (χ^2=11.250; p<0.01), and by 15% (χ^2=12.755; p<0.001). As far as the Silhouette Test is concerned, the examined females estimated their body mass adequately to reality at the first stage (χ^2=80.667; p<0.001) and at the second stage (χ^2=19.549; p<0.001). At the third stage the proportion of females who estimated themselves adequately and inadequately was even. However, at the fourth stage the number of females who estimated their body mass inadequately prevailed (χ^2=4.592; p<0.05).

Table 10. The adequacy of a subjective estimation of body mass in declarative aspect

| Adequacy | Method | Stage of cure | N | Number of adequate estimates | | | Test* | | |
				O	E	O - E	χ^2	df	p
Declarative BMI vs. Objective BMI	The Assessment Scale	①	150	85	75.0	10.0	2.667	1	0.102
		②	113	42	56.5	-14.5	7.442	1	0.006
		③	80	25	40.0	-15.0	11.250	1	0.001
		④	49	12	24.5	-12.5	12.755	1	<0.001
	Silhouette Test	①	150	130	75.0	55.0	80.667	1	<0.001
		②	113	80	56.5	23.5	19.549	1	<0.001
		③	80	39	40.0	1.0	0.050	1	0.823
		④	49	17	24.5	-7.5	4.592	1	0.032

* O - value observed
E - value expected.

The test for dichotomous variables – the Cochran Test, was used to study whether during the weight loss therapy the adequacy of a subjective body mass estimation in respect of a declarative aspect was changing. The results showed that the variability was significant in both the Assessment Scale of a Body Mass (Q=21.578; p<0.001), and the Silhouette Test (Q=43.108; p<0.001). Upon the reduction in body weight, the adequacy of an estimation was decreasing, on the other hand, the inadequacy was increasing (table 11).

Table 11. Changes in the adequacy of a subjective assessment of body mass during the weight loss therapy, in declarative aspect

Method	Stage of cure	Percentage of adequacy	Cochran Test *		
			Q	df	p
The Assessment Scale	①	65.3	21.578	3	< 0.001
	②	38.8			
	③	28.6			
	④	24.5			
Silhouette Test	①	89.8	43.108	3	< 0.001
	②	67.3			
	③	51.0			
	④	34.7			

* N = 49.

As far as a sensory aspect is concerned (table 12), in the case of the Assessment Scale of a Body Mass, the participants estimated their body mass significantly inadequately to reality at all stages of the therapy: at the first stage (χ^2=27.303; p<0.001), at the second stage (χ^2=24.858; p<0.001), at the third stage (χ^2=28.800; p<0.001) and at the fourth stage (χ^2=22.224; p<0.001). In the case of the Silhouette Test an adequate body mass estimation significantly prevailed at the first stage (χ^2=22.427; p<0.001) and at the second stage (χ^2=3.903; p<0.05). At the third stage (χ^2=5.000; p<0.05) and at the fourth stage (χ^2=10.796; p<0.01) participants estimated themselves significantly inadequately to reality.

The test of data with the use of the Cochran Test showed that (table 13) during the weight loss therapy the adequacy of body mass estimation in respect of a sensory aspect was not changing significantly in the case of the Assessment Scale of a Body Mass. During the whole research process the number of inadequate estimations prevailed and maintained at a constant level. The number of adequate estimations decreased slightly. In the case of the Silhouette Test the adequacy of a subjective body mass estimation was changing significantly (Q=25.114; p<0.001) during the therapy. The number of adequate estimations was decreasing, and the number of inadequate estimations was increasing.

Table 12. The adequacy of a subjective estimation of body mass in sensory aspect

Adequacy	Method		Stage of cure	N	Number of adequate			Test*		
					O	E	O - E	χ^2	df	p
Declarative BMI vs. Objective BMI	The Assessment Scale	①		150	43	75.0	-32.0	27.307	1	< 0.001
		②		113	30	56.5	-26.5	24.858	1	< 0.001
		③		80	16	40.0	-24.0	28.800	1	< 0.001
		④		49	8	24.5	-16.5	22.224	1	< 0.001
	Silhouette Test	①		150	104	75.0	29.0	22.427	1	<0.001
		②		113	67	56.5	10.5	3.903	1	0.048
		③		80	30	40.0	-10.0	5.000	1	0.025
		④		49	13	24.5	-11.5	10.796	1	0.001

* O - value observed.
 E - value expected.

Table 13. Changes in the adequacy of a subjective assessment of body mass during the weight loss therapy, in sensory aspect

Method		Stage of cure	Percentage of adequacy	Cochran Test *		
				Q	df	p
The Assessment Scale		①	28.6			
		②	26.5	2.935	3	0.402
		③	20.4			
		④	16.3			
Silhouette Test		①	71.4			
		②	57.1	25.114	3	<0.001
		③	36.7			
		④	26.5			

* N = 49.

In the case of an imaginable aspect it was showed that (table 14) in both the Assessment Scale of a Body Mass and the Silhouette Test the number of inadequate body mass estimations prevailed over the number of adequate estimatios. The difference was statistically significant at all research stages: at the first stage (the Assessment Scale of a Body Mass: χ^2=89.707; p<0.001; the Silhouette Test: χ^2=58.907; p<0.001), at the second stage (The Assessment Scale of a Body Mass: χ^2=63.938; p<0.001; the Silhouette Test: χ^2=42.133;

p<0.001), at the third stage (the Assessment Scale of a Body Mass: χ^2=57.800; p<0.001; the Silhouette Test: χ^2=36.450; p<0.001) and at the fourth stage (the Assessment Scale of a Body Mass: χ^2=37.735; p<0.001; the Silhouette Test: χ^2=31.041; p<0.001).

Table 14. The adequacy of a subjective estimation of body mass in imaginable aspect

Adequacy	Method	Stage of cure	N	Number of adequate			Test*		
				O	E	O - E	χ^2	df	p
Declarative BMI vs. Objective BMI	The Assessment Scale	①	150	17	75.0	-58.0	89.707	1	<0.001
		②	113	14	56.5	-42.5	63.938	1	<0.001
		③	80	6	40.0	-34.0	57.800	1	<0.001
		④	49	3	24.5	-21.5	37.735	1	<0.001
	Silhouette Test	①	150	28	75.0	-47.0	58.907	1	<0.001
		②	113	22	56.5	-34.5	42.133	1	<0.001
		③	80	13	40.0	-27.0	36.450	1	<0.001
		④	49	5	24.5	-19.5	31.041	1	<0.001

* O - value observed .
E - value expected.

The test of data with the use of the Cochran Test showed that (table 15) during the weight loss therapy the adequacy of a subjective body mass estimation was not changing significantly in either the Assessment Scale of a Body Mass or the Silhouette Test. In both cases the number of inadequate estimations was relatively constant. In the case of the Assessment Scale of a Body Mass the number of adequate estimations was decreasing slightly. In the case of the Silhouette Test the number of adequate estimations was fluctuating – the largest number of adequate estimations appeared when the reduction of body weight was by 10 %.

Table 15. Changes in the adequacy of a subjective assessment of body mass during the weight loss therapy, in imaginable aspect

Method	Stage of cure	Percentage of adequacy	Cochran Test *		
			Q	df	p
The Assessment Scale	①	12.2	2.308	3	0.511
	②	10.2			
	③	8.2			
	④	6.1			
Silhouette Test	①	14.3	5.364	3	0.147
	②	18.4			
	③	20.4			
	④	10.2			

* N = 49.

In the case of a perceptive aspect it was showed that (table 16) at all stages of the weight loss therapy the inadequacy of a subjective body mass estimation prevailed in the Assessment Scale of a Body Mass. The results were statistically significant at the following stages: the second stage (χ^2=6.451; p<0.05), the third stage (χ^2=18.050; p<0.001) and the fourth stage (χ^2=12.755; p<0.001). In the case of the Silhouette Test participants gave significantly more adequate body mass estimations than inadequate ones at the first stage (χ^2=64.027; p<0.01) and at the second stage (χ^2=19.549; p<0.01). In the case of the last two stages the tendency reversed – the number of inadequate estimations prevailed over the number of adequate estimations. At the fourth stage the result reached a statistical variability (χ^2=5.898; p<0.05).

Table 16. The adequacy of a subjective estimation of body mass in perceptive aspect

Adequacy	Method	Stage of cure	N	Number of adequate estimates			Test*		
				O	E	O - E	χ^2	df	p
Declarative BMI vs. Objective BMI	The Assessment Scale	①	150	71	75.0	-4.0	0.427	1	0.514
		②	113	43	56.5	-3.5	6.451	1	0.011
		③	80	21	40.0	-9.0	18.050	1	<0.001
		④	49	12	24.5	-2.5	12.755	1	<0.001
	Silhouette Test	①	150	124	75.0	49.0	64.027	1	<0.001
		②	113	80	56.5	23.5	19.549	1	<0.001
		③	80	34	40.0	-6.0	1.800	1	0.180
		④	49	16	24.5	-8.5	5.898	1	0.015

* O - value observed .
  E - value expected.

The test of data with the use of the Cochran Test showed that (table 17) during the weight loss therapy a subjective body mass estimation was changing significantly in the Assessment Scale of a Body Mass (Q=18.677; p<0.01). From the beginning of the therapy to the moment of reaching the reduction in body weight by 10% the number of adequate estimations was decreasing, and the number of inadequate estimations was increasing. At the fourth stage the proportion of adequate estimations to inadequate ones was identical as in the third stage. In the Silhouette Test the adequacy of a subjective body mass estimation was changing significantly (Q=51.283; p<0.01), too. At the next stages of the therapy the number of adequate estimations was decreasing successively, and the number of inadequate estimations was increasing.

Table 17. Changes in the adequacy of a subjective assessment of body mass during the weight loss therapy, in perceptive aspect

Method	Stage of cure	Percentage of adequacy	Cochran Test *		
			Q	df	p
The Assessment Scale	①	59.2	18.677	3	<0.001
	②	34.7			
	③	24.5			
	④	24.5			
Silhouette Test	①	89.8	51.283	3	<0.001
	②	73.5			
	③	38.8			
	④	32.7			

* N = 49.

5. The Consistency of Particular Body Image Aspects with Respect to the Adequacy of a Subjective Body Mass Estimation

The Cochran Test for dichotomous variables was used to compare whether particular body image aspects are consistent with each other in respect of the adequacy of a subjective body mass estimation. The table below (table 18) shows the results of analyzing the data from the Assessment Scale of a Body Mass.

At the beginning of the therapy body image aspects were inconsistent with each other. Some significant differences appeared between the following aspects: a declarative aspect and a sensory one (Q=31.500; p<0.001), a declarative aspect and an imaginable one (Q=64.222; p<0.001), a declarative aspect and a perceptive one (Q=4.261; p<0.001), a sensory aspect and an imaginable one (Q=21.125; p<0.001), a sensory aspect and a perceptive one (Q=15.077; p<0.001), an imaginable aspect and a perceptive one (Q=50.276; p<0.001). The examined females declared the most adequate estimations of their body mass in the case of a declarative aspect, then, a perceptive aspect, and finally, a sensory aspect. The least adequate estimations of body mass appeared in the case of an imaginable aspect.

At the second stage of the therapy significant differences in respect of the adequacy of body mass estimation appeared between the following aspects: a declarative aspect and a sensory one (Q=4.800; p<0.05), a declarative aspect and an imaginable one (Q=20.632; p<0.001), a sensory aspect and an imaginable one (Q=21.125; p<0.01), a sensory aspect and a perceptive one (Q=6.760; p<0.01), an imaginable aspect and a perceptive one (Q=22.730; p<0.001). In the case of a declarative aspect and a perceptive one, the estimations become even. It means that participants estimated their body mass adequately, similarly as in the case when they estimated their body mass on the basis of their sight in the mirror.

Table 18. Differences between the aspects of a body image in the case of an adequacy of subjective assessment of body mass, during the weight loss therapy (te Assessment Scale)

Stage	Aspect	Estimate		N	Cochran Test		
		adequate	inadequate		Q	df	p
①	declarative vs. sensory	65	85	150	31.500	1	< 0.001
		107	43				
	declarative vs. imaginable	65	85		64.222	1	< 0.001
		133	17				
	declarative vs. perceptive	65	85		4.261	1	< 0.001
		79	71				
	sensory vs. imaginable	107	43		21.125	1	< 0001
		133	17				
	sensory vs. perceptive	107	43		15.077	1	< 0.001
		79	71				
	imaginable vs. perceptive	133	17		50.276	1	< 0.001
		79	71				
②	declarative vs. sensory	71	42	133	4.800	1	0.028
		83	30				
	declarative vs. imaginable	71	42		20.632	1	< 0.001
		99	14				
	declarative vs. perceptive	71	42		0.032	1	0.857
		70	43				
	sensory vs. imaginable	83	30		10.667	1	0.001
		99	14				
	sensory vs. perceptive	83	30		6.760	1	0.009
		70	43				
	imaginable vs. perceptive	99	14		22.730	1	< 0.001
		70	43				
③	declarative vs. sensory	55	25	80	6.231	1	0.013
		64	16				
	declarative vs. imaginable	55	25		17.190	1	< 0.001
		74	6				
	declarative vs. perceptive	55	25		1.143	1	0.285
		59	21				
	sensory vs. imaginable	64	16		7.143	1	0.008
		74	6				
	sensory vs. perceptive	64	16		2.273	1	0.132
		59	21				
	imaginable vs. perceptive	74	6		13.235	1	< 0.001
		59	21				

Table 18. (Continued).

Stage	Aspect	Estimate		N	Cochran Test		
		adequate	inadequate		Q	df	p
④	declarative vs. sensory	37	12	49	2.667	1	0.102
		41	8				
	declarative vs. imaginable	37	12		7.364	1	0.007
		46	3				
	declarative vs. perceptive	37	12		0.000	1	1.000
		37	12				
	sensory vs. imaginable	41	8		3.571	1	0.059
		46	3				
	sensory vs. perceptive	41	8		2.667	1	0.102
		37	12				
	imaginable vs. perceptive	46	3		7.364	1	0.007
		37	12				

At the third stage of the therapy significant differences appeared between the following aspects: a declarative aspect and a sensory one ($Q=6.31$; $p<0.05$), a declarative aspect and an imaginable one ($Q=17.190$; $p<0.001$), a sensory aspect and an imaginable one ($Q=7.143$; $p<0.01$), an imaginable aspect and a perceptive one ($Q=13.235$; $p<0.001$).

At the fourth stage of the therapy significant differences appeared between the following aspects: a declarative aspect and an imaginable one ($Q=7.364$; $p<0.01$), and an imaginable aspect and a perceptive one ($Q=7.364$; $p<0.01$).

The data from the Silhouette Test (Table 19) were analyzed in the same way as above. At the first stage of the weight loss therapy there were significant differences in respect of a subjective body mass estimation between the following aspects: a declarative aspect and a sensory one ($Q=17.789$; $p<0.001$), a declarative aspect and an imaginable one ($Q=100.038$; $p<0.001$), a sensory aspect and an imaginable one ($Q=74.051$; $p<0.001$), a sensory aspect and a perceptive one ($Q=10.526$; $p<0.01$), and an imaginable aspect and a perceptive one ($Q=96.000$; $p<0.001$).

At the second stage of the therapy significant differences appeared between the following aspects: a declarative aspect and a sensory one ($Q=6.259$; $p<0.05$), a declarative aspect and an imaginable one ($Q=52.563$; $p<0.001$), a sensory aspect and an imaginable one ($Q=41.327$; $p<0,001$), a sensory aspect and a perceptive one ($Q=6.259$; $p<0.05$), and an imaginable aspect and a perceptive one ($Q=49.471$; $p<0.001$).

At the third stage of the therapy significant differences appeared between the following aspects: a declarative aspect and a sensory one ($Q=5.400$; $p<0.05$), a declarative aspect and an imaginable one ($Q=21.125$; $p<0.001$), a sensory aspect and an imaginable one ($Q=9.966$; $p<0.01$), and an imaginable aspect and a perceptive one ($Q=15.207$; $p<0.001$).

At the fourth stage of the therapy there was statistically significant difference between the following aspects: a declarative aspect and an imaginable one ($Q=9.000$; $p<0.01$), a sensory aspect and an imaginable one ($Q=5.333$; $p<0.05$), and an imaginable aspect and a perceptive one ($Q=8.067$; $p<0.01$).

Table 19. Differences between the aspects of a body image in the case of an adequacy of subjective assessment of body mass, during the weight loss therapy (Silhouette Test)

Stage	Aspect	Estimate		Stage	Cochran Test		
		adequate	inadequate		Q	df	p
①	declarative vs. sensory	20	130	150	17.789	1	< 0.001
		46	104				
	declarative vs. imaginable	20	130		100.038	1	< 0.001
		122	28				
	declarative vs. perceptive	20	130		2.571	1	0.109
		26	124				
	sensory vs. imaginable	46	104		74,051	1	< 0.001
		122	28				
	sensory vs. perceptive	46	104		10.526	1	0.001
		26	124				
	imaginable vs. perceptive	122	28		96.000	1	< 0.001
		26	124				
②	declarative vs. sensory	33	80	133	6.259	1	0.012
		46	67				
	declarative vs. imaginable	33	80		52.563	1	< 0.001
		91	22				
	declarative vs. perceptive	33	80		0.000	1	1.000
		33	80				
	sensory vs. imaginable	46	67		41.327	1	< 0.001
		91	22				
	sensory vs. perceptive	46	67		6.259	1	0.012
		33	80				
	imaginable vs. perceptive	91	22		49.471	1	< 0.001
		33	80				
③	declarative vs. sensory	41	39	80	5.400	1	0.020
		50	30				
	declarative vs. imaginable	41	39		21.125	1	< 0.001
		67	13				
	declarative vs. perceptive	41	39		1.667	1	0.197
		46	34				
	sensory vs. imaginable	50	30		9.966	1	0.002
		67	13				
	sensory vs. perceptive	50	30		1.000	1	0.317
		46	34				
	imaginable vs. perceptive	67	13		15.207	1	< 0.001
		46	34				

Table 19. (Continued).

Stage	Aspect	Estimate		Stage	Cochran Test		
		adequate	inadequate		Q	df	p
④	declarative vs. sensory	32	17	49	1.600	1	0.206
		36	13				
	declarative vs. imaginable	32	17		9.000	1	0.003
		44	5				
	declarative vs. perceptive	32	17		0.077	1	0.782
		33	16				
	sensory vs. imaginable	36	13		5.333	1	0.021
		44	5				
	sensory vs. perceptive	36	13		1.000	1	0.317
		33	16				
	imaginable vs. perceptive	44	5		8.067	1	0.005
		33	16				

6. Satisfaction with Ones Own Body

To determine a participant's emotional attitude towards her body, the average from all six detailed scales was assigned to one out of two categories: a positive attitude and a negative attitude. The Cochran Test was used to study the data transformed in the above mentioned way.

The test results proved that during the weight loss therapy in respect of a declarative aspect an emotional attitude towards body was changing significantly ($Q=31.299$; $p<0.001$) (table 20). At the beginning of the therapy most of participants assessed their body more positively than negatively. With the passage of time the number of positive assessments was increasing, and the number of negative assessments was decreasing.

Table 20. Changes in the emotional attitude towards ones own body during the weight loss therapy, in declarative aspect

Stage of cure	Percentage of positive estimates	Cochran Test *		
		Q	df	p
①	63.3	31.299	3	<0.001
②	75.5			
③	93.9			
④	95.9			

* N = 49.

The Friedman's chi^2 Test was used to study the variability of the assessment of the dimensions during the therapy. As it is presented in a table below (table 21), at the particular stages of the research the average ranks concerning a general satisfaction with ones own body and its particular dimensions were decreasing, which means that the number of positive assessments was increasing. During the therapy participants' satisfaction increased significantly in respect of all dimensions: attractiveness ($\chi^2=82.14$; p<0.001), charm ($\chi^2=52.05$; p<0.001), agility ($\chi^2=59.79$; p<0.001), shapeliness ($\chi^2=71.80$; p<0.001), proportionality ($\chi^2=40.58$; p<0.001), and firmness ($\chi^2=29.19$; p<0.001). In connection with the above, a general satisfaction (which is a total assessment from all detailed scales) with body increased significantly ($\chi^2=91.25$; p<0.001), too.

Table 21. The assemssment of each dimension of body imane during the weight loss therapy, in declarative aspect

Dimension	Stage of cure*				Friedman Test **		
	①	②	③	④	χ^2	df	p
attractiveness	3.39	2.82	2.21	1.58	82.142	3	< 0.001
charm	3.09	2.69	2.32	1.90	52.051	3	< 0.001
agility	3.18	2.83	2.29	1.70	59.791	3	< 0.001
shapeliness	3.34	2.76	2.30	1.61	71.803	3	< 0.001
proportionality	3.01	2.78	2.37	1.85	40.581	3	< 0.001
firmness	2.92	2.64	2.48	1.96	29.191	3	< 0.001
general satisfaction	3.61	2.88	2.18	1.33	91.251	3	< 0.001

* Average ranks.
** N = 49.

As far as a sensory aspect is concerned, an emotional attitude towards body was changing significantly (Q=22.444; p<0.001) during the therapy (table 22). At the beginning of the therapy there were more participants who declared a positive attitude towards their body than those who declared a negative attitude. The proportion maintained until the end of the research.

Table 22. Changes in the emotional attitude towards ones own body during the weight loss therapy, in sensory aspect

Stage of cure	Percentage of positive estimates	Cochran Test *		
		Q	df	p
①	75.5			
②	77.6			
③	95.9	22.444	3	<0.001
④	98.0			

* N = 49.

During the therapy participants' satisfaction was changing significantly in respect of all dimensions: attractiveness (χ^2=42.228; p<0.001), charm (χ^2=37.432; p<0.001), agility (χ^2=40.96; p<0.001), shapeliness (χ^2=62.03; p<0.001), proportionality (χ^2=44.644; p<0.001), and firmness (χ^2=17.045; p<0.01). Automatically, a general satisfaction with body increased significantly (χ^2=56.882; p<0.001) (table 23).

Table 23. The assemssment of each dimension of body imane during the weight loss therapy, in sensory aspect

Dimension	Stage of cure*				Friedman Test **		
	①	②	③	④	χ^2	df	p
attractiveness	3.03	2.84	2.20	1.93	42.228	3	< 0.001
charm	2.84	2.78	2.51	1.88	37.432	3	< 0.001
agility	2.91	2.90	2.34	1.86	40.960	3	< 0.001
shapeliness	3.08	2.98	2.33	1.61	62.030	3	< 0.001
proportionality	2.95	2.83	2.41	1.82	44.644	3	< 0.001
firmness	2.74	2.72	2.48	2.05	17.045	3	0.001
general satisfaction	3.16	3.01	2.32	1.51	56.882	3	< 0.001

* Average ranks.
** N = 49.

As it is seen in the above table, at the particular stages of the research the average ranks concerning a general satisfaction with body and its particular aspects were decreasing significantly, which means that the number of positive assessments increased significantly.

As far as an imaginable aspect is concerned, during the whole therapy there were more people who declared a positive emotional attitude towards their body than those who declared a negative emotional attitude. A positive attitude towards body intensified significantly upon the reduction in body weight (Q=8.250; p<0.05) (table 24).

Table 24. Changes in the emotional attitude towards ones own body during the weight loss therapy, in imaginable aspect

Stage of cure	Percentage of positive estimates	Cochran Test *		
		Q	df	p
①	89.8			
②	93.9			
③	98.0	8.250	3	0.041
④	98.0			

* N = 49.

As it is seen in the table below (table 25), at the particular stages of the research the average ranks concerning a general satisfaction with body and its particular aspects changed significantly only in respect of the following categories: charm (χ^2=8.243; p<0.05) and shapeliness (χ^2=8.958; p<0.05).

Table 25. The assemssment of each dimension of body imane during the weight loss therapy, in imaginable aspect

Dimension	Stage of cure*				Friedman Test **		
	①	②	③	④	χ^2	df	p
attractiveness	2.57	2.53	2.63	2.27	5.155	3	0.161
charm	2.57	2.61	2.61	2.20	8.243	3	0.041
agility	2.34	2.60	2.63	2.43	3.793	3	0.285
shapeliness	2.47	2.64	2.67	2.21	8.958	3	0.030
proportionality	2.59	2.59	2.59	2.22	6.719	3	0.081
firmness	2.39	2.58	2.62	2.41	2.651	3	0.449
general satisfaction	2.48	2.64	2.72	2.15	7.582	3	0.055

* Average ranks.
** N = 49.

As far as a perceptive aspect is concerned, an emotional attitude towards body was changing significantly (Q=40.880; p<0.001) during the therapy (table 26). At the beginning of the therapy there were more people who declared a positive attitude towards their body than those who declared a negative attitude. Upon the reduction in body weight, the number of people with a positive attitude towards their body increased, and the number of people who assessed themselves in a negative way decreased.

Table 26. Changes in the emotional attitude towards ones own body during the weight loss therapy, in perceptive aspect

Stage of cure	Percentage of positive estimates	Cochran Test *		
		Q	df	p
①	53.1			
②	71.4	40.880	3	<0.001
③	91.8			
④	95.9			

* N = 49.

All the following dimensions were subject to a significant change: attractiveness (χ^2=83.547; p<0.001), charm (χ^2=54.401; p<0.001), agility (χ^2=42.88; p<0.001), shapeliness (χ^2=78.72; p<0.001), proportionality (χ^2=59.458; p<0.001), and firmness (χ^2=32.327; p<0.001). A general satisfaction with body (table 27) increased significantly (χ^2=85.752; p<0.001), too.

Table 27. The assemssment of each dimension of body imane during the weight loss therapy, in perceptive aspect

Dimension	Stage of cure*				Friedman Test **		
	①	②	③	④	χ^2	df	p
attractiveness	3.46	2.87	2.06	1.61	83.547	3	< 0.001
charm	3.18	2.65	2.30	1.87	54.401	3	< 0.001
agility	3.13	2.72	2.24	1.90	42.880	3	< 0.001
shapeliness	3.42	2.90	2.00	1.68	78.720	3	< 0.001
proportionality	3.22	2.82	2.16	1.80	59.458	3	< 0.001
firmness	2.99	2.68	2.42	1.91	32.327	3	< 0.001
general satisfaction	3.66	2.77	2.08	1.49	85.752	3	< 0.001

*.Average ranks.
**.N = 49.

As it is presented above, at the particular stages of the research the average ranks concerning a general satisfaction with body and its particular aspects decreased significantly, which means that the number of positive assessments increased significantly.

7. The Consistency of Particular Body Image Aspects in Respect of Satisfaction with Body

The Wilcoxon signed-rank Test was used to study the differences between body image aspects in respect of satisfaction with body. A general satisfaction (which is a total assessment from all six detailed scales) with body was analyzed. The test results in respect of each research stage are presented in a table below (table 28).

At the first stage of the therapy, there were significant differences in respect of satisfaction with body between the following aspects: a declarative aspect and a sensory one (Z=-3.095; p<0.01), a declarative aspect and an imaginable one (Z=-9.460; p<0.001), a sensory aspect and an imaginable one (Z=-9.345; p<0.001), a sensory aspect and a perceptive one (Z=-4.474; p<0.001), and an imaginable aspect and a perceptive one (Z=-9.455; p<0.001). There were no differences between a declarative aspect and a perceptive one in respect of satisfaction.

At the second stage of the therapy, there were significant differences between the following aspects: a declarative aspect and a sensory one (Z=-1.988; p<0.05), a declarative aspect and an imaginable one (Z=-7.890; p<0.001), a sensory aspect and an imaginable one (Z=-8.015; p<0.001), a sensory aspect and a perceptive one (Z=-3.703; p<0.001), and an imaginable aspect and a perceptive one (Z=-8.018; p<0.001). At this stage of therapy there were no significant differences between a declarative aspect and a perceptive one, either.

Table 28. Differences between the aspects of a body image during the weight loss therapy, in the case of the emotional attitude towards ones own body

Stage	Aspects	N	M1	M2	Average rank -	Average rank +	Wilcoxon Test Z	Wilcoxon Test p
①	declarative vs. sensory	150	20.62	19.75	51.38	64.69	-3.095	0.002
	declarative vs. imaginable	150	20.62	14.49	25.58	72.65	-9.460	< 0.001
	declarative vs. perceptive	150	20.62	20.97	60.57	54.66	-1.689	0.091
	sensory vs. imaginable	150	19.75	14.49	27.14	70.59	-9.345	< 0.001
	sensory vs. perceptive	150	19.75	20.97	63.46	53.60	-4.474	< 0.001
	imaginable vs. perceptive	150	14.49	20.97	72.18	19.19	-9.455	< 0.001
②	declarative vs. sensory	113	19.22	18.79	38.97	41.47	-1.988	0.047
	declarative vs. imaginable	113	19.22	14.47	26.65	54.20	-7.890	< 0.001
	declarative vs. perceptive	113	19.22	19.87	50.60	39.13	-1.959	0.050
	sensory vs. imaginable	113	18.79	14.47	15.23	53.83	-8.015	< 0.001
	sensory vs. perceptive	113	18.79	19.87	46.81	40.85	-3.703	< 0.001
	imaginable vs. perceptive	113	14.47	19.87	52.06	20.75	-8.018	< 0.001
③	declarative vs. sensory	80	17.88	16.95	25.00	29.13	-3.333	0.001
	declarative vs. imaginable	80	17.88	13.58	15.90	35.98	-6.697	< 0.001
	declarative vs. perceptive	80	17.88	17.76	29.95	30.98	-0.569	0.569
	sensory vs. imaginable	80	16.95	13.58	7.21	35.61	-6.640	< 0.001
	sensory vs. perceptive	80	16.95	17.76	28.74	23.89	-2.339	0.019
	imaginable vs. perceptive	80	13.58	17.76	35.56	14.70	-6.669	< 0.001
④	declarative vs. sensory	49	16.10	15.41	18.65	19.94	-1.875	0.061
	declarative vs. imaginable	49	16.10	13.18	15.17	19.87	-4.726	< 0.001
	declarative vs. perceptive	49	16.10	16.18	18.07	15.12	-0.132	0.895
	sensory vs. imaginable	49	15.41	13.18	8.93	21.89	-4.488	< 0.001
	sensory vs. perceptive	49	15.41	16.18	19.15	17.21	-2.016	0.044
	imaginable vs. perceptive	49	13.18	16.18	22.64	17.10	-4.693	< 0.001

At the third stage of the therapy there were differences in respect of satisfaction with body between the following aspects: a declarative aspect and a sensory one (Z=-3.333; p<0.01), a declarative aspect and an imaginable one (Z=-6.697; p<0.001), a sensory aspect and an imaginable one (Z=-6.640; p<0.001), a sensory aspect and a perceptive one (Z=-2.339; p<0.05), and an imaginable aspect and a perceptive one (Z=-6.669; p<0.001). There were no significant difference only between a declarative aspect and a perceptive one, either.

At the last stage of the therapy there were significant differences in respect of satisfaction with body between the following aspects: a declarative aspect and an imaginable one (Z=-4.726; p<0.001), a sensory aspect and an imaginable one (Z=-4.488; p<0.001), a sensory aspect and a perceptive one (Z=-2.016; p<0.05), and an imaginable aspect and a perceptive one (Z=-4.693; p<0.001). There were no significant differences between a declarative aspect and a perceptive one, and between a declarative aspect and a sensory one.

As it is seen in the table above, at all stages of the therapy there was a similar regularity – body image aspects differed from each other significantly in respect of satisfaction with body. A declarative aspect and a perceptive aspect constituted an exception. At all stages a general satisfaction with body was similar in the case of the above mentioned aspects. In addition, at the last stage of the therapy participants assessed their satisfaction with body in a similar way. They followed the knowledge of their body and body awareness.

8. The Imaginary Picture of One's Own Body

The examined females were asked about details concerning an appearance of a figure they were supposed to imagine. The majority of participants (from 94% to 97% - depending on a research stage) declared that an imagined figure corresponded to their image from the past. The examined females assessed the age and body mass of an imagined figure. BMI was calculated on the basis of the above mentioned assessment.

It was observed that an imagined figure's age differed from the examined female's age. The t-Student test was used to show that the above mentioned difference was significant at the following stages: the first stage t=(149)=11.612; p<0.001, the second stage: t(149)=11.612; p<0.001, the third stage: t(149)=12.169; p<0.001, and the fourth stage: t(149)=8.466; p<0.001 (table 29).

Additionally, it was stated that there was difference between an imagined figure's BMI and an objective BMI of the examined person. The difference was significant at the following stages: the first stage: t(149)=17.774; p<0.001, the second stage: t(149)=13.883; p<0.001, the third stage: t(149)=13.362; p<0.001, and the fourth stage: t(149)=7.510; p<0.001 (table 30).

Table 29. Certificate age versus imagined age

Stage of cure	Age	N	M	SD	Test		
					t	df	p
①	certificate	150	42.97	13.557	13.234	149	< 0.001
	imagined		31.81	12.704			
②	certificate	113	43.42	13.146	11.612	112	< 0.001
	imagined		32.96	12.927			
③	certificate	80	42.93	12.990	12.169	79	< 0.001
	imagined		31.05	12.288			
④	imagined	49	43.45	13.348	8.466	48	< 0.001
	certificate		31.47	11.988			

Table 30. Objective BMI versus imagined BMI

Stage of cure	BMI	N	M	SD	Test		
					t	df	p
①	objective	150	37.17	6.429	17.774	149	< 0.001
	imagined		27.86	6.344			
②	objective	113	35.50	6.254	13.883	112	< 0.001
	imagined		28.10	4.966			
③	imagined	80	34.03	5.966	13.362	79	< 0.001
	objective		27.36	5.331			
④	objective	49	32.44	5.789	7.510	48	< 0.001
	imagined		27.46	4.628			

DISCUSSION

The weight loss therapy was effective in the case of most women who took part in the presented research. Over 50% of the females who were examined (80 women) reduced their initial body weight by 10%. It should be regarded as a success because even a minor, but permanent reduction in the body weight brings tangible benefits in the case of obese people. Some particular medical parameters improve, for example: blood pressure, the level of cholesterol, triglicerides and glucose. The physical efficiency of the body, physical condition and quality of life improve also (Kinzl, 2001; Wadden et al., 2001; Hamilton, 2002; Besteghi,

2002; Zahorska – Markiewicz, 2005; Berkel et al., 2005; Wing, Phelan, 2005; Buddeberg-Fischer et al., 2006).

A subjective body mass estimation of the examined women was conducted in respect of each aspect of the body image separately. There are four body image aspects: a declarative aspect, a sensory aspect, an imaginary aspect and a perceptive aspect. A positive correlation coefficient was observed between the above mentioned aspects. However, the changes in respect of estimating the body weight varied during the weight loss therapy.

As far as a declarative aspect, a sensory aspect and a perceptive aspect are concerned, a subjective body mass estimation was changing significantly upon an objective reduction in the body weight. At the beginning of the research the examined women described themselves as obese women. However, after some time they estimated their body mass as decreasing.

In respect of a subjective body mass the consistency between the aspects appeared at all stages of the therapy, which is not an obvious phenomenon. Some scientific reports indicate that visual and somatic sensory stimuli are not always integrated with respect to experiencing ones own body (Lacey, Birtchnell, 1986; Lautenbacher et al., 1993).

The adequacy of a subjective body mass was analyzed, i.e. the consistency of a subjective body mass with an objective body mass estimation. As far as a declarative aspect, a sensory aspect and a perceptive aspect are concerned, both the decrease in the adequacy and the increase in the inadequacy of the estimation were observed upon the reduction in the body mass. The inadequacy – in most cases – meant that a subjective body mass was underestimated in comparison with an objective body mass. The aspects differed from each other only in respect of the inadequacy degree. However, the difference blurred with time.

The results concerning the adequacy of the body mass estimation turned out to be inconsistent with expectations. It was expected that women participating in the weight loss therapy will be more aware of their appearance with time. The increase of the body awareness was associated with: weighting systematically, talking about the therapy, focusing on the body, doing physical exercises, and dieting. However, it turned out that the above mentioned factors did not influence the adequacy of perceiving the body weight. Quite the opposite, the inconsistency between a subjective estimation and the actual state increased. The phenomenon can be explained by the fact that a positive emotion that was caused by an objective reduction in the body weight had a significant effect on underestimating the body size. This case presents an affective distortion or the effect of looking through rose-tinted spectacles.

Researches of other authors confirm that an emotional condition has an effect on the estimation of the body mass. For example, dissatisfaction with the body resulting from feeling obese influences the overestimation of the body mass regardless of the actual body mass (Cash, Hicks, 1990; Sands, 2000).

In the conducted research, in the following aspects: a declarative aspect, a sensory aspect and a perceptive aspect, the differentiation of changes in respect of the adequacy of a subjective body mass estimation was observed. This differentiation depended on the research method which was used. As far as the Assessment Scale of a Body Mass is concerned, the number of inadequate estimations prevailed over the number of adequate estimations as early as after a minimal reduction in an initial body weight by 5%. As far as the Silhouette Test is concerned, a crucial moment in this respect was when an initial body mass decreased by

10%. The differences are probably connected with different categories of stimuli which are used in each method mentioned above. The Assessment Scale of a Body Mass refers to a conceptual dimension and uses the labels representing the body mass. The Silhouette Test is based on visual representations of the body size and shape. The estimation of the body, including its mass, undergoes distortions more often and faster at a conceptual level (a semantic code) than at a visual level (a pictorial code).

Using the labels representing the body mass favors the underestimation. It can be caused by an equivocal understanding of terms and an avoidance of identifying with pejorative terms. The comparison of the body mass with figures that are drew favors a greater adequacy of an estimation. It seems that the basic reason for this situation is a significant adequacy of the presented stimuli and larger range of a scale. Undoubtedly, for this reason, among other things, the Silhouette Test is one of the most often used methods of analyzing the body image (Leonhard, Barry, 1998; Rand, Resnick, Macgregor, 1999; Williamson et al., 2000; Rinderknecht, Smith, 2002; Stunkard, Zelten, Platte, 2002).

Generally, in everyday life people refer to an intellectual sphere rather than a visual sphere in respect of their body. The knowledge about the body is derived mainly from analyzing sensory sensations (stimuli coming from the body) and cognitive impressions (readings of weighing scales, the size of the clothing we buy, the knowledge about our body mass). In addition, the integration of information coming from the others with the knowledge about ones own appearance takes place. Even looking in the mirror is often of fragmentary character, i.e. it is not directed at the assessment of a particular body part or feature. It can be assumed that the knowledge about ones own body, including the appearance, is based mainly on the opinions concerning an appearance, and rarely on the facts. Only selected contents appear in the field of an actual consciousness. The contents are useful due to their significance for a person – his/her needs, self-assessment and tasks he/she wants to realize. It means that a general estimation of the body mass can be inadequate to the reality significantly, which was observed in the presented research. The lack of the accuracy of the estimation of ones own actual appearance occurred in this case.

An incomplete awareness of ones own appearance is also supported by circumstantial reports of other authors and confessions of obese people who experienced their time of "discovery" concerning their excess weight. For example, NATPOL PLUS research showed that 70% of males and 60% of females between 20 and 74 have BMI over 25. And, only 37% of them are aware of this fact, especially, younger women, younger people, better-educated people and people from cities (Babinska et al., 2004).

The above mentioned issue can be also illustrated by a response of a patient: "You know, I caught a glimpse of myself in the mirror this morning, and I was surprised at how fat I have become. It made me feel that it's time to get some of this weight off." * (Stunkard, Mendelson, 1967, p. 1297)

The literature on the subject that is presented in this study lacks data which would enable to state why in some group of people – including at least some part of obese people – the inadequacy of the body mass estimation occurs. Valtolina with his team (1998) conducted a research which helped answer the question above partially. Valtolina showed that in fact obese women underestimated their body mass in respect of the whole body and its particular parts like the head, the breast, the stomach and the hips. In the case of slim women the degree of underestimation was lower in respect of the whole body, the head and the breast, on the other hand, slim women overestimated the size of their stomach and hips. The authors of the research suggest that distortions were caused by the projection of a phantom body which refers to previous experiences of a person. A phantom body here is understood as an outline of a physical body that is fossilized and stored in mind. In the case of people with the proper body mass who gained weight in a short time, an actual body image differs from a phantom body that people got used to in an obvious way. It can cause difficulties in setting the borders of ones "bodily self". Moreover, it can cause ambivalent emotions. Consequently, perhaps it can cause repeated overeating. The present knowledge about the body image does not give the grounds for the determination of what occurs first – overeating and putting on weight or changes of a sense of a bodily identity.

All described aspects of the body image (a declarative aspect, a sensory aspect and a perceptive aspect) turned out to be relatively consistent with each other in respect of a subjective body mass estimation, the adequacy of the estimation and changes occurring during the weight loss therapy. The lack of significant differences between the aspects suggests that all the aspects work in accordance with a conscious processing of external and internal stimuli.

The issue above is supported by the fact that the participants of the weight loss therapy often justified their estimation with noticeable and objective changes concerning the reduction in body weight. As far as a declarative aspect is concerned, the participants stressed the number of kilograms they got rid off. As far as a sensory aspect is concerned, the participants stressed a positive feelings resulting from, for example, becoming fitter, the feeling of lightness, the reduction in the feeling of satiety. As far as a perceptive aspect is concerned, the participants referred to an observable reduction in fatness and measurement of particular parts of the body, wearing clothes which were close-fitting for many years.

The fourth aspect of the body image – an imaginable aspect – differed from other aspects in respect of a subjective body mass estimation, its adequacy and the variability during the weight loss therapy. During the whole therapy the examined people defined an imaginary picture of their body as average in respect of the body mass. Regardless of the research method, the estimation of an imaginary person's body mass was inadequate, and the fact did not change significantly during the whole weight loss therapy. As far as the next research stages are concerned, the number of inadequate estimations was relatively constant, and the number of adequate estimations was decreasing slightly. The imaginary age was significantly lower than the actual age of the examined people, and the imaginary body mass was significantly lower than the actual objective body mass of the examined people.

Despite an objective reduction in body mass, the constancy of the body image suggests that an imaginary aspect of the body image is resistant to sensory stimuli, visual stimuli and new information. In the case of most examined people the image of the body remained unchanged in respect of both the age and the body mass. This image seems to be a completely separate quality, which is consistent with the definition of an image. An image is defined as: "a picture in mind; it's one out of three subclasses of consciousness, beside sensations and feelings; it's a mental representation of a previous sensory experience, its copy" (Reber, 2000, p.847).

Researchers expresses different opinions on whether an image is a faithful copy of an experience. Some researchers think that most imaginary operations that are conducted in a pictorial code are based on the change of proportions between particular elements of an image, and the displacement of an original image or the attribution of new properties to the elements of an image (Zdankiewicz – Scigala, Matuszewski, 2000). Other authors suggest that an actual body image includes the elements of a former, past body image. Its parts are transported to the reality and have a direct effect on an attitude towards oneself and an external expression. It happens outside a person's consciousness (Waxler, Liska, 1975 by Cohen, 1984).

Irrespective of the fact whether an actual image is a part of a former information or its distortion, images results from a person's experience – it is a common point of view. This viewpoint was also confirmed by the conducted research. At all research stages over 95% (143 people) of the females participating in the research imagined a figure resembling their own figure. In most cases it was a picture of self from the past.

The analysis of the consistency of particular body image aspects showed that in the case of the examined females the most adequate estimation was the body mass estimation in a declarative aspect, then, in a perceptive aspect, and finally, in the sensory aspect, although there were no significant changes. The least adequate was the body mass estimation in an imaginary aspect of the body image. Moreover, as far as the first three body image aspects are concerned, the body mass estimation and its adequacy was changing during the weight loss therapy. In the case of an imaginary body image aspect, the estimation remained unchanged.

The literature on the subject that is presented in this study lacks an unambiguous point of view concerning the constancy of the body image. The inconsistency of the results obtained by different authors is partially explained with the methods that were used. For example, Marten Smets (1997) thinks that the estimation of the body image is problematic because of the fact that most of the methods examine a memory image instead of a perceptive image. These dimensions often coincide with each other. However, the dimensions do not depend on each other.

Another reason that is independent and probable may be referring to different body image aspects in particular researches. Even if a method examines a memory image it may come from different periods of a person's life. A memory image in an imaginary aspect seems to be the oldest and fossilized. A declarative, sensory or perceptive memory would be more fresh and more susceptible to influences and changes (Bąk-Sosnowska, Zahorska-Markiewicz, Trzcieniecka-Green, 2004).

The presented research included also the analysis of the examined peoples' satisfaction with their body during the weight loss therapy. A general satisfaction with the body was assessed. Moreover, satisfaction with particular body dimensions was assessed. The dimensions were as follows: attractiveness, charm, agility, shapeliness, proportionality and firmness. The Scale of Satisfaction with One's Own Body (own instrument) was used. The method differs from generally used tools which focus on the assessment of a general satisfaction with the body image and its efficiency rather than the body qualities.

As far as a declarative, sensory and perceptive aspects of the body image are concerned, the majority of the examined people assessed their body in a more positive rather than a negative way. A positive emotional attitude toward the body was found both in a general and detailed assessment, which is inconsistent with a general knowledge and scientific reports on the subject of the satisfaction with the body in obese people. It is assumed that obese people have a negative attitude towards their body. Moreover, it is assumed that, especially in obese women, the body image is more negative than in people with the proper body weight (Wadden, Stunkard, 1985; Fila, Terelak,1994; Basdevant, Le Barzic, Guy – Grand, 1996; Adami et al., 1997; Carpenter et al., 2000; Larsson, Mattsson, 2001; Friedman et al, 2002; Glebocka, Wisniewska, 2005). An additional significance has the fact of overeating because people with binge eating disorders, irrespective of whether they are slim or obese, feel a stronger dislike for their body than people without a compulsive overeating (Cash, 1993; Adami et al., 1998; Becker, 2001).

The researches by Cash and Hicks (1990) showed that a subjective feeling of an excessive weight, and not its objective level, influences a psychological general feeling that is connected with an appearance. The strongest effect on the satisfaction with the body have both a general shape of the body and the hip measurement, and not the body fat level or the overweight level (Valtolina, 1998).

During the period of body mass reduction up to a 10% decrease in an initial body weight, the number of positive assessments concerning the body image was increasing significantly, whereas the number of a negative assessments was decreasing. Later, until the end of the therapy the number of both assessments remained at a constant level. Undoubtedly, an objective reduction in the body weight was not the only factor that caused the increase in the satisfaction with the body. Moreover, both the significant increase in the number of positive assessments and the decrease in the number of negative assessments had occurred after the minimal body weight reduction which did not change the appearance significantly. Researchers studying the issue confirm that an emotional attitude toward the body depends on lots of factors. The researchers suggest that the correlation between a subjective and an objective assessment of an attractiveness is very low in females (Feingold, 1992). A current mood is considered to be a significant factor (Sands, 2000; Glebocka, Kulbat, 2005) which can generate both opinions on ones own body and its appearance and actions concerning the body (for example, body care, body adornment, etc.). Frederickson and Roberts (1997 by Jestes, 2004) proved that the adjustment of a physical appearance to the cultural standards of beauty affects the increase in the satisfaction with the body in females positively.

As far as the conducted research is concerned, the increase in the satisfaction with the body depended on a general self-satisfaction resulting from a successful realization of the objective, i.e. the reduction in the body weight. However, the general satisfaction with the body was increasing only until the 10% reduction in an initial body weight was reached by the examined people. Later, during the therapy, the general satisfaction with the body was at a constant level. The result proves that the satisfaction with the body results from the body mass (both an objective weight and a subjective weight) only partially. The unsolved issue is why the satisfaction with the body remained unchanged from the certain moment. Perhaps, the changes are of non-linear but saltatory character. It would be possible to check in people who reduce their body weight by more than 15%.

It was also observed that at the first three stages of the therapy a sensory aspect differed significantly from both a declarative aspect and an imaginary aspect in respect of the level of the satisfaction with the body. The level of satisfaction in a sensory aspect was relatively higher than in a declarative aspect or in an imaginary aspect. After the 15% body weight reduction, a sensory aspect differed significantly only from an imaginary aspect. During the whole weight loss therapy, a declarative aspect and a perceptive aspect were relatively consistent with each other in respect of the satisfaction with the body.

A relative satisfaction with the body – based on feelings coming from the body – is a popular phenomenon in obese people. It is known from a clinical practice that lots of obese people feel their body as: "well-shaped", "agile" and "fit". It results from the lack of perceptible pains or limits resulting from being obese, and being accustomed to an excess weight. Additionally, positive feelings coming from the body are stimulated by both the feeling of satiety and the action of substances secreting after a meal (for example glucose or endorfins).

All the above aspects of the body image (a declarative aspect, a sensory aspect and a perceptive aspect) differed from an imaginary aspect significantly during the whole therapy. As far as an imaginary aspect is concerned, an average assessment of satisfaction with the whole body and its particular parts was significantly higher. Moreover, the assessment was increasing with the reduction in the body weight. The number of positive assessments increased, and the number of negative assessments decreased. However, only two analyzed categories changed significantly. The categories were as follows: "charm" and the body "shapeliness". After the reduction in an initial body weight by 10%, the level of the satisfaction with the body did not changed significantly in an imaginary aspect, as in the case of the other aspects.

CONCLUSION

In the case of estimating both the body mass and the level of satisfaction with the body, an imaginary body image aspect differed from the other aspects (a declarative aspect, a sensory aspect and a perceptive aspect) in the examined people. It means that the imaginary picture of the body differed significantly from: thinking about the body, feeling the body and perceiving the body in the mirror.

The imaginary picture of ones body turned out to be slimmer and younger than an objective body mass and the age of the examined people. In most cases, the imaginary picture of the body was a copy of an examined person's past appearance.

The differences that were observed between the particular aspects indicate that images play an important role in functioning of the body image. Taking the role of images into consideration may contribute to the explanation of the differences in the results that are obtained in respect of studying the body mass estimation in obese people. Moreover, it may also indicate that diagnostic methods that use a pictorial code are more accurate in respect of studying the body image than the methods which are based on a semantic code.

REFERENCES

Adami G.F., Bauer B., Gandolfo P. and Scopinaro N. (1997). Body image in early – onset obese patients. *Eating and Weight Disorders, 2* (2), 87 – 93.

Adami G.F., Gandolfo P., Campostano A., Meneghello A., Ravela G. and Scopinaro N. (1998). Body Imane and Body Weight In Obese Patients. *International Journal of Eating Disorders, 24* (3), 299 – 306.

Babińska Z., Bandosz P., Zdrojewski T. and Wyrzykowski B. (2004). Epidemiologia otyłości i otyłości brzusznej w Polsce, Europie Zachodniej i USA. *Kardiologia w Praktyce, 3,* 3 – 7.

Basdevant A., Barzic Le M., and Guy – Grand B. (1993). *Les obésités.* Paris: Ardix Médical.

Bak – Sosnowska M., Trzcieniecka – Green A. and Zahorska – Markiewicz B. (2004). Ekspresja obrazu własnego ciała u osób otyłych, na podstawie analizy porównawczej rysunku człowieka i rysunku siebie. *Psychoterapia, 3* (130), 37 – 44.

Becker E.., Margraf J., Turke V., Soeder U. and Neumer S. (2001). Obesity and mental illness in a representative sample of young women. *International Journal of Obesity and Related Metabolic Disorders, 25* (supl 1*)*, 5-9.

Bell C., Kirpatrick S. and Rinn R. (1986). Body image of anorectic, obese and normal females. *Journal of Clinical Psychology, 42,* 431 – 439.

Berkel L.A., Carlos-Poston W.S., Reeves R. S. and Forey J.P. (2005). Behavioral interventions for obesity. *Journal of the American Dietetic Association, 105* (5 Pt 2), 35 – 43.

Besteghi L., Di Domizio S., Sartini A., Pasqui F., Baraldi L., Forlani G., Melchionda N., Marchesini G., Natale S., Manini R. and Chierici S. (2002). Effects of cognitive-behavioural therapy on health -related quality of life in obese subjects with and without binge eating disorder. *International Journal of Obesity, 26* (9), 1261 – 1267.

Buddeberg-Fischer B, Klaghofer R, Krug L, Buddeberg C, Muller MK, Schoeb O. and Weber M. (2006). Physical and psychosocial outcome in morbidly obese patients with and without bariatric surgery: a 4 1/2-year follow-up. *Obesity Surgery, 16* (3), 321 - 330.

Butters J.W. and Cash T.F. (1987). Cognitive – behavioral treatment of women's body – image dissatisfaction. *Journal of Consulting and Clinical Psychology, 55* (6), 889 – 897.

Carpenter K.M., Hasin D.S., Allison D.B. and Faith M.S. (2000). Relationships between obesity and DSM-IV major depressive disorder, suicide ideation, and suicide attempts: results from a general population study. *American Journal of Public Health, 90* (2), 251 - 257.

Cash T.F. (1993). Body image attitudes among obese enrollees in a commercial weight – loss program. *Perceptual and Motor Skills, 77* (3 Pt 2), 1099 – 1103.

Cash T.F. and Hicks K.L. (1990). Being Fat versus Thinking Fat: Relationships with Body Image, Behaviors and Well – Being. *Cognitive Therapy and Research, 14* (3), 327 – 341.

Cohen B. (1984). The Psychology of Ideal Image as an Oppressive Force In the Limes of Women. www. healingthehumanspirit.com

Craig P. and Caterson I. (1990). Weight and perceptions of body image in women and men in a Sydney sample. *Community Health Study, 14* (4), 373 – 383.

Epstein S. (1990). Cognitive-experiential Self-theory. In L. Pervin (Ed.), *Handbook of personality theory and research: Theory and research* (165 - 192). New York: Guilford Publications, Inc.

Etcoff N. (2002). *Przetrwają najpiękniejsi*. Warszawa: CIS/ WAB.

Feingold A. (1992). Good – looking people, are not we think. *Psychological Bulletin, 111*, 304 – 341.

Fila M. and Terelak J. (1994). Otyłość jako źródło stresu psychologicznego w funkcjonowaniu człowieka. *Przegląd Psychologiczny*, XXXVII, (1-2), 105 – 126.

Friedman K.E., Reichmann S.K., Costanzo P.R. and Musante G.J. (2002). Body image partially mediates the relationship between obesity and psychological distress. *Obesity Research, 10* (1), 33 – 41.

Furhnam A. and Alibhai N. (1983). Cross – cultural differences in the perception of female body shapes. *Psychological Medicine, 13*, 829 – 837.

Gardner R.M., Gallegos V., Martinez R. and Espinoza T. (1991). Mirror feedback and judgments of body size. *Journal of Psychosomatic Research, 33*, 603 – 607.

Glebocka A. and Kulbat J. (2005). Czym jest wizerunek ciała? In A. Glebocka and J. Kulbat (Ed), *Wizerunek ciała. Portret Polek* (9 – 28). Opole: Wydawnictwo Uniwersytetu Opolskiego.

Glebocka A. and Wisniewska A. (2005). Psychologiczny portret kobiet otyłych. In A.Glebocka and J.Kulbat (Ed), *Wizerunek ciała. Portret Polek* (63 – 78). Opole: Wydawnictwo Uniwersytetu Opolskiego.

Greenwald A. (1986). Samowiedza i samooszukiwanie. *Przegląd psychologiczny, 2*, 291 – 303.

Greenwald, A. (1997). Self-knowledge and self-deception: Further consideration. In M. S. Myslobodsky (Ed.), *The mythomanias: An inquiry into the nature of deception and self-deception* (pp. 51-71). Mahwah, NJ: Erlbaum.

Grilo C.R., Masheb R.M., Brody M., Burke – Martindale C.H. and Rothschild B.S. (2005). Binge eating and self-esteem predict body image dissatisfaction among obese men and women seeking bariatric surgery. *The International Journal of Eating Disorders, 37* (4), 347 – 351.

Hamilton M. (2002). Strategies for the management of patients with obesity. *Treatments in Endocrinology, 1* (1), 21 – 36.

Harwas – Napierała B. and Trempała J. (2002). *Psychologia rozwoju człowieka*. Warszawa: PWN.

Jestes D. (1993). Body image: how you see it, how you don't. www.clearinghouse.mwsc.edu/ manuscripts/93.asp

Kinzl J.F., Trefalt E., Fiala M., Hotter A. Biebl W. and Aigner F. (2001). Partnership, sexuality, and sexual disorders in morbidly obese women: consequences of weight loss after gastric banding. *Obesity Surgery, 11*(4): 455 – 458.

Lacey H.J. and Birtchnell S.A. (1986). Body image and its disturbances. *Journal of Psychosomatic Research, 30* (6), 623 – 631.

Larsson U.E. and Mattsson E. (2001). Perceived disability and observed functional limitations in obese women. *International Journal of Obesity and Related Metabolic Disorders, 25* (11), 1705 – 1712.

Lautenbacher S., Roscher S., Strian F., Pirke K. and Krieg J. (1993). Theoretical and empirical considerations on the relation between "body image", body scheme and somatosensation. *Journal of Psychosomatic Research, 37* (5), 447 – 454.

Leonhard M. and Barry N. (1998). Body Image and obesity: effects of gender and weight on perceptual measures of body image. *Addictive Behaviors, 23* (1), 31 – 34.

Mandal E. (2004). The influence of youth magasines on mood and self – image of Polish girls in early and late adolescence – The role of self – affirmation mechanisms in the integration of attractiveness, intellectual and interpersonal competence. *Polish Psychological Bulletin, 35* (4), 217 – 224.

Mlodkowski J. (1998). Wyobraźnia. In Wl. Szewczuk (Ed), *Encyklopedia psychologii (*1019 – 1024). Warszawa: Fundacja Innowacja.

Molinari E. and Riva G. (1995). Self-others perception in a clinical sample of obese women. *Perceptual and Motor Skills, 80* (3 Pt 2), 1283 – 1289.

Nawaz H, Chan W., Abdulrahman M., Larson D. and Katz D.L. (2001). Self-reported weight and height: implications for obesity research. *American Journal of Prevention Medicine, 20* (4), 294 – 298.

Offman H. and Bradley S. (1992). Body image of children and adolescents and its measurement. A overview. *Canadian Journal of Psychiatry, 37,* 417 – 422.

Rand C., Resnick J. and Macgregor A. (1999). A comparison of body size evaluations of obesity surgery patients and general population adults. *Obesity Research, 7* (3), 281 – 287.

Rinderknecht K. and Smith C. (2002). Body – Image perceptions among urban native american youth. *Obesity Research, 10* (5), 315 – 327.

Reber A. (2000). *Słownik psychologii.* Warszawa: Scholar.

Samuels M. and Samuels N. (1975). *Seeing with the Mind's Eye.* New York: Random House.

Sanchez-Villegas A.., Madrigal H., Martinez-Gonzalez M.A., Kearney J., Gibney M.J., de-Irala J.A. and Martinez J.(2001). Perception of body image as indicator of weight status in the European union. *Journal of Human Nutrition and Dietetics, 14* (2), 93 – 102.

Sands R. (2000). Reconceptualization of Body Image and Drive for Thinness. *International Journal of Eating Disorders, 28* (4), 397 – 407.

Smeets M. (1997). The rise and fall of body size estimation research in anorexia nervosa: a review and reconceptualization. *European Eating Disorders Review, 5,* 75 – 95.

Stoke R. and Recascino Ch. (2003). Women's Perceived Body Image: Relations with Personal Happiness. *Journal of Woman and Aging, 15* (1), 17 – 30.

Stunkard A.J. and Mendelson M. (1967). Obesity and the Body Image: Characteristics of Disturbances in the Body Image of Some Obese Persons. *American Journal of Psychiatry, 123,* 1296 – 1300.

Stunkard A.J. and Wadden T. (1992). Psychological aspects of severe obesity. The American *Journal of Clinical Nutrition, 55,* 524 – 532.

Stunkard A.J., Zelten J.F. and Platte P. (2002). Body Image in the Old Amish: A people separate from „the world". *International Journal of Eating Disorders, 28* (4), 408 – 414.

Thompson K. (2002). Interview. www.athealth.com

Valtolina G.G. (1998). Body size estimation by obese subjects. *Perceptual and Motor Skills, 86* (3 Pt 2), 1363 – 1374.

Wadden T.A., Sarwer D.B., Womble L.G., Foster G.D., McGuckin B.G. and Schimmel A. (2001). Psychosocial aspects of obesity and obesity surgery. *Surgical Clinics of North America*, *81* (5), 1001 - 1024.

Wadden T.A. and Stunkard A.J. (1985). Social and psychological consequences of obesity. *Annales of Internal Medicine*, *103*, 1062 – 1067.

Waller G. and Barnes J. (2002). Preconscious processing of body image cues. Impact on body percept and concept. *Journal of Psychosomatic Research*, *53*, 1037 – 1041.

Williamson D.A., Womble L.G., Zucker N.L., Reas D.L., White M.A., Blouin D.C. and Greenway F. (2000). Body image assessment for obesity (BIA – O) development of a new procedure. *Internationnal Journal of Obesity*, *24* (10), 1326 – 1332.

Wing R.R. and Phelan S. (2005). Long-term weight loss maintenance. The *American Journal of Clinical Nutrition*, *82* (supl 1), 222 – 225.

Zahorska – Markiewicz B. (2005). *Nauka i praktyka w leczeniu otyłości*. Kraków: ArchiPlus.

Zdankiewicz – Scigała E. and Maruszewski T. (2000). Wyobrażenia jako pierwsza forma doświadczenia generowanego przez jednostkę. In J. Strelau (Ed.), *Psychologia*t. II (183 – 203). Gdańsk: GWP.

In: Life Style and Health Research Progress ISBN: 978-1-60456-427-3
Editors: A. B. Turley, G. C. Hofmann © 2008 Nova Science Publishers, Inc.

Chapter IX

An Innovative Approach to Promote a Healthy Lifestyle for Persons with Chronic Conditions in Brazil

Mercedes Trentini[1] and Lygia Paim*[2]*

[1] Professor – Universidade do Contestado; Rua Jardim dos Eucalíptos,
912; Campeche, 88 063 270; Florianópolis, SC, Brazil
[2] Professor – Universidade do Vale de Itajaí; Rua Rui Barbosa,
14 – Apto 301; Agronômica, 88 025 300; Florianópolis, SC, Brazil

ABSTRACT

The purpose of the chapter is to present results obtained from the contribution of an innovative research approach about the lifestyle of persons in chronic conditions. The Brazilian population has undergone substantial changes in the number of individuals who are exposed to different illnesses. There has been a reduction of transmitted diseases, but, at the same time, an increase in chronic degenerative diseases. Chronic diseases are considered to be a result of a disorderly lifestyle, however, the life style they live is not only the individuals' fault. Yet, individuals can only take on greater responsibility for their lifestyles if they have access to education and economic support to make healthy decisions. It is up to health professionals to take on part of the responsibility, since those diseases require continued assistance to support people not only with the medicinal and clinical treatment, but mainly in preparing them to manage their lifestyles. A new qualitative research approach was developed by the authors of this abstract in 1999, and it was named Converging Assistance Research (Pesquisa Convergente Assistencial – PCA). The approach maintains a strict link with daily health practices. This study was conducted by searching 100% of the studies on lifestyle carried out with people with chronic condition in Southern Brazil and used the PCA as a methodological reference. The results showed that there were changes in two dimensions: 1) direct changes in people's life styles such as, a) minimizing feelings of loneliness and seeking occupational

---

* Mercedes Trentini: Tel. + 55 84 3237 4518; Email: mertini@terra.com.br
* Lygia Paim: Email: lypaim@matrix.com.br

and leisure activities; b) increased well-being and improved self-esteem; c) reducing of stress, anxiety and depression; d) access to help support the new reality of the new life relationships; e) replacement of stereotyped movements; f) intensified relationships with peers; g) changing from learning to continuous learning; 2) changes in the approach of health professionals; a) acting modes from the individual to the collective; b) contents originating from themes generated by people in chronic conditions as well as political, social, and technical themes related to the rights assured by the Health Services; c) interpreting news and technological innovations focused on improving the qualification in the lifestyles of people in chronic situations. Conclusion: PCA has been contributing effectively to improving the lifestyles of individuals in chronic conditions and in the way the professional care is given to those individuals.

Keywords: lifestyle, chronic diseases, nursing care.

INTRODUCTION

This chapter addresses the contribution from an innovative research approach that includes changes in the lifestyles of persons in chronic health conditions. The underlying notion of engaging new daily practices is a value of centrality among those who get involved with the idea of building qualification for a new style of living and being healthy. The pursuit for producing changes, being an intention that adds value to the new practices, is present in the Converging Assistance Research (Pesquisa Convergente Assistencial – PCA), for the progress of its strategies. As a basic strategy in the PCA, what stands out is that the researcher takes part in both the investigation itself and in the practice of assistance in a simultaneous fashion throughout the research development process. This two-way strengthening between research and the practice of assistance, characterized as the PCA, generates transformation and new knowledge, substantiates affinities regarding the common intention of encouraging change and compose new solid ways of health action know-how. Furthermore, being an outline that requires and maintains a democratic scenario of activity, the PCA in the Brazilian Health context has been used with great diversity of research issues, including those pertaining to changes in chronic health conditions, which strengthens the crossings to reach new healthy lifestyles.

Being a type of investigation guided towards solving problems in the practice of assistance, the PCA is aimed at making changes, and the synthesis of its process, thus articulated, brings the introduction of innovations in health practices, which may lead to expressive theoretical constructions in the daily lives of the situations that are researched. Also, because of this bridge with hands-on actions, the involvement of the researcher with other people who are representatives of the researched situation determines, during the research progression process within the practice, a mutual cooperation relationship. PCA has been sought and interpreted mainly due to its character of bringing changes, which makes it compatible with the issues of transformations to lifestyles and work that are increasingly required in the field of living and being healthy nowadays.

In the experience of its authors, in just over a decade of studies and practices the PCA has become one of many ways to take an innovative approach and make the research available in the daily activities of health professionals, especially in Brazilian nursing. This is mostly due to the articulation of two processes: research and health assistance practice that are inherent to the design proposed for this type of investigation called Converging Assistance Research (Pesquisa Convergente Assistencial – PCA). The PCA differential lies exactly in the intention to integrate throughout its process assistance practice, which requires proximity and distancing specificities in the field of know-how so as to research and provide assistance with movement reciprocity and progress simultaneity in the intentional articulation of both processes. The PCA takes into consideration this articulation and makes it fundamental in its outline. Additionally, because of this characteristic, the production of knowledge within the strictness of the PCA is in tune with an investigation that is compatible with the desired and sought after changes when the issue is present in chronic conditions and the changes required for a more healthy style of living.

Investigative practices with PCA in Brazil have resulted in confluences towards assistance, which is now ruled by a health system called Unified Health System (Sistema Único de Saúde – SUS) with democratic proposals and principles with which PCA is tuned and committed to. This way, driven within the PCA design, the investigation also becomes a bridge that allows highlighting the socialization of know-how and the construction of concrete changes to health practices. The Unified Health System (SUS) is the policy that guides health professional practices in Brazil, it was created in 1988 and regulated in 1990 by Law 8.080 that sets forth the conditions for promoting, protecting and recovering health, as well as the organization and operation of health services [1]. The Unified Health System (SUS) has influenced the Brazilian health scenario especially through the change it has imprinted in the ways of guidance, conception, and execution of health assistance in the country. The SUS consists of a system in which all would gain the right to Health assistance, at all levels of care, with the population having access to the Services organized into a Care Offer Network. It is an achievement by the Brazilian people that originates from the democratic process that sustains the following basic principles: equity, integrity, comprehensiveness, decentralization, and social participation. Thus, the SUS should assure universal and equal access opportunities to actions and services to promote, protect and recover health attention according to the needs presented by its patients.

The SUS is structured as a proposal to establish health democracy in the country, where health is regarded as the result of people's life conditions. It is an achievement of government and society responsibility via economic and social policies. It is a human and citizenship right, since the State must assure access to assets and services: the idea that Health is everyone's right and a State duty is a basic principle of sanitary reform [2]. For the SUS to be successful, general government policies are needed and the health sector structured and organized with the objective of producing positive effects on the health of persons and of the collectivity. In order that the proposal for Sanitary Reform is complied with, it is crucial to implement the SUS basic principles in its entirety.

The SUS, as presented, is a system formed by various segments at the three government levels – Union, States and Municipalities – and by the contracted private sector as a single body; it is unique due to its common philosophy and systematic, and should serve everybody in an integral, decentralized, rational, effective and efficient, and democratic way. It is a process that is constantly being enhanced and adapted [2].

Although advancements have been made in health since regulation of the SUS, there is still a conservative aspect that is expressed by the gap between conception and execution of transforming actions in health practices, that is, its basic principles are not yet being totally implemented in practice. A large portion of the Brazilian population depends on the SUS health actions, which has not shown to be sufficiently structured to operate meeting the intense demands, especially those that require prevention and health promotion actions. Therefore, a reform of the ethical and social base principles has been establishing itself, and by nature, it promises changes that will slowly bring into perspective the desirable health care model.

In Brazil, the average life expectancy age increased by three years during the 1980's, and the proportion of the elderly in the population has been increasing considerably. In 1970, the percentage of the population over 60 years of age was of 5.1%; in 1990, it raised to 7.2% [3]. It is estimated that by 2015, the number of people over 60 years of age will reach 15% of the Brazilian population. Studies show that 85% of the Brazilian elderly suffer from at least one chronic disease, and 15% suffer an average of five diseases [3].

The Brazilian population has undergone substantial changes in the number of individuals who are exposed to different illnesses. While there was a decrease in population groups vulnerable to transmissible infectious diseases, there has been an increase in groups vulnerable to degenerative chronic diseases [4].

Chronic conditions involve both non-transmissible and some transmissible diseases. Non-transmissible diseases include cardiovascular and neurological diseases, nephropathies, cancer, diabetes, depression, among others, and the transmissible ones include mainly leprosy, tuberculosis, and HIV-AIDS, which until recently was synonymous to death. The inclusion of mental disorders and physical handicaps broaden the group of diseases identified as chronic conditions, examples of which are depression and schizophrenia that usually become chronic. Regarding disabilities determined by chronic conditions, depression deserves special attention, as it is estimated that by 2020 it will be second only to heart diseases [5].

Chronic conditions have been increasing significantly all over the world, with no social class distinction. In 2000, non-transmissible conditions represented 46% of the total global load of diseases in the world [5].

It is believed that the majority of chronic diseases is a consequence of a disordered lifestyle, however, individuals are not the only ones responsible for the lifestyles they lead. The truth is, individuals can only take on the proper responsibility for their lifestyles if they have access to education and economic support to make healthy decisions. Governments are co-responsible, along with its citizens, for keeping and improving health in the populations, especially the vulnerable groups. These populations include poor people who also have limited choices about what they eat, their housing conditions, and limited access to education and health care. However, health professionals also have a share of the responsibility, as chronic conditions are long lasting and require continued assistance strategies to provide support for patients not only in clinical and medication treatment, but mainly in preparing them to manage their own lifestyles.

Unhealthy consumption patterns, such as smoking, excessive ingestion of food, and especially unhealthy habits, such as inactivity, alcohol and illegal drug abuse, high risk sexual practices, and uncontrolled social stress predominantly lead to the appearance of chronic conditions [5].

Nevertheless, these negative lifestyle changes are spreading in the world and must be treated very seriously where chronic health problems are concerned. Every harmful behavior is recognized and a factor that leads to vulnerability to several chronic problems, including cardiovascular diseases, diabetes and strokes. Increasingly, dietary intake is being recognized as a fundamental driver of chronic health problems [5].

The prevalence in obesity has increased dramatically during the last 30 years. Obesity is associated with an increased risk of type 2 diabetes mellitus, dyslipidemia, hypertension, liver diseases, obtrusive sleep apnea, and certain types of cancer. The physiopathology of obesity is very complex, and involves genetic, behavioral and environmental factors. Today, the treatment options include changes to behavior and lifestyles that incorporate weight reduction, dieting and physical activities [6]. The majority of chronic conditions can be prevented, as well as their complications. Among the main strategies, at the micro level, to minimize the appearance of chronic conditions, early detection of the vulnerability of people and education aimed at encouraging healthy living practices is included, however, not always do health professionals make the most of the opportunities to inform the community about health promotion and disease prevention strategies.

A study carried out in Texas revealed that health professionals' work regarding prevention of diabetes only included controlling glucose levels and providing strategies for patients to go on diets, undertake physical exercises and use the medication correctly. Patients, however and beside that, also concern themselves more with conciliating their chronic conditions, when these coexist with their life structure especially in the social aspect, than with the physiopathology itself [7].

The activity of some health professionals is not articulated with the health policies and generates problems such as dehumanization of care, lack of commitment, low solving rate of activities, besides the lack of a list of offerings to assure patient access and acceptance [8]. On the other hand, the professionals are facing a crisis regarding their accomplishments and satisfaction, both as professionals and citizens. This way, it becomes necessary to make those professionals responsible for the quality of care they provide in this living work, in a role that places their knowledge as technological options producing effective initiatives to serve patients and their problems [9].

In order to accomplish this, the professionals must develop relationships with the patients, making it necessary to understand those people's needs to maintain and preserve their symbols. This will only be materialized through an inter-subjective relationship. Believing that the others are an infinite possibility of being makes the dialog to require a large amount of commitment, hope, and mainly, trust [10, 11].

The creation of relationships between patients and workers implies in taking on a new conception of health initiatives, that is, a change of attitude, both by the health worker and the patient. Traditionally, health education initiatives were centered around guidance and providing information regarding what is good and what is not, in order to maintain a healthy life, the patient was just someone taking part in the Health Service, mainly as a receiver of information and care. It is evident that within this view of health education no relationships will be built, but the opposite, a space is created in which the initiatives are channeled to a single direction that goes from the active professional to the passive patient. In this aspect, by incorporating assistance in the simultaneity with the investigation process, the PCA creates relationships both among the professionals and among these and the health action patients, therefore promoting the knowledge on how to research and care.

The truth is that the relationship between the lifestyle and chronic conditions has been researched for several years, by many researchers, however, the health professionals' experience shows that despite the knowledge built, it has not helped the population taking on a healthy lifestyle very much. This fact made the PCA authors raise a few questions such as: Is the practice of professionals regarding chronic conditions based on scientific evidence? Are researchers making interpretations with no practical evidence, that is, away from those people who live their daily lives with their chronic conditions? Is the nursing practice contributing to enforcing the national health policy set forth in the National Humanization Plan? After all, what research and health practice strategies could integrate theoretical and practical conceptions in such a way that, together with the research process, a promotion and prevention process could be conducted at the same time?

CONVERGING ASSISTANCE RESEARCH (PESQUISA CONVERGENTE ASSISTENCIAL – PCA): A NEW IDEA

The construction of this new idea that is, the Converging Assistance Research (Pesquisa Convergente Assistencial – PCA) started in 1990s after a set of experiences in the 1980s. The idea was tested during ten years with studies conducted in health institutions that made part of the Public Health Service Network (SUS) [12]. This type of research features its property to articulate with health assistance practice for this reason has been named Converging Assistance Research (Pesquisa Convergente Assistencial – PCA) [13]. The PCA uniqueness consists in maintaining throughout its process a close relationship with assistance practice with the purpose of finding alternatives to either solve or minimize problems, make changes and/or introduce innovations in the context of practice in which the investigation takes place. Therefore, the PCA is intended to be developed in the same physical and time space of a determined practice, and include the health professionals from that setting, such as those involved in the researching team. Together, they simultaneously develop research and health practices within that context, but with additions of critical and creative characteristics and the intention of bringing qualifying changes for that assistance.

The Converging Assistance Research (Pesquisa Convergente Assistencial – PCA) approach was developed by Trentini and Paim and published for the first time in 1999 [13]. Since then, this methodology has been used to research the nursing practice by several nurses in their research projects, including graduation dissertations and thesis, concentrating more in the Southern Region of Brazil – SC.

The fact that the PCA requires the incorporation of assistance activities in the research process and vice-versa, this does not imply the attribution of identical characteristics in the process developed by those two activities because each one's logic is preserved: research and assistance practice. After all, each one maintains its own identity, that is, both PCA and assistance have their borderlines delimited regarding the typification of knowledge to which it binds in its ethical aspects, to the scientific rigor and the aim of their respective activities as it pertains to it [12]. Therefore, the PCA strongly contributes to humanizing health assistance by being developed during the immersion of the researcher in the assistance, which makes it a partner in the humanization process. This way it interferes in refreshing the quality of education activities for the professionals and the health care. The PCA subjects (patients and professionals) are the same ones that are considered in the Federal Government National Humanization Plan [11].

The PCA Is Supported by the Following Assumptions [13]

- The context of assistance practice evokes innovation, solution alternatives to minimize or solve adverse situations, renewing the practices to overcome or maximize favorable situations. This requires commitment by the professionals to include the research projects in their assistance activities by bringing together the know-how to think and to do.
- The context of assistance practice is potentially a fertile ground for issues open to research studies.
- The space of relationships between research and assistance gives life simultaneously to the live work in the field of assistance practice and in scientific investigation.
- PCA implies the commitment of benefiting the assistance context during the investigation process, at the same time benefiting with straightforward access to information originating from this context.
- The health professional is a potential researcher of issues they deal with on a daily basis, which allows for a critical attitude that is appropriate to the growing intellectual dimension in the work they perform.

The articulation of the PCA with assistance practice takes place mainly in an attendance way, even more intensive in the information gathering phase, when participants and researchers are involved both in the assistance and research.

The subject matter connects theory and practice and has been object of reflection for many nursing professionals who discussed the possibility for the nurse to care, teach and research in an associated way [14] [15]. They stated that processing of these integrated actions would require a specific research methodology. The PCA has shown in its process a methodology that partly addresses such specificity. Thus, when a researcher decides to use the PCA methodology, he/she should be convinced of his/her interest in entering the field of assistance practice. This way, the researcher makes a pledge to building new knowledge that renews assistance practices in the field being studied.

The PCA acquires greater importance for its methodological feature of proximity an distancing before the know-how to assist. In this proximity and distancing between the PCA and assistance there are exchanges of reciprocate information along both processes that constitutes a special movement. This critical, intentional movement constitutes an interactive bridge and appears clearly outlined, both in methodological moments whose dominance is participation in care, and in the moments in which research has the greater dominance. At the central point of this critical movement between distancing and proximity of research and assistance is exactly the high point of autonomy of each process. During the research, the similarities and differences between such processes become visible and making the bridge between them is the common basis to build new knowledge from this assistance practice. Therefore, in this research approach there are common moments for the distinct scientific systems of assisting and researching, different logics that, during field research, both encompass the meaning of synthesis in the system to build new renewing knowledge of focused assistance.

The PCA is being configured as a tool that is typified by the immersion of the researcher in assistance practice, making this immersion the peculiar force of convergence that is essential to characterize the investigation method, hereby presented. Then the PCA implemented by studies with people in chronic health conditions in this field has been displaying results that influence lifestyles and cause evolutionary changes to the concrete reality of the scenarios through the dialog between the fields: of assistance practice and of the scientific investigation itself.

The PCA Is Typified by the Following Criteria

- Essentiality – the overlaying of the processes of assistance practice and investigation in a continuous dialogic action.
- Connectivity – the demand for actions of commitment between the researcher and the assistance team in rebuilding the "think and do" relationship.
- Interfaciality – the production of changes in assistance practice in the face of the investigative issues and vice-versa.
- Immersibility – the insertion of the researcher and his/her project as a present part in assistance activities aimed at the construction of shared and appropriate changes for new knowledge in both instances.

Ethics in Converging Assistance Research
(Pesquisa Convergente Assistencial – PCA)

The assurance of pragmatic effectiveness of ethical codes, the morality of research with human beings are aspects as relevant in the PCA as in any other research modality. Bioethical discussions are presented to analyze and suggest solutions to enforce a cultural and moral plurality in the complex societies of the contemporary world. However, bioethical questions are embedded, as in every research, by the best practices recognized by the Ethical Research Committees (Comitês de Ética em Pesquisa – CEP).

It is the responsibility of the researcher in PCA to consider the ethical aspects, in which he/she is involved as a research agent in their morality, which is one of the fundamental assurances of ethics in the research being developed. One noble value among others resides in cultivating respect and dignity in the relationships, mainly in the diverse modes of thinking and acting of those involved in the research throughout the researching process. Sharing information and responsibilities with the continuous return of research results are stressed, encompassing everyone that was included in it.

The commitment of the PCA researcher then presents itself extended in its assistance aspect. In it, note the combination of other professionals in direct assistance to subjects by the researcher ethics with those health service professionals, which serves as a locus for investigation. It is not about just including those professionals in the research team, but a commitment with its development. Therefore, it is the researcher's responsibility to promote feelings of participation, encouragement, cooperation with the benefits to human development from collective work. Following in this aspect of assistance when the researcher immerses himself/herself in the practice with the subjects, responsibility is imposed in the sensitive entry into this assistance locus connected to a health institution with its own ethical rules operationally set forth. The specific PCA ethic requires further that the researcher makes his/her work plan compatible with the already existing assistance ethics in the health services. The answers to the ongoing investigative questions get exposed to the local organization which will assume and include them while considering its benefits and the relevance of this inclusion.

Eventually, the researcher is ethically supported by the moral legitimacy of the research and the assistance codes of ethics and makes support provisions for those involved in the PCA in order to keep them encouraged to make decisions for changes following the research in the daily routine of their activities.

Summary of the Considerations Regarding: Detailed Vulnerabilities and Ethical Strictness

- Conflict in the research and practice theoretical reference;
- Confidentiality implied in the small and selective number of subjects;
- Ethical dilemmas: work on what the subject expresses himself/herself;
- The welcoming and pleasure feelings that generate suffering at the end of the research;
- The estimated continued benefits;
- Work on what the subject has left deep in the memory to avoid suffering (intensely variable/sensitive zone);
- The research problem never arises from single and individual thinking, it emerges from day-to-day practice;
- The idea of the problem sounds familiar among the team members;
- The importance and relevance of the research subject matter emerge from the practice itself;
- Project development includes the members of the Assistance team;
- The aggregation of the team around the problem issue substantiates political and ethical aspects;
- The assistance team shares the building and the advancement of knowledge;
- A research team may arise from the assistance team;

- Exercise criticism with validity and effectiveness as a duty, easy, hasty criticism spreads irresponsibly and gets lost with time;
- Criticism encompasses the entire project course;
- Determination of the problem corresponds to socialization of the idea;
- The widely presentation of the project encourages the promotion of studies in the assistance team;
- Making the research information available to the research team and the health team reenergize the collective competence;
- The PCA results provide visibility to other PCA proposition.

Outline of Studies about Lifestyle in the Context of Chronic Conditions – Using the PCA

In the present study, where the use of the PCA is concerned in order to compose a sample of the studies focusing on the lifestyles of patients in chronic conditions, a search was conducted in the website of the nursing graduate programs at the Federal University of Santa Catarina (Universidade Federal de Santa Catarina – UFSC) for thesis and dissertations that focused on lifestyle. The subjects in some of these researches were the persons in critical conditions themselves, and in others were nursing professionals involved in caring for people in such conditions. Five hundred and thirty five (535) studies were found among doctorate thesis and masters dissertations in nursing approved in the period from 2000 to 2006 at the Federal University of Santa Catarina (Universidade Federal de Santa Catarina – UFSC) – Brazil. Of this total, 41 (7.66%) were characterized as studies on lifestyle. Of the 41 studies, 16 (39.02%) used the PCA as methodological reference, and were reviewed. Therefore, 100% of the studies that used the PCA and focus on lifestyle with chronic patients and/or nurses were the sample for this revision.

Revision to the mentioned sources followed the procedure below: identification of the focus of each study through the title and key words; then the abstract was read in order to identify the methodological reference used. The 16 full studies were accessed at the University (UFSC) library and read entirely, with special attention to the results obtained, which were summarized and stored in a file. A further reading was made of the results to detect the changes obtained in the lifestyles of the research participants, considering that the PCA specificity is to find alternatives to solve or minimize problems, make changes and/or introduce innovations in the context of the practice where the investigation takes place.

The results regarding the changes were grouped into two main categories, each one with sub-categories, as shown below.

1) Changes to the lifestyle of persons in chronic conditions

    a) Minimization of negative feelings; stress and anxiety and domination between married couples.

    b) Maximization of occupational and leisure activities; well being, self esteem, access to support/aid and relationships; broadening of learning to learn; reconciliation of break ups resulting from the stress imposed by the chronic conditions; relationship with peers; awareness of rights to referral and claims addressed to obtaining improved citizenship and dialog relationship between married couples.

2) Changes to the approach by Professionals regarding care.

   a) Operational ways from the individual to the collective.
   b) Political, social and technical subject matters connected to the assured rights in the Health System
   c) The PCA in the building of innovations.

Changes as Results

The changes in lifestyles of patients and the changes in the behavior of nursing professionals are two major and best results obtained up to the present in the studies with individuals in chronic conditions using the PCA. The challenges faced by those professionals in this field of chronic conditions include an evolutionary search for the elements of growing qualification by accessing new health styles and lifestyles.

The PCA adds contributions to the changes to people's lifestyles, thus, its delimitation includes theory and practice, which helps the researcher to also act as a carer in the assistance practice. The progress of the PCA in the proposition itself and the uses that have been made of it point to the relation of commitment the PCA imposes in establishing the changes resulting from its process. In general, those changes are caused intentionally by the researcher activities, especially from his/her immersion in the nursing practice with the PCA subjects. The changes to the lifestyles of persons in chronic conditions bring through modulation results that were presented in the research reports read and could be organized and classified for this study: 1) Minimization of suffering; 2) Maximization of well being; 3) Awareness of growing behavioral replacements. The PCA process also brings, as a consequence, changes to the behavior of researchers regarding nursing practices. Although in the PCA investigations this objective is not intentional, it is reached regardless of the strategies used for this purpose. However, nurses and research subjects in PCA undergo changes and rethink their techniques, methods, nursing practice activities, reaching a new level with increased quality in creativity, documentation and methodological approaches in their professional routines. In every movement there is a dialectic relationship between assistance and research activities in order to promote changes in both.

Converging Assistance Research (PCA)
Conducted with Patients in Chronic Conditions

Changes to the lifestyle of persons in chronic conditions today correspond to one of the greatest challenges for care professionals in this area of activity. The paradigm breaks are increasingly becoming a sign in this beginning of the 21st Century, which brings changes to life habits and intended alterations in favor of health and daily activities.

Nursing research has been following up and assuming subject matters and methodological choices, with new trends and even with more creativity expression. In this building of knowledge, a greater possibility of disclosure, socialization, and accessibility to new care and the adoption of new styles for a healthy living appears.

Some reports from research using the PCA show a path between their results, which appears as a transition from minimizing suffering, going through behavior replacements to maximizing well being. The topic classified as minimization is a part of the category "negative feelings", translated as human burnout expressed by patients with negative perceptions of themselves. With the progression of joint learning resulting from care in PCA, those perceptions are replaced with new behaviors. Those behaviors are reaffirmed and made available in ideas from the patients for renewal and acquisition of new ways of thinking about life and health in their concrete situations they live in there.

In the movement of research results, this chapter shows the negative feeling expressed by: stated sadness; manifested low self esteem; anxieties and insomnia with no association to the cause; feelings of powerlessness in the face of resolutions about the self; feelings of isolation, loneliness. These feelings have emerged from the patients investigated by the PCA.

The PCA researcher bases his/her activity of practices in the findings of the strict research process being implemented. The practice with persons in chronic conditions has focused mainly in the fundamental activities in health education, which included: a) acknowledgement of and care with the body within possibilities and limitations; b) body movement in individual exercising and in socializing with walks; c) dance and singing together; d) learning micro techniques for stretching; e) pushups and other appropriate movements. Those procedures not only provide health to the body in its physical structure and functions but also provide soothing of symptoms and signs that could exacerbate and overload those patients, whose conditions are irreversible since they are chronic.

One result that implies in the maximization of the quality of relationships is the situation of treating "relationships between married couples". This relationship, when it is negative (gender domination) appeared as a health vulnerability that could favor various ways of becoming ill. For issues of health promotion and disease prevention, the PCA has been used in the corporate field and gave place to learning a new lifestyle. The involvement of researcher and subjects in this matter was instigating and brought to light the domination between married couples (husband dominating over the wife) [16]. During the evolution of the research in the assistance phase, the negative relationship was minimized and domination was replaced by a symmetrical relationship between the married couples. Proceeding with the research on practice, the researcher encouraged the acknowledgement of their gender relationships and the situation was maximized with a marital relationship qualified as being healthy.

The core idea that added results to the conduction of the mentioned PCA is that the gender relationships imply determining elements for a healthy living and that recomposing democratic aspects of those relationships promotes health [16].

Care, as part of the PCA, potentializes the legitimacy of doing and approximates theoretical and practical dimensions of the nursing profession in search of a life quality aimed at new styles of living. The health professionals face the shifting and extension of models that surpass the exclusive biological outlook and build activities that consider social sciences with human values. In the interest of changes to people's lifestyles, the PCA, in its practical dimension, has proved more effective when implemented with groups. With this, the PCA has been seeking changes to processes pertaining to assistance practices and reaching some stages of differentiation with results in lifestyles. There are evidences that the quality of relationships in groups in chronic conditions has added value to the building of new research and assistance practices.

Several PCA studies have been conducted with patients in diabetes mellitus conditions [17] [18] [19] [20]. Most of them revealed that the lifestyles of those people are under the desirable. A large part amongst those taking oral medication manifested the fear of taking insulin; showed social isolation; did not accept the condition of diabetes, which resulted in anger and problems in family and work relationships. It is very common in the culture of people with diabetes in Brazil to reject the use of insulin, since some people claim they are not skilled to apply it and do not want to depend on others for such. Others believe that who needs to inject insulin is at the final stage of the disease, and also believe that insulin is addictive.

The patients also showed difficulty and resistance to adapt to a new lifestyle, since the condition of diabetes requires changes of habits and the acquisition of new responsibilities, such as for example, trying to learn what diabetes actually is, why the treatment regime is needed, learning to live with diabetes and learning to control the possible complications inherent to this chronic condition. Research has also shown that the patients maintained habits of consuming tobacco, alcohol, legal and illegal drugs, and consuming foods that are not recommended for diabetic individuals.

The food regime was mentioned as the greatest difficulty faced by patients, for some it was due to financial conditions; for others, the difficulty to resist a plentiful table and also the lack of family support. Those factors were seen as an impossibility to make a suitable diet viable. In communities outside the large urban centers, there is also the belief that reducing the amount of food and/or consume foodstuffs with low carbohydrate content means losing strength and not being able to perform daily activities.

Among patients there was a feeling manifested that diabetes is a disease of the body, therefore it can be healed and/or controlled with medication; others believe it is a disease of the mind. It is supposed then that it is related to stressful situations. There are some who believe diabetes is a "karma" or a "bad spell", that is, there is a superstition influencing their ways of thinking [21] [20].

The majority of patients presented serious physical complications – visual and renal impairment; foot integrity compromising; diabetic autonomous cardiovascular neuropathy; and sexual impairment [18]. Besides, the patients reported they suffer prejudice and discrimination from society and also suffer with the precarious health institutions attending conditions.

Health policies in Brazil are well structured in theory and have legal power, but unfortunately are not yet effective in their practices with the same technological coverage in the distributions among the several regions of the country. In theory, the Unified Health System (Sistema Único de Saúde – SUS) assures access to health services to all the Brazilian population, although it is not structured well enough to cope with all that demand. Regarding healing treatment, people of higher acquisition power usually contract private health insurance. Patients with lower social economic conditions depend solely on the public system offerings that, in some regions, is practically inoperative, with patients spending months in line waiting for specialized treatment. The Unified Health System proposition includes the Promotion of Health according to the Ottawa Conference, however, the population usually does not have access, or has limited access to preventive measures. This is related to the precarious results, including aggravation of chronic conditions.

As to treatment, it was identified that patients not only seek help in the professional system, they also treat themselves with teas from a variety of herbs, ingest their own urine and chicken bile. They visit "healers", and undergo spiritual surgery as well as "spells". Regarding the last item, one patient reported and example of a spell: "take a piece of sugar cane as tall as the person, with the root, remove the leaves and wash thoroughly, place the cane under the mattress on the side you sleep. When the cane dries up, throw it into a river and it takes the diabetes away" [17].

The Converging Assistance Research (PCA) has greatly contributed to redirect the lifestyles of those patients due to the fact that the PCA encompasses research and assistance practice activities. This convergence leads to the issues emerged from the subjects in the process and their cultural expressions are acknowledged and brought into assistance through health education. According the aforementioned results, assistance included mainly health education that was being implemented as patients related the problems. Education was developed with patients gathered in groups with workshops and, when necessary, complemented with individual activities. In most studies the subject matters discussed emerged from the patients and served as a basis for planning and executing the nursing activities on the next meeting, thus building the PCA thematic continuity.

By the end of the project, researchers were able to identify the changes that took place, as shown by the conclusions of one researcher [17]. Through health education during the PCA process, it was found that feelings, behaviors, attitudes, values and beliefs were minimized or replaced or maximized so as to create a new lifestyle, which will help to live with diabetes in a more healthy way.

The practical part of the PCA that took place with the patients during the workshops allowed the participants to broaden their knowledge about the chronic complications of diabetes, about the resources available for prevention and treatment, as well as thinking of strategies to face the already initiated complications. The education activity allowed sufferers of diabetes a new look over the issue of chronic complications of the disease. The autonomy the patients with diabetes show in prevention and early detection of complications and quick and efficient intervention, when initiated, reduces the deeper damage to health in the individual with diabetes [18].

The PCA has also been used in studies with patients with chronic cardiovascular problems [22, 23, 24]. Although cardiovascular conditions include several coronary artery diseases, congestive heart failure, hypertension, among others, the daily problems of patients with different pathologies face are similar. The situations researched are presented here as a whole, having in common the lifestyle of those patients threatened with a variety of problems that, in this chapter, have been grouped into three categories: 1) losses; 2) threats; 3) challenges.

The research subjects reported losses in physical capacity, in keeping their jobs, in social relationships, and financial status. The chronic conditions are long in duration, since the majority of them remain throughout people's lives, which implies in losses in income with permanent emotional and financial burdens with treatment. The losses related to physical capacity for restricting daily activities affect those persons' autonomy, generating dependency due to the limitations in the daily routine. They also affect their work and social relationships since they affect their role in the family and in society. Abandoning something that is pleasurable, such as the habitual food, even if not the healthiest to follow a food regime. Those situations of loss, many times considered as deprivations, have a negative effect in those persons' lifestyles.

Patients also consider the chronic condition as a threat due to the perception of frailness and dependency in the performance of an organ in their body and the possibility of being away from the beloved ones. The threat involves lack of control due to the unforeseeable nature of something that is about to happen represented by the complications they are subject to and the need to maintain a new model of fulfill commitments in the family environment, at work and with themselves.

The chronic condition as a challenge to continue with the treatment is referred to as the need to take on new habits, cover the financial costs, seek resources and the possibility of appearing side effects from the medication. Medical follow-up, the exaggerated amount of exams, or even being hospitalized demand time and energy to maintain all the commitments, beside exposure to risks and dependency on professional care. Dieting and exercising are seen as challenges as they require new knowledge, change of habits, and the belief in a future well being. Stress also results from the chronic condition, as it has impact, imposing significant changes in those persons' lifestyles.

The articulation of research activities and nursing assistance practice in those studies occurred via workshops where there was an opportunity for patients to speak out about their life and health condition. This part corresponded to the research data. The practical assistance part of the PCA has comprised an educational process that takes place in parallel with the production of research data. For each group of problems presented there was a break for discussion, reflection, and gathering of the information required by the researchers.

The educational practice makes it possible to promote an interrelation between the research subjects and the exchange of experiences they live. With educational practice, it was possible to drive awareness for research subjects to change their way of facing the losses, threats and to face the challenges in a healthier way [24].

The PCA approach has been also very useful to study the lifestyle of the elderly with chronic pain and Alzheimer's [25]. The PCA assistance practice consisted in the use of several therapeutic techniques. One of them used exercises in water which contributed to minimize pain in patients [26]. Playful body activities were also practiced, body expression dancing, recreational games, "capoeira", trekking, gymnastics, yoga, among others [23]. The playful body activities provided a variety of body movements, differing from the hegemony in the traditional physical education programs. Patients maximized their understanding and perception of their own bodies, physical fitness, and the relationship with their peers.

Stimulation of playful activities has brought feelings of joy and happiness in the elderly, feelings which were observed by the researcher and reported by the research subjects.

The playful workshops included the creation of a space for freedom and satisfaction in playing with others, playing together, as very seldom do adults allow themselves any play during their lives. It was found that "playing together" has emerged, among the patients, a true relationship that made them feel valued, loved and understood. Those aspects are much more important for health than the repetitive activities performed in health clubs. In those workshops, the patients spontaneously expressed their perceptions, their values, their needs and still tried to help their peers. These collective experiences encouraged new ways of behave in relation to life and health, and showed a will to make significant changes in their lifestyles.

Currently there are new ways of considering chronic conditions. Treatment is not based on the origin of a specific health condition, but in the requirements imposed by the problem [5]. Regarding chronic conditions, the requirements are similar, regardless of their origin, therefore the care strategies are also similar. Attempting to live the healthiest lifestyle as possible is what there is in common in people with chronic conditions, no matter what kind of disease. To accomplish this goal, these people must be stimulated to take on their lives independently and to take, as partners in their care, health professionals.

Converging Assistance Research (PCA) Performed with Nursing Professionals

Beside the changes to patient lifestyles, the PCA has also contributed to the change of behavior of some nursing professionals when they are subjects of research and carers of persons in chronic conditions. Based on the problems identified in the nursing care, studies were developed using the PCA in different settings in search of consistency with the Brazilian Unified Health System principles.

The intention of researchers in the mentioned studies was based on the assumption that the nurses could work as multipliers in the change of lifestyles for persons with chronic diseases. For such, the researchers needed authentic information about the context of the current practices, including the relationship between nurses and patients [27]. With these new concepts for caring in nursing acquired during the research process, nurses included in their ways of caring an educational process as well. To implement such a complex project of bringing together two activities such as research and assistance in their individual characteristics, they have decided to use the PCA approach as it considers the relationship between those processes.

The PCA does not support own techniques to collect and analyze data or establish a specific approach as a theoretical reference for assistance. Thus, each researcher feels free to choose, as long as he/she remains faithful to the PCA purposes and principles. All those studies used several information gathering techniques, such as individual interviews with nurses, observation, and mainly discussion in small groups. At the same time that they involved the nurses in the education process, they recorded statements regarding questions, the way they assisted the patients, how they behaved and the difficulties faced, among others

[8] [28]. This way, the research activities and the practice activities, in this case the educational practices overlapped and seemed to be the same activity. However, researchers differentiated them by observing the PCA indication for essentiality by assuring the dialogic for respect toward individuality of each overlapping process.

The PCA contributed to the change in the nurses' mode of activity regarding assistance, going from an almost, exclusively individual activity to a collective involvement. This change is also due to the fact that the opportunity has been given to reveal their problems and difficulties and the possibility of renewing their professional practice during the research process. This fact is evident in the considerations made in the researcher reports: this research approach, beside providing an outlook of the nurses work situation, generated changes in the entire assistance methodology developed with the diabetic persons in the community [8]. The nurses became aware that, in order to help patients gain a healthy lifestyle, they should introduce a radical change to the way the nurses interacted with them. They went from imperative attitudes to democratic ones, and developed care methods to reach the collective by abandoning the reductionist health outlook focused exclusively in the biological dimension and migrating to an extended conception of health. [29, 30]. It was evident that there were skill inadequacies of the nursing professionals to stimulate patients to follow a healthy lifestyle; fact which could lead patients to abandon treatment and only return when the complications arise. However, in studies like these, whose approach makes use of the PCA, there is a compromise between researchers and assistance nurses, for this reason, nurses could be awakened to acknowledge and avoid a gap between practice and research.

Political, Social and Technical Issues Connected to the Assured Rights in the Health System

Others, using the Converging Assistance Research (Pesquisa Convergente-Assistencial – PCA) developed with nurses revealed that not always did health institutions fulfill their duties regarding the offer of continued education. When this occurs, it is at times done superficially, centered around technical skills only, fragmented and with no political compliance to the current health policy. Rarely are recently admitted health professionals aware of the UnifiedHealth System (Sistema Único de Saúde – SUS) guiding principles for a really significant approach, with all its dimensions and resulting implications [31].

The activity of some health professionals occurs in a way that is unarticulated from the health policies, generating several problems in the daily routine of services, dehumanization, lack of commitment, poor capacity of resolution for the activities. Workers are living through a crisis regarding their fulfillment and satisfaction as professionals and citizens. For such, it is necessary to make those professionals responsible for the quality of assistance they offer, placing their knowledge as technological options producing effective activities to serve patients and their problems [9].

As nurses verbalized situations they have experienced regarding the promotion of a healthy lifestyle, there was room for critical reflection about the problems observed in patients. This is one of the PCA differences, when compared with other types of research. As it can be seen in the PCA, the research subjects are also subjects in the education practice.

This research-assistance process has contributed to build awareness of the group of nurses regarding the need to redirect their practice in order to be consistent with the Unified Health System (Sistema Único de Saúde – SUS) principles, therefore the change in the way of thinking of health and the way of nurses caring has become evident [30].

During the Converging Assistance Research process, some nurses understood that they could not provide assistance to people unless by hearing what they have to say and it would also not be convenient to invent assistance models without knowing what people consider as being their priority. Listening to them and having them listen to themselves is the start of every and any change to be encouraged [32]. In collective health, more trends to know about health indicators were identified than modes of intervening in reality. In fact, collective health would play the role of a social player advocating for life, since in practice more respect to private property is perceived than to citizens' health [33]. This situation has appeared every day in health institutions life in Brazil, which is expressed in the population insecurity, in the type of care, and in the crisis of fulfillment and satisfaction as citizens and professionals in the group of health sector professionals [9].

The Converging Assistance Research (PCA) Ahead in Building Technological Innovations

The PCA served as a valuable instrument for a group of nurses to translate and apply an assistance technology to the families of patients in critical conditions [30]. The collection of data was carried out with the technical nursing team as the subject of research through interviews, active observation and group discussion. The research data shows that there is a distance between the sector nurses and the patient families, that is, the presence of the family was being ignored by the nurses, which was considered a problem.

The objective of the discussion with this group of nurses was to reflect upon the data obtained and decide on strategies to be followed to solve the problem of distancing. They reached a consensus to translate and implement a technological tool whose main principle was welcome people. This study also made clear that the PCA goes beyond research results because the researcher is committed to also practicing assistance during the study process. In this study, assistance took place with the group of nurses that resulted in the awareness of the nursing team to extend the paradigm that they had been using to another one that would also include the area of social relationships [30].

Advances of the Converging Assistance Research (PCA) in Other Areas of Lifestyle and Health

In the research records (PCA) with persons in chronic conditions in the scope of the sample assessed, no investigation was found with children and adolescents as study subjects. This is a gap to be filled, given the compatibility the PCA opens up for these situations.

As with adults, this reality is also experienced by children and adolescents. Recent epidemiological studies have documented trends about the increase in obesity and the consumption of legal and illegal drugs among adolescents. Faced with evidence that the cardiovascular risk factors have appeared to be persistent in adult life, this could become an epidemic of cardiovascular diseases in the future. This way, the health professionals must take on the responsibility for prevention, detection and intervention regarding risk factors in adolescence, including hyperlipidemia, hypertension, obesity and drug abuse.

Promoting health, changing lifestyle, including an adequate diet to maintain the desired body weight, avoiding risky behaviors must be incorporated in people's daily lives. Intervention directed at adolescents must take into account its social profiles, particularly the family, school and community. Adolescents must be empowered through education and the development of skills to take on responsibility for their own health behaviors [34].

Overweight and obesity in children has become epidemic, the number of overweight children in the United States has doubled in the last three decades. Internationally, approximately 22 million children around the world are overweight, which may lead to metabolism abnormalities and this, in turn, to chronic conditions [35].

Co-morbidities associated with obesity and overweight are similar in children as in the adult population. High blood pressure, dyslipidemia, and the high prevalence of factors associated with insulin resistance and type 2 diabetes appear as frequent co-morbidities in the overweight and obese pediatric population. Obesity in childhood, particularly in adolescents, is a predicting factor of obesity in adult life. Morbidity and mortality in the adult population increase in individuals who were overweight as adolescents, even after eliminating the overweight during adult life [36] [6].

Skeletal problems, especially in the spine, have also been detected in children and adolescents. The overload from the weight of backpacks and incorrect postural habits constitute risk factors for chronic conditions related to the skeletal system. The weight of backpacks was researched in a population of 240 children aged between 11 and 14 years, in the 5th and 6th grades, correlating it to the children's body weight. The findings showed a reverse relation between the children's weight and the backpack weight that leads to postural overload and osteomuscular disorders [37].

Researchers examined the relation between self-reported positive events and blood pressure in 69 children and adolescents with average age of 11.7 years. The co-relational analysis showed a reverse relation between positive events and diastolic blood pressure, which suggests that adolescents who experienced more positive events in life had lower diastolic pressure. The hierarchic regression analysis revealed that physical activity, sodium- and potassium-based diets, family hypertension history had a prediction of 24.6% in the variance of systolic pressure and 34.6% in the variance of diastolic pressure. Besides, the "positive events" variable had an additional prediction of 4.3% in the variance of diastolic arterial pressure. Those results suggest that the increased perception of positive events in life works as an absorber in higher blood pressure in adolescents [38].

CONCLUSION

The Converging Assistance Research (Pesquisa Convergente Assistencial – PCA) approach is configured as follows: 1) innovative investigation approach by bringing together health professional subjects overlapping in convergence, theory, research and assistance practice; 2) a means of building relationships between the research and assistance practice processes; 3) a qualified projection of interventions summarized in changes.

The results obtained through the PCA in the various investigations dealt with in this chapter show the differential in this innovative approach to maintain an effective articulation between research and assistance practice so as to contribute with changes to the lifestyles of individuals in chronic health conditions.

REFERENCES

[1] Brasil. Lei N° 8.080, de 19 de setembro de 1990. Dispõe sobre as condições para a promoção, proteção e recuperação da saúde, a organização e o funcionamento dos serviços correspondentes e dá outras providências. Diário Oficial da República Federativa do Brasil, 19 de Set 1990.

[2] Neto, ER. Reforma sanitária e o sistema único de saúde: suas origens suas propostas, sua implantação, suas dificuldades e suas perspectivas. In: Brasil, MS. *Incentivo à participação popular e controle social no SUS*. Textos técnicos para conselheiros de saúde. Brasília: Ministério da Saúde IEC, 1994; 48-62.

[3] Néri, AL. A pesquisa em gerontologia no Brasil: análise de conteúdo de amostra de pesquisa em psicologia no período de 1975-1976. *Texto Contexto Enferm*, 1997 Maio-Agosto; 6 (2), 69-105.

[4] Monteiro, CA; Iunes, RF; Torres, AM. A evolução do país e de suas doenças: síntese, hipóteses e implicações. In: Monteiro CA, editores. *Velhos e novos males da saúde no Brasil: a evolução do país e de suas doenças*. 2. ed. São Paulo: Hucitec; 2000; 34-52.

[5] Organização Mundial da Saúde (OMS). Cuidados inovadores para condições crônicas: componentes estruturais de ação relatório mundial 2003. Brasília: OMS; 2003.

[6] Meninger, JC et al. Genetic and enviromental influences on cardiovascular disease, risk factors in adolescents. *Nurs. Res*, Dec.1998 44 (1), 11-8.

[7] Hunt, LM; Arar, NH; Larme, AC. Constrasting patient and practitioner perspectives in type II diabetes management. *WJNR,* Dec.1998 20 (6), 656-682.

[8] Moretto, EFS. A enfermagem e o SUS: da realidade à possibilidade [Dissertação]. Florianópolis: UFSC/Programa de Pós-graduação em Enfermagem; 2000.

[9] Nasser, ESQC. O que dizem os símbolos? São Paulo: Paulus; 2003.

[10] Brasil. Humaniza SUS. Política nacional de humanização: a humanização como eixo norteador das práticas de atenção a gestão em todas as instâncias do SUS. Brasília: Ministério da Saúde; 2004.

[11] Trentini, M; Paim, L. Pesquisa Convergente-assistencial: um desenho que une o fazer e o pensar na prática assistencial de saúde-enfermagem. 2 ed. Florianópolis: Insular; 2004.

[12] Trentini, M; Paim, L. Pesquisa em enfermagem: uma modalidade convergente-assistencial. Florianópolis: *UFSC.* 1999.

[13] Neves, EA; Dias, LP; Silva, AL. Pesquisar para assistir. *Rev. da Esc. de Enfermagem da USP*. Número especial 1992 26, 119-124.

[14]   Boyd, CO. Toward a nursing practice research method. *Adv. Nurs. Sc, Dic.* 1993 16 (2), 9-25.

[15]   Madureira, VF. A visão masculina das relações de por no casal heterossexual como subsídio para a educação em saúde na prevenção de DST/AIS [Tese]. Florianópolis: UFSC/Programa de Pós-graduação em Enfermagem; 2005.

[16]   Beltrame, V. O cuidado cultural compartilhado em grupo com pessoas na condição crônica de diabetes mellitus [Dissertação]. Florianópolis: UFSC/Programa de Pós-graduação em Enfermagem; 2000.

[17]   SandovaL, RDCB. Grupo de convivência de pessoas com diabetes mellitus e familiares percepção acerca das complicações crônicas e conseqüências sociais crônicas [Dissertação]. Florianópolis: UFSC/Programa de Pós-graduação em Enfermagem; 2003.

[18]   Francioni, FF. Grupo de convivência: uma alternativa para o processo de aceitação do viver com diabetes mellitus [Dissertação]. Florianópolis: UFSC/Programa de Pós-graduação em Enfermagem; 2000.

[19]   Mattosinho, MMS. Itinerário terapêutico do adolescente com diabetes melitus tipo 1 e seus familiares [Dissertação]. Florianópolis: UFSC/Programa de Pós-graduação em Enfermagem; 2005.

[20]   SILVA, DMGV. A construção da experiência de viver com diabetes mellitus [Tese]. Florianópolis: UFSC/Programa de Pós-graduação em Enfermagem; 2000.

[21]   Natividade, MSL. Os estressores decorrentes do processo de viver de pessoas com doença arterial coronariana [Dissertação]. Florianópolis: UFSC/Programa de Pós-graduação em Enfermagem; 2004.

[22]   Bonetti, A. O coração e o lúdico: vivências corporais para um viver mais saudável de pessoas com doenças aterosclerótica coronariana [Dissertação]. Florianópolis: UFSC/Programa de Pós-graduação em Enfermagem; 2006.

[23]   Bastos, DS. Cuidados de pessoas portadoras de hipertensão arterial [Dissertação]. Florianópolis: UFSC/Programa de Pós-graduação em Enfermagem; 2002.

[24]   Pelzert, MT. Assistência cuidativa humanística de enfermagem para familiares cuidadores de idosos com doença de Alzhaimer a partir de um grupo de ajuda mútua [Tese]. Florianópolis: UFSC/Programa de Pós-graduação em Enfermagem; 2005.

[25]   Martins, P. O significado de uma terapia em meio aquático para o idoso com doença articular degenerativa [Dissertação]. Florianópolis: UFSC/Programa de Pós-graduação em Enfermagem; 2005.

[26]   Moretto, MA. A política e a prática nas umidades básicas de saúde [Dissertação]. Florianópolis: UFSC/Programa de Pós-graduação em Enfermagem; 2000.

[27]   Paini JP. Diálogo vivido como cuidado humanizado no processo educativo de enfermagem [Dissertação]. Florianópolis: UFSC/Programa de Pós-graduação em Enfermagem; 2000.

[28]   Manfrini, GC. O cuidado às famílias rurais com base na teoria do desenvolvimento da família [Dissertação]. Florianópolis: UFSC/Programa de Pós-graduação em Enfermagem; 2005.

[29]   Nascimento, EFP. Acolhimento no espaço das relações na unidade de terapia intensiva [tese]. Florianópolis: UFSC/Programa de Pós-Graduação em Enfermagem; 2003.

[30] Moretto, EFS. Os enfermeiros e o SUS. Passo Fundo: UPF, 2001.

[31] Merhy, EE. O SUS e um dos seus dilemas: mudar a gestão e a lógica do processo de trabalho em saúde (um ensaio sobre a micropolítica do trabalho vivo). In: Fleury, S, editor. *Saúde e democracia: a luta do CEBES*. São Paulo: Lemos Editorial; 1997; 125-141.

[32] Trentini, M; Paim L. Pesquisa e assistência experiências com grupos de estudo na enfermagem. Curitiba: Champangnat; 2003.

[33] Campos, GWS. Análise crítica das contribuições da saúde coletiva à organização das práticas de saúde no SUS. In: FLEURY, S, editor. *Saúde e democracia: a luta do CEBES*. São Paulo: Lemos Editorial; 1997; 113-124.

[34] Mccrindle, BW. Cardivascular risk factors in adolescents: relevance, detection, and intervention. *Adolesc. Med*, Feb. 2001 12 (1), 147-62.

[35] Deckelbaum, RJ; Williams, CL. Childhood obesity: the health issue. *Adolesc. Med*, Feb. 2001 12 (1), 110 -25.

[36] Orbach, P; Lowenthal DT. Evaluation and treatment of hypertension in active individuals. *Med Sci Sports Exerc*, Oct.1998 30 (10), 354-66.

[37] Vitta, A; Madrigal, C; Sales VS. Peso corporal e peso do material escolar transportado por crianças em idade escolar. *Fisioterapia em Movimento*, Abr/Jun 2003 16 (2),61-72.

[38] Caputo, JL; Rudolph, DL; Morgan, DW. Influence of positive life events on blood pressure in adolescents. *J. Behv. Med*, Apr. 1998 21 (2), 115-29.

Reviewed by
Márcia Lisboa RN, PhD.
Professor – Universidade Federal do Rio de Janeiro
Email: marcialis@terra.com.br
And by
Enedina Soares RN, PhD.
Professor – Universidade Federal do Estado do Rio de Janeiro
Email: soaresene@ig.com.br

In: Life Style and Health Research Progress
Editors: A. B. Turley, G. C. Hofmann

ISBN: 978-1-60456-427-3
© 2008 Nova Science Publishers, Inc.

Chapter X

Gender Differences in Proneness to Depression among Hungarian College Students

Ferenc Margitics and Zsuzsa Pauwlik

Department of Psychology at College of Nyíregyháza, Hungary

ABSTRACT

Aims: Our research aimed to find out what role the risk mechanisms, as described in Goodman and Gotlib's (1999) model (genetic-biological, interpersonal, social learning related cognitive and stress related factors), play in the development of increased risk for depression in the case of men and women.

Methods: The genetic-biological factors were examined with certain temperament characteristics, the interpersonal factors with parental educational purpose, educational attitudes, educational style and parental treatment. In the case of factors related to social learning we looked at the dysfunctional attitudes and the attributional style. As far as the stressors are concerned, we observed the quality of family atmosphere, and the number of the positive and negative life events of the preceding six months and their subjective evaluation. Six hundred and eighty-one students took part in the research (465 female and 216 male).

Results: Our research results show that all of the increased risk mechanisms, namely the genetic-biological, interpersonal, social learning related cognitive, and stress related factors are connected with the development of vulnerability to depression, explaining 41.4% of the depression symptoms' variance in the case of women, and 36.5% in the case of men. Harm avoidance, a genetic-biological factor, proved to be the most significant risk mechanism, irrespective of the sexes. From among the environmental factors – irrespective of the sexes – one stress-related factor, the subjective evaluation of negative life experiences, which implies an increased sensitivity to stress, proved to be the strongest risk mechanism. While the above factors played an important role in the development of vulnerability to depression in both sexes, the social learning related cognitive and interpersonal risk mechanisms differed in their degree in women and men. In the case of women, the social learning-related mechanisms proved to be stronger and higher impact risk factors than in the case of men. The effect of interpersonal factors seemed to be relatively the weakest in the development of increased risk for depression.

Limitations: The results of our research cannot be generalised to represent present day 18- to 23-year-old Hungarian youth due to the limitations of our sample.

Conclusion: The mental hygienic interpretation of our research findings is that in the future there should be more emphasis put on the personality development of college and university students, especially on the development of such competencies which aid them in effectively coping in their struggle with the depressive mood.

Keywords: depression symptoms, risk transmitting mechanisms, gender differences.

1. INTRODUCTION

The results of psychiatric epidemiological research show that depression has become one of the most common illnesses of our time. Based on Hungarian and international data, nearly 20 percent of adults have, at least once in their life, experienced a depressive episode and the prevalence of chronic depression is over 10 percent.

According to the results of research using self-rating scales, depressive syndrome is also very frequent in samples taken from the Hungarian population. Thirty-four percent of women and 19% of men interviewed reported symptoms of depression, which in the case of women reached 11.8% whereas in the case of men 5.5% of the serious clinical level [2,3]. A study carried out by Margitics [4] among college students showed mild, subclinical level of depression in 36.6% of the samples (40% of women, 29.3% of men) and moderate depression in 6.7% (8.4% of women, 3.4% of men).

Several well-documented studies carried out in the field of psychiatric epidemiology have proved a higher prevalence of depression among women. A great number of studies have dealt with the differences between the genders in the cases of chronic minor depression and dysthymia [5]. These studies consistently found that the proportion of prevalence is 2:1. Kessler et al [6], in minor depression, Angst and Merikangas [5] in short repetitive depression, found a consistently higher prevalence among women than among men. On the other hand, they did not find major differences between the genders in the prevalence of mania, neither in epidemiological research [7], nor in clinical studies [8].

The question arises of whether the proportion of prevalence is the same between the genders if the age of the study population is examined as well. Kessler at al [9] compared retrospective age-of-onset reports in a representative cross-sectional research with reports across subsamples of different age respondents. Group scales gained after the study of data distribution showed that differences between the genders relating to depression surfaced at the age of 11-15 and remained consistently higher later on.

Over the years several theories have been made to explain these differences between the genders. For instance, the female role theories argue that chronic stress connected to traditional female roles may cause higher prevalence of depression among women [10]. According to the rumination theory, women are more likely to deal with a problem longer than men and, as a result, the temporary symptoms of disphory turn to major parts of depression [11]. Both perspectives assume that the higher prevalence of clinically more significant depression among women is, at least partly, the result of their higher persistence.

Goodman and Gotlib [12] suggest the separation four mechanisms within an integrative model with the help of which the increased risk for depression can be explained. Two of these mechanisms are primarily genetical-biological while the other two are cognitive-interpersonal: the first mechanism focuses on the genetic factors, on the heritability of depression, the second is connected to innate dysfunctional neuroregulatory mechanisms, the third mechanism focuses on the confused interpersonal relations and dysfunctional cognitions related to social learning, the fourth mechanism includes the stressful context of a child's life; thus it can be connected to the stress load of a child

According to Goodman and Gotlib [12], all four above mentioned mechanisms are possible mechanisms of the increased risk for depression, but it is not quite clear to what extent they are responsible for the development of risk, or furthermore how they interact with each other. It is possible that one or more are present at the same time.

A substantial amount of literature discusses the consistent genetic transmission of depressive disturbance in the case of adults. According to the studies, which examined twins, families and adopted people, the risk for depression in the case of first grade relatives of those suffering from affective disturbance is 20-25%, in contrast to the 7% of risk level among the average population [13]. The genetic analysis of behaviour has proved numerous correlations with the high possibility of inheritance for depression [14]. Among other factors, temperament [15], behavioral inhibition and timidity [16], neuroticism [17] and sociability [18] may increase vulnerability to depression and be special factors in connection with inheritance. The results of modern temperament studies indicate that a tendency to avoid harm may be considered as the basic factor of biological vulnerability to depression which appears as a characteristic feature as early as in childhood. Harm avoidance refers to an inherited pattern which may appear in the form of passive avoidance and fear of the uncertain [19]. According to studies carried out by Hansen et al. [20], harm avoidance and low self-directedness are in harmony with the degree of depression.

A great number of studies have examined the connection between interpersonal factors and depression. In his studies, Parker [21] noted that those suffering from neurotic depression had received less parental attention, and higher maternal overprotection. In non-clinic groups the signs of depression were also related to less parental attention, and showed a slight correlation with parental overprotection. According to Parker's [22] research results, the correlation between lower parental care and depression was independent of the degree of depression. In his later studies Parker [23] argued that the kind of parental care which is characterised by low attention and high overprotection is linked to the high risk of neurotic disturbance (depressive neurosis, social phobia, anxiety neurosis), while the additional risk for psychotic disturbance is low or completely non-existent. In research carried out by Mackinnon and his colleagues [24] on non-clinic samples, lack of parental care was the number one risk factor of depression, as opposed to overprotection. Narita and his colleagues [25] carried out a study of Japanese samples and found that low parental care was always connected with depression at any age and the connection between depression and overprotection was obvious, also.

Problematic parental care related to cognitive functions and styles may have a negative effect on children's development. Dysfunctional attitudes may have a significant role in the development of depression. The unbalanced gradation of these attitudes with abilities and possibilities may also lead to the development of symptoms of depression. If a person has high expectations of himself and his surroundings in many fields of life, and is not able to meet the expectations of his context, he may then easily have a negative self-evaluation which can directly lead to hopelessness, which in turn can cause the development of symptoms of depression [26]. According to Beck, those characterised with dysfunctional attitudes are more likely to develop depression. These attitudes may not automatically cause illness when they are present separately. Furthermore, some of these insets might be an important drive in society, but their accumulation or high level may create a tendency for pathological development [27].

In Garber's and Hilsman's cognitive diathesis-stress model, in addition to dysfunctional attitudes, another cognitive factor, the negative attributional style, may also play a key role in the appearance of depressive symptoms. It is assumed that copying significant others, parental refusal and uncontrollable stressful events may be responsible for the development of the negative cognitive style. According to Metalsky, Halberstadt and Abramson's studies [29], students with a negative, pessimistic attributive style were more distressed than those who had a more optimistic attributive style. According to Peterson et al. [30], this negative attributional style is connected to physical illnesses; people who can be described with this attributional style do not care about themselves and their negative lifestyle may lead to illness. According to Abramson, Metalsky and Alloy [31], the pessimistic attributional style alone is not an adequate cause of depression. It becomes important when the individual encounters strong or frequent negative events. In their opinion, in the development of depression the extent a person believes his life can be influenced is more important than how he interprets unpleasant events. The belief that he is able to tackle problems increases his resistance to depression.

Those who have suffered from depression are more vulnerable to stressful life events than those who do not have such a history of depression. According to Brown and Harris' vulnerability theory, depression occurs in an interaction between the individual and his environment. The joint appearance and interaction of predispositional factors and external events (provoking factors) are needed for its evolvement. Predispositional factors can be certain personality characteristics (self-evaluation, self-power, conflict solving strategies, degree of distress endurance, relationship ability etc.), traumatic family prehistory, disturbed personality development, and the deficiency of the social criteria system. Life events work as provoking factors, and external events, as stressors, contribute to the manifestation of depression. However, the interpretation of life events is unique, and it depends on the antecedents of personality development. Negative life events do not cause depression, but they may contribute to the development of depression.

The aim of this paper is to find out what role the risk mechanisms, as described in Goodman and Gotlib's [12] model (genetical-biological, interpersonal, social learning related cognitive and stress related factors), have in the development of increased risk for depression in the case of men and women. (Due to methodological difficulties we left out the innate dysfunctional neuroregulatory risk-transfer mechanisms.) The genetical-biological factors were examined with certain temperament characteristics, the interpersonal factors with parental educational purpose, educational attitudes, educational style and parental treatment. In the case of factors related to social learning we looked at dysfunctional attitudes and attribution style. As far as stressors are concerned, we observed the quality of family atmosphere, and the number of positive and negative life events of the preceding six months and their subjective evaluation.

2. METHOD

Participants

Data was collected among college students at the College of Nyíregyháza, in a county seat in the north-eastern part of Hungary. We collected data randomly at every faculty and participation was voluntary and it was done with their consent. Students filled out the questionnaires individually at lectures with the guidance of the researchers.

700 students took part in the research and 681 of them provided valuable data (465 female and 216 male). According to their majors, the following students participated in the study: 225 undergraduate BA students, 125 undergraduate BSc students, 125 business students, 74 students studying to be infant teachers, 70 studying to be social teachers and 62 students of arts (visual arts and music).

The average age was 19.98 (standard deviation 1.51) the median value was 20 years.

Measures

To study depression we applied an abridged version of the 13 item multiple-choice questionnaire of the Beck Depression Inventory [34, 35]. The inventory studies the following components of depressive syndromes: sadness, pessimism, sense of failure, dissatisfaction, guilt, fear of punishment, self-harm, indecisiveness, social withdrawal, self-image change, work difficulty, fatigability and anorexia.

To study genetical-biological factors we applied the Hungarian version of Cloninger's Temperament and Character Inventory adapted by Rózsa and his colleagues [19]. The temperament dimension measuring scales of the questionnaire were the following: novelty seeking, harm avoidance, reward dependence and persistence.

To study interpersonal factors (effects of family socialisation) we applied the Goch's Family Socialisation Questionnaire [36, 37]. The following scales of the questionnaire were used in the study: maternal educational aims (independence – autonomy, as an educational aim; conformity – conformity as an educational aim), maternal educational attitudes (consistent, manipulative or inconsistent attitude) and maternal educational style (supportive or punitive style).

To study interpersonal factors we applied the Hungarian adaptation of Parker and his colleagues' questionnaire on Parental Treatment [38]. The following dimensions of parental treatment were examined: maternal care, maternal overprotection, maternal control, paternal care, paternal overprotection and paternal control.

The study of cognitive factors related to social learning: We used the Hungarian adaptation of Weismann's Dysfunctional Attitude Scale to examine dysfunctional attitudes [39, 40]. The questionnaire examines the following attitudes: need for external recognition, need to be loved, need for achievement, perfectionism, rightful increased expectations towards context, omnipotence (increased altruism orientation), external control –autonomy.

The attributive style was examined by using Abramson and his colleagues' Attributional Style Questionnaire [41]. The attributive style was valued on the following factors: internal or external attribution, stable or instable attribution, specific or global attribution. The research participants were asked to form judgements about the following situations: judgment of performance (exam failure) and judgment of loss (breaking up a relationship with a close friend).

To study stressors we applied the Goch's Family Socialisation Questionnaire [36, 37]. The following scale of the questionnaire was used in the research: the type of family atmosphere (conflict oriented family atmosphere).

To study stressors we applied the High School Life Experience Questionnaire of Cohen and his colleagues, adapted by Csorba and his colleagues for the Hungarian context [42].The questionnaire focused on the frequent, mainly negative, but sometimes partly positive, life events of the preceding six months. The questionnaire measured the following dimensions: number of positive life events, score of positive life events, number of negative life events, score of negative life events.

3. RESULTS

The Connection between Genetical-Biological Factors and Depression

The presence of biological vulnerability was examined by the use of Cloninger's Temperament and Character Inventory. Linear regression analysis was used in observing the relationship between certain temperament scales (novelty seeking, harm avoidance, reward dependence, persistence) as independent variables, and the values measured by Beck's Depression Inventory, as dependent variables.

Table 1. summarizes the connection between depression and certain temperament scales of the different sexes.

Table 1. The regression of depression on genetical-biological factors

Predictor	β	t	p<
Women: $F_{total}=73,670$; $p<0,000$			
Harm avoidance	0.511	12.124	0.000
Novelty seeking	0.165	3.910	0.000
Men: $F_{total}=30,994$; $p<0.000$			
Harm avoidance	0.431	7.099	0.000
Reward dependence	-0.158	-2.543	0.012

In both sexes, about the same proportion of depression variance is explained by the genetic-biological factors (24.2% of women, 22.5% of men). In both sexes, we have found a very tight connection between depression and harm avoidance. Harm avoiding people are more likely to be pessimistic, careful, timid, stressed, distressed, afraid of danger, risks, tend to be worried, reserved, hampered and are easily exhausted [19]. Furthermore, in the case of women, novelty seeking had a positive correlation with depression. Novelty seekers are impulsive, and they are open to new things, but lose their patience easily. They are irresolute, they quickly get bored with what they are doing, they are irritable and unstable. Extravagant behaviour, lack of restraint and untidiness may also characterise them [19]. In the case of men, reward dependence had a significant negative correlation with depression. Less reward dependent people are indifferent to social signals, and are more liable to being socially isolated, emotionally cold and pragmatic [19].

The Connection between Interpersonal Factors and Depression

As far as interpersonal factors were concerned, we were primarily interested in the role of parents in the family socialisation process. Among the effects of family socialisation we focused on the parent's educational aims (education for self-sufficiency - autonomy as an educational aim, education for conformity – conformity as an educational aim), educational attitudes (consistent educational attitude, manipulative educational attitude, and inconsistent educational attitude), educational styles (supportive style, punitive style), and parental treatment (care, overprotection and control). With linear regression analysis we examined the connection between the above mentioned variables, as independent variables, and the values measured by Beck's Depression Inventory, as dependent variables.

Table 2 shows the connection between depression and certain interpersonal factors of the sexes.

Table 2. The regression of depression on certain interpersonal factors

Predictor	β	T	p<
Women: $F_{total}=19,944; p<0,000$			
Parents' manipulative educational attitude	0.188	3.734	0.000
Paternal care	-0.156	-3.273	0.001
Maternal control	-0.134	-2.974	0.003
Parents' inconsistent educational attitude	0.108	2.020	0.044
Men: $F_{total}=12.615; p<0.000$			
Paternal care	-0.204	-2.733	0.007
Parents' inconsistent educational attitude	0.186	2.493	0.013

The interpersonal factors explain nearly the same rate the variance of depression in both sexes. Though in the case of women the rate is somewhat higher (15.3 %) than in the case of men (11.1 %). In both cases depression was closely connected to the parents' inconsistent educational attitude and the lack of paternal care. In the case of women, the parents' manipulative attitude and the lack of maternal care also contributed to the risk of developing depression.

The Connection between Depression and
Social Learning Related Cognitive Factors

From the cognitive factors related to depression, we examined dysfunctional attitudes (need for acknowledgement, love, achievement, perfectionism, rightfully increased expectations towards the context, omnipotence, external control – autonomy) and the attributional style (internal or external, stable or unstable, specific or global attribution). With the help of linear regression analysis we examined the connection between the above mentioned variables, as independent variables, and values measured by Beck's Depression Inventory, as dependent variables.

Table 3 shows the connection between depression and certain social learning factors of the sexes.

Table 3. The regression of depression on certain social learning factors

Predictor	β	t	p<
Women: F_{total}=45.717; p<0.000			
External control-autonomy	0.289	6.920	0.000
Performance: specific or global	0.256	6.079	0.000
Performance: stable or instable	0.161	3.841	0.001
Men: F_{total}=11.402; p<0.000			
External control-autonomy	0.213	3.282	0.000
Loss: specific or global	0.173	2.538	0.012
Performance: specific or global	0.163	2.258	0.019

In the case of women, the cognitive factors related to social learning explained a greater variance of depression than in the case of men (women: 22.5 %, men: 12.8 %). In both sexes, among the dysfunctional attitudes, depression showed a close connection with external control attitude. A person with external control attitudes feels he does not have control over his life, instead things just happen to him. While examining the attributional styles we found that women perceive the causes of losing control over their judgment of performance deficit as stable ("it will always be that way") and global, such that has an effect on every aspect of their life. Men, on the other hand, see the cause of both control loss and performance deficit as global.

The Connection between Depression and Stress Related Factors

When examining the connection between stress and depression we looked at the quality of family atmosphere (its conflict load on the individual's life up to the time of investigation) and the number of positive and negative life events in the preceding six months and their subjective evaluation (the degree of positive or negative effect). With the help of linear regression analysis, we examined the connection between the above mentioned variables as independent variables, and values measured by Beck's Depression Inventory, as dependent variables.

Table 4 shows the connection between depression and certain stress related factors of the sexes.

Table 4. The regression of depression on certain stress related factors

Predictor	β	t	p<
Women: F_{total}=63.668; p<0.000			
Evaluation of negative life events	0.374	8.689	0.000
Conflict oriented family atmosphere	0.188	4.358	0.000
Men: F_{total}=17.658; p<0.000			
Evaluation of negative life events	0.331	4.772	0.017
Conflict oriented family atmosphere	0.170	2.494	0.013

In the case of women, stress related factors explained a greater variance of depression (women: 21.6%, men: 14.2%). In both sexes depression was closely, significantly connected to both the subjective evaluation of negative life experiences in the preceding six months, and the conflict oriented family atmosphere.

The Role of the Examined Factors in the Development Of Depression

In the following model we included all those variables which showed a strong correlation with depression when examining the different factors (table 5).

The result of regression analysis shows that in the case of women the examined risk mechanisms explained a greater variance of depression than in the case of men (women: 41.4%, men: 36.5%).

The genetic-biological factors of risk mechanisms were stronger in the case of men, since two temperament factors, harm avoidance and reward dependence, proved to be greater risk factors. In the case of women this was only true for harm avoidance.

The interpersonal factors as risk mechanisms did not prove a significant correlation with depression. In the case of women, only the inconsistent parental educational attitude, while in the case of men, the lack of paternal care proved to be risk factors.

Out of the social learning related cognitive factors, one of the negative attributional styles, the experience of control loss as stable ("it will always be that way") proved to be a great risk factor. This acted as a distorting factor for women when judging performance deficit and it had the same effect for men when judging loss. Furthermore, in the case of women we were able to prove the role of another social learning related risk factor, the external control attitude.

Out of the stress related factors, only the subjective evaluation of negative life experiences proved to be a risk factor.

**Table 5. The regression of depression on those variables
which had a strong correlation with depression during the research**

Predictor	β	t	p<
Women: F_{total}=61.561; p<0.000			
Harm avoidance	0.340	8.886	0.000
Evaluation of negative life events	0.244	6.153	0.000
Performance: specific or global	0.166	4.342	
External control-autonomy	0.151	3.831	0.000
Parents' inconsistent educational attitude	0.145	3.806	0.002
Men: F_{total}=25.651; p<0.000			
Harm avoidance	0.365	6.260	0.000+
Evaluation of negative life events	0.267	4.623	0.000
Loss: specific or global	0.158	2.774	
Reward dependence	-0.154	-2.709	0.006
Paternal care	-0.152	-2.602	0.008

4. DISCUSSION

The aim of this present study was to show the differences between the sexes in their predisposition to depression, using a non-clinical sample. We examined what role those factors which are considered increased risk mechanisms (genetic-biological, interpersonal, social learning relater cognitive and stress related factor) play in the development of increased risk for depression in women and men.

The results of the study show that all of the increased risk mechanisms, thus the genetical-biological, the interpersonal, the social learning related cognitive and stress related factors, are connected to the development of predisposition to depression and they explain 41.4% of the depression symptoms' variance in the case of women, and 36.5% in the case of men.

According to the results of our study, harm avoidance, a genetic-biological factor, proved to be the most significant risk mechanism, irrespective of the sexes. Cloninger [43] believes that of the temperament factors, harm avoidance is the most important one as it has a control influence on the other two, and it appears first during ontogenesis. Reward dependence, another temperament factor, was also a risk factor for men. It is in harmony with the results of other studies [19] according to which the ability of emotional reaction is generally not affected by depression, only a specific disturbance of emotional reactions to joyful stimuli can be detected, which may be the result of a malfunctioning reward system. Besides these, the other risk mechanisms – interpersonal, cognitive and stress related factors- also have an important role in the development of increased risk to depression in men and women, though to a different degree, higher for women and lower for men. When examining twins, Kendler et al. [44] found that while the development of clinical, major depression was connected primarily to additive genetic factors, the development of milder, sub-clinical forms of depression was influenced mainly by environmental factors. The results of our research, carried out with a non-clinical sample, prove that although harm avoidance, as a genetic-biological factor, showed the strongest correlation with depression symptoms, it was the environmental factors which were more dominant on the whole.

From among the environmental factors – irrespective of the sexes- one stress related factor, the subjective evaluation of negative life experiences, which implies an increased sensitivity to stress, proved to be the strongest risk mechanism. Nowadays a great number of theorists believe that there are many environmental factors which increase the risk of vulnerability to depression, and that these are inherited. For example, Plomin [45] argues that genetic factors contribute to the difference of variables such as poor parental care or the reaction to stressful life events. In 1978, Brown and Harris [46] already pointed out the fact that sensitivity to stress is genetically transmitted. According to the results of our research, this transmitted factor, which lies behind the harm avoiding behaviour, may be the genetic-biological mechanism. Harm avoidance means the inherited pattern of behavioural inhibition, which may manifest itself in passive avoiding behaviour and in fear of uncertainty. Several studies [19] have pointed out that certain groups of children, even before acquiring social experiences, are more diffident, more uncertain and tense in unknown situations than their peers; they avoid new stimuli, do not adapt easily to changes and their mood is often gloomy and negative. These factors may increase vulnerability to depression by leading children towards choosing or avoiding certain types of environment and making them selectively react to certain aspects of their environment. As a result, the child perceives the world with a bias and reacts more sensitively to environmental stress. This may even be related to the fact that the negative, pessimistic attribution style, a factor related to social learning, also plays a major role in the development of predisposition to depression in both sexes. One of its characteristic marks, the experience of control loss as stable ("it will always be that way"), showed a specific relationship with depression symptoms. This, however, appeared in different areas in the sexes. The relationship was found in the area of achievement in the case of women, while it was detected in the area of loss in the case of men. Joiner and Wagner [47] found moderate proof that the negative attributional style may be a predictor of increasing depressive symptoms in children and adolescents.

While both the genetic-biological and stress related risk mechanisms played an important role in the development of vulnerability to depression in both sexes, the social learning related cognitive and interpersonal risk mechanisms differed in their degree in women and men. Besides the pessimistic attribution style, the external control attitude – another social learning related risk mechanism – had an important role in the development of increased risk for depression. According to Fiske and Taylor [48], when defining a person's self-evaluation and self-image, the extent the individual considers himself effective in a given situation and how much control and influence he believes he may have over it are very important. Therefore, the perception of control is an important aspect of how an individual behaves in a certain situation. A person with external control attitude feels he does not have control over his life, things just happen to him. The resulting passive, inert state, according to Seligman [49], may develop the implicit belief that he has no control over his life and whatever he does has no impact on the course of actions in his life. This might make him passive, his motivation may decrease and he may be liable to depression.

The effect of interpersonal factors seemed to be relatively the weakest in the development of increased risk for depression. The biological and cognitive factors for liability to depression are formed in the interaction of the personality and the environment, primarily within the social context created by the parents. The dissonance between the child's temperament and the expectations and requirements of the social context may act as a predispositional factor for the development of depression [19]. According to our research findings, such a factor for women can be the inconsistent parental educational attitude, and, in the case of men, the lack of paternal care.

5. CONCLUSION

The mental hygienic interpretation of our research findings is that in the future there should be more emphasis put on the personality development of college and university students, especially on the development of such competencies which aid them in effectively coping in their struggle with the depressive mood. According to Bugán [50], mental hygiene opportunities and methods may be built into the tertiary curricula either in a direct or in a non-direct way. The direct methods mean the incorporation of mental hygiene information in course content, while indirect methods may include the formation of profession socialisation groups - which could act as effective mental hygienic transmitters in the development of the professional personality - and the development of mental hygienic ambulance services at colleges and universities. Bagdy and Bugán [51] found the formation of profession socialisation groups, which functioned as effective mental hygienic transmitters in the development of the professional personality, effective at universities.

REFERENCES

[1] Kiss, H.G., and Szabó, A., and Rihmer, Z. (1998). A depresszió. Egy népbetegség korszerű megközelítése. [Depression. The modern approach of an endemic.] *Praxis*, 7, 7-13.

[2] Kopp, M., and Szedmák, S., and Lőke, J., and Skrabski, Á. (1997). A depressziós tünetegyüttes gyakorisága és egészségügyi jelentősége a mai magyar lakosság körében. [The frequency and health importance of depression symptoms among the Hungarian population today.] *Lege Artis Medicine*, 7, 136-144.

[3] Kopp, M., and Csoboth, CS., and Purebl, Gy. (1999). Fiatal nők egészségi állapota.]Young women's health status.] In: Pongrácz, T. and Tóth I.,Gy. (Szerk.): *Szerepváltozások* [Role changes.] (pp.239-259). Budapest: TÁRKI.

[4] Margitics F. (2005). A diszfunkcionális attitűdök, megküzdési stratégiák és az attribúciós stílus összefüggése a szubklinikus depressziós tünetegyüttessel főiskolai hallgatóknál. [Interrelations between dysfunctional attitudes, coping strategies and

attributional style and subclinical depressive syndrome at college students.] *Mentálhigiéné és Pszichoszomatika*, 6, 95-122.

[5]   Angst, J., and Merikangsamm, K. (1997). The depressive spectrum: Diagnostic classification and course. *Journal of Affective Disorders*, 45, 31-39.

[6]   Kessler, R.C., and Zhao, S., and Blazer, D.G., and Swartz, M.S. (1997). Prevalence, correlates and course of minor depression and major depression in the NCS. *Journal Affective Disorders*, 45, 19-30.

[7]   Kessler, R.C., and Wittchen, H.U., and Abelson, J.M., and McGonagle, K.A., and Schwarz, N., and Kendler, K.S. et al. (1998). Methodological studies of the Composite International Diagnostic Interview (CIDI) in the US National Comorbidity Survey Int. J. Methods. Psychiatr. Res. 7, 33-55.

[8]   Goodwin, F.K., and Jamison, K.J. (1990). *Manic-Depressive Illness*. New York : Oxford University Press.

[9]   Kessler, R.C., and McGonagle, K.A., and Nelson C.B., and Hughes M., and Swartz, M.S., and Blazer D.G. (1994). Sex and depression in the National Comorbidity Survey II: Cohort effect. *Journal Affective Disorders*, 30, 15-26.

[10] Mirowsky, J., and Ross, C.E. (1989). Social Cases of Psychological Distress. New York: Aldine De Gruyter.

[11] Noel-Hoeksema, S. (1990). Sex differences in unipolar depression: Evidence and theory. *Psychological Bulletin*, 101, 259-282.

[12] Goodman, S. H., and Gotlib, I. H. (1999). Risk for psychopathology in the children of depressed mothers: A developmental model for understanding mechanisms of transmission. *Psychological Review*, 3, 458-490.

[13] Tsuang, M.T., and Faraone, S.V. (1990). *The genetics of mood disorders*. Baltimore: John Hopkins University Press.

[14] Loehlin, J.C. (1992). *Genes and environment in personality development*. Beverly Hills, CA: Sage.

[15] Goldschmith, H.H., and Buss, K.A., and Lemery, K.S. (1997). Toddler and childhood temperament: Expanded content, stronger genetic evidence, new evidence for the importance of environment. *Developmental Psychology*, 33, 891-905.

[16] Cherny, S.S., and Fulker, D.W., and Corley, R.P., and Plomin, R., and DeFries, J.C. (1994). Continuity and change in infant shyness from 14 to 20 months. *Behavior Genetics*, 24, 365-379.

[17] Tellegen, A., and Lykken, D.T., and Bouchard, T.J., and Wilcox, K.J., and Segal, N.L., and Rich, S. (1988). Personality similarity in twins reared apart and together. *Journal of Personality and Social Psychology*, 54, 1031-1039.

[18] Plomin, R., and Emde, R.N., and Braungart, J.M., and Campos, J., and Corley, R., and Fulk, D.W. et al. (1993). Genetic change and continuity from fourteen twenty months: The MacArthur Longitudinal Twin Study. *Child Development*, 64, 1354-1376.

[19] Rózsa S., and Kállai, J., and Osváth, A., and Bánki M. Cs. (2005). *Temperamentum és karakter: Cloninger pszichobiológiai modellje. A Cloninger-féle temperamentum és karakter kérdőív felhasználói kézikönyve*. [Temperament and character. Cloninger's psychobiologycal model. The handbook of the Cloninger Temperament and Character Inventory.] Budapest: Medicina Könyvkiadó Rt.

[20] Hansenne, M., and Reggers, J., and Pinto, M., and Kjiri, K., and Ajamier, A., and Ansseau, M. (1999). Temperament and character inventory and depression. *Journal of Psychiatric Research*, 33, 31-36.

[21] Parker, G. (1979). Parenthal characteristics in relation to depressive disorders. *British Journal of Psychiatry*, 134, 138-147.

[22] Parker, G. (1981). Parental representations of patients with anxiety neurosis. *Acta Psychiatrica Scandinavica,* 63, 33-36.

[23] Parker, G. (1983). Parental „affectionless control" as an antecedent to adult depression. A risk factor delineated. *Archives of General Psychiatry*, 40, 956-960.

[24] Mackinnon, A.J., and Henderson, A.S., and Andrews, G. (1993). Parental „affectionless control" as an antecedent to adult depression: a risk factor refined. *Psychological Medicine*, 23, 135-141.

[25] Narita, T., and Sato, T., and Hirano, S., and Gota, M., and Sakado, K., and Uehara, T. (2000). Parental child-rearing behavior as measured the Parental Bonding Instrument in a Japanese population: factor structure and relationship to a lifetime history of depression. *Journal of Affective Disorders*, 57, 229-234.

[26] Kopp, M., and Skrabski, Á. (1995). *Alkalmazott magatartástudomány.* [Applied science of behavior.] Budapes: Corvinus Kiadó.

[27] Beck, Á.T., and Rush, A.J, and Shaw, B.F., and Emery, G. (2001). *A depresszió kognitív terápiája.* [The cognitive therapy of depression.] Budapest: Animula.

[28] Garber, J., and Hilsram R. (1992). Cognition, stress, and depression in children and adolescents. *Child and Adolescent Psychiatric Clinics of North America*, 1, 129-167.

[29] Metalsky, G.I., and Halberstadt, L.J., and Abramson, L.Y. (1987). Vulnerability to depressive mood reactions. *Journal of Personality and Social Psychology*, 52, 386-393.

[30] Peterson, C., and Semmel, A., and von Baeyer, C., and Abramson, L.Y., and Metalsky, G.I., Seligman, M.E.P. (1982). The Attributional Style Questionnaire. *Cognitive Therapy and Research,* 6, 287-299.

[31] Abramson, L Y., and Metalsky, G.I., and Alloy, L.B. (1989). Hopelessness depression: a theory –based subtype of depression. *Psychological Review*, 96, 358-372.

[32] Brown, G.W., and Harris, T. (1986). Establishing Causal Links, The Bedford College Studies of Depression. In H. Kasching (Ed). *Life Events and Psychiatric Disorders* (pp.125-129) London-Cambridge: University Press.

[33] Kessler, R.C., and Magee, W.J. (1993). Childhood adversities and adult depression: Basic patterns of association in a US National Survey. *Psychological Medicine*, 23, 679-690.

[34] Beck, A.T., and Beck R.W. (1972). Screening depressed patients in family practice. A rapid technique. *Postgraduate Medicine*, 52, 81-85.

[35] Margitics, F. (2005). Prediszponáló tényezők kapcsolata a szubklinikus depressziós tünetegyüttessel főiskolai hallgatóknál. [Interrelation between predisposition factors and sub clinical depression syndrome at college students.] *Psychiatria Hungarica*, 20, 211-223.

[36] Goch, I. (1998). *Entwicklung der Ungewissheitstoleranz. Die Bedeutung der familialen Socialization.* Regensburg: Roderer.

[37] Sallay, H., and Dabert, C. (2002). Women's perception of parenting: a German-Hungarian comparison, *Applied Psychology in Hungary*, 3-4, 55-56.

[38] Tóth, I., and Gervai, J. (1999). Szülői Bánásmód Kérdőív (H-PBI): a Parental Bonding Instrument magyar változata. [Perceived parental styles: the Hungarian version of the Parental Bonding Instrument (H-PBI).] *Magyar Pszichológiai Szemle*, 54, 551-566.

[39] Weismann, A.N., and Beck, A.T. (1979). *The Dysfunctional Attitude Scale*. Thesis, University of Pennsylvania.

[40] Kopp, M. (1994). *Orvosi pszichológia*. [Medical psychology.] Budapest: SOTE Magatartástudományi Intézet.

[41] Atkinson, R.L., and Atkinson C.R., and Smith E.E., and Bem D.J. (1995): *Pszichológia*. [Psychology.] Budapest: Osiris.

[42] Csorba, J., and Dinya, E., and Párt, S., and Solymos, J. (1994). Életesemény kutatás és serdülőkor. A középiskolás életesemény kérdőív bemutatása. [Life event research and adolescence. The Hungarian version of the Junior High Life Experiences Survey.] *Magyar Pszichológiai Szemle*, 50, 67-83.

[43] Cloninger, C.R. (1987). A systematic method for clinical description and classification of personality variants. *Archives of General Psychiatry*, 44, 573-588.

[44] Kendler K.S., and Kessler R.C., and Walters, E.E., and Maclean, C.J., and Sham P.C., and Neale M.C. et al.(1995). Stressful live evens, genetic liability and onset of an episode of major depression in women. *American Journal of Psychiatry*, 152. 833-842.

[45] Plomin R. (1994). *Genetics and experience: The interplay between nature and nurture*. Thousand Oaks, CA: Sage.

[46] Brown, G.W., and Harris, T. (1978). *Social origins of depression*. New York: Free press.

[47] Joiner, T.E., and Wagner, K.D. Attributional style and depression in children and adolescents: A meta-analytic review. *Clinical Psychology Review*, 15, 777-789.

[48] Fiske, S. T., and Taylor S. E. (1984). *Social cognition*. New York: Random House.

[49] Seligman, M.E.P. (1992). Wednesday's children. *Psychology Today*, 25, 61-67.

[50] Bugán, A. (1999). Mentálhigiénés lehetőségek és módszerek a felsőoktatásban. [Facilities and methods in the mental hygienic in the higher education.]: E. Bagdy (Szerk.): *Mentálhigiéné. Elmélet, gyakorlat, képzés, kutatás* [Mental hygienic. Theory, practice, education, research.] (pp.135-140). Budapest: Animula.

[51] Bagdy, E., and Bugán, A. (1997): A pszichológiai csoportmunka, mint a személyiség fejlődésének színtere és eszköze. [The psychological teamwork as the scene and method of the personal development.] In: E. Bagdy (Szerk.) *A pedagógus hivatásszemélyiség*. [Professional personality of pedagogues.] (pp.55-85). Debrecen: KLTE.

Reviewed by Antal Bugán, PhD., Department of Psychology, University of Debrecen

In: Life Style and Health Research Progress
Editors: A. B. Turley, G. C. Hofmann

ISBN: 978-1-60456-427-3
© 2008 Nova Science Publishers, Inc.

Chapter XI

Adherence to Treatment in Social Phobia Patients: Predictors Factors

Mariangela Gentil Savoia[*1] and Márcio Bernik[2]

[1]Anxiety Clinic, Institute of Psychiatry, University of São Paulo Department of
Psychiatry and Medical Psychology, Santa Casa Medical School
[2] Anxiety Clinic, Institute of Psychiatry, University of São Paulo
Department of Psychiatry, University of São Paulo

ABSTRACT

Adherence to treatment may be considered the coincidence degree observed between the patient's behavior and healthcare professional's therapeutic recommendations. Several cognitive-behavioral mechanisms are likely to interfere with this process. Low-level treatment compliance shows to be related to situations requiring long-term treatments or those of preventive nature, or else, when patients´ lifestyles are affected by alterations. From either the behavioral and economic points of view, long-term perceived rewards show lower reinforcement strength. Objective: The present study was intended to examine predictive factors related either to pharmacological with selective serotonin reuptake inhibitor and cognitive-behavioral treatments in patients with Social Phobia. Method: Evaluation of the following items as possible predictive factors in treatment adherence included personality traits, personality disorders, social abilities and comorbidity depression in 144 patients with patronized scales. Results: Social abilities were not included into the proposed adherence treatments. A correlation between depression, dependent personality trait, and anti-social and borderline personality disorders were observed when based on the proposed adherence treatments findings. Conclusion: Study findings suggest that significant factors in those patients´ treatment adherences were their personality characteristics and symptoms of depression.

[*] Author responsible for correspondence: Dra. Mariângela Gentil Savoia; Ambulatório de Ansiedade, Instituto de Psiquiatria, Hospital das Clínicas da FMUSP. R. Dr. Ovídio Pires de Campos, 785 CEP: 05403.010 Tel/Fax: 00 55 11 30696988; mangy.savoia@globo.com; amban@amban.org.br

Keywords: Social phobia, treatment adherence, predictive factors.

INTRODUCTION

Adherence to treatment may be considered as the coincidence degree observed between the patient's behavior and the therapeutic recommendations prescribed by the health care professional (Epstein et Cluss, 1982). Adherence is a relevant factor able to influence results attained by clinical trials and clinical practice. Any study disregarding those variables could underestimate the results of the proposed treatment. In addition to that, if the non-adherent patients are not taken in consideration into the initial investigation design, the final sampling may not be significant, thus a less important impact will be observed in the study conclusions. This way, the investigator must continuously evaluate the patient's adherence to treatment and deal with desistance when analyzing the achieved findings; also, the number of desisting subjects should be previously estimated in order in favor of the sample size calculation.

Adherence should not be considered as a characteristic or trait inherent to the patient's personality, but accepted as a cluster of several different self-care behaviors (Glasgow et al., 1985). According to Skinner (1989) this would be a type of modeled behavior and maintained by its consequences, only those occurring in the past. In this way, it is easier to understand why a treatment offers a symptomatic relief associated to the highest levels of adherence, if compared to an eminently prophylactic treatment, since the prevention actions are associated to future complications.

Social phobia is a psychiatric disorder affected by several factors related to low adherence levels, common to general disease occurrences and treatments indicated below. In addition to those "universal" factors, there are also factors related to different psychiatric diseases and most importantly to disease peculiarities as social contact avoidance, which may render difficulties for the therapist-patient interaction. Thus, the analysis off the adherence to social phobia treatment is extremely relevant when dealing with this disorder.

It is important that the adherence to the treatment be evaluated at the initial stage of the treatment, since a good adherence to the treatment is a predictor of long-term adherence. (Jordan et al., 2000). This evaluation may be performed using either direct or indirect methods. The indirect methods are those mostly adopted and include from self-reports instruments such as interviews, evaluation scales, structured questionnaires to clinical and laboratory results estimates. Generally, the indirect methods tend to overestimate the adherence level. Patient reports could eventually include the patient's bias i.e., he/she may consider the adherence level adequate, just for experiencing a symptomatic relief, or fear of negative repercussions by reporting to the therapist his/her inadequate adherence levels. On the other hand, the good clinical and laboratory results may be observed even though the patients may have presented an inadequate treatment adherence.

As an advantage, besides evaluating adherence, some indirect measures are likely to interfere in the treatment course and cause the patients behavior changes as those occurring during the feedback technique used to control the diabetes patient's glycemic levels (Malerbi, 2000). If by one hand, the patient is instructed to actively act in his/her own treatment making decisions, such as, change the insulin dose based on the observed glycemic value found, on the other hand, unsatisfactory values constantly observed may represent an averse stimulus and function as a punishment for his/her self-monitoring.

The direct methods generally reflect a better treatment adherence but also presents a number of limitations since they show to be more expensive and of a more restrictive application, as for example, electronic bottle caps measurements, pills count, and management of medical prescriptions and medical drugs stored in pharmacies. Observational methods as third-party observers may be employed although such methods could cause of behavioral changes what constitute an important bias.

The following " universal" factors which could influence treatment adherence include :

- Patient's characteristics: a lower adherence level to treatment is observed among adolescent subjects but shows a tendency to improve with age (Jordan et al., 2000) and marital status, since these variables might influence the adherence to food diets (Dunbar-Jacob et al., 1996). Some types of comorbidities may also negatively influence the adherence to treatment, such as substance abuse and intercurrent psychiatric events. Information regarding either the disease or treatment may also influence the patient's adherence.
- Treatment: usually, higher complexity treatments generate lower adherence levels. (Haynes, 1976).
- Disease: aspects such the presence or absence of symptoms, their regression at treatment onset, the preventive character, the need for the patient to be submitted to medical control at regular intervals, duration, acute or chronic diseases, degree of attack (gravity, functional impairment), all of them are important factors in the treatment adherence.
- Healthcare Professional: the professional's ability in reaching, attending, and communicating with the patient and provide him/her with information on the disease and treatment will certainly generate better results. The therapeutics' setting of realistic objectives for the treatment and attentive therapeutic process follow thru, will certainly contribute for a better treatment adherence.

Among the reasons reported by the psychiatric patients to justify the non-adherence, are: disease denial, missed medications, lack of control over his/hers own life, medication adverse effects, forgetfulness, euphoria absence, (in bipolar disorder patients) and the belief in the disease's spontaneous resolution (Kech et al., 1996).

A study carried out by Kech et al., 1988 divided the psychiatric patients into adherent to treatment, partially adherent, and non-adherent. These patients were followed up during 12 months and evaluations performed after that period showed that the adherent patients presented a higher functional improvement when compared to their pre-treatment status, which did not occurred to the partially adherent patients (that adhered to some stages of the proposed treatment); or to the non-adherent patients. No differences could be observed between partially and non-adherent patients after the 12-month follow up period.

Related literature shows that measures able to attain a higher impact level in adherence to treatment are intended to increase the number of the patient's attendance to medical and therapist consultations and their understanding about the disease and treatment. Such interventions may be of educational, behavioral, and affective character. Therapist-patient interaction may be considered as a very important factor influencing patient's adherence to treatment; similar influences are observed when different psychological techniques are adopted. In a study with hypertension subjects, (Lipp et al., 1991) and notwithstanding the adopted approach, coadjuvant psychological techniques succeeded to reach a good rapport and bounding between patient and therapist, thus enabling improvement to the levels of adherence to treatment in this chronic and difficult-to-control disease.

Generally, adherence shows a tendency to be more unsatisfactory in chronic diseases and those requiring long term care. This statement is also compatible with psychiatric disorders; thus, the adherence to treatment in individuals with psychiatric disorders is of a lesser degree than that observed in patients with physical diseases. (Cramer et Rosenheck, 1998). Some studies have described the existing relationship between the disease's severity to inadequate adherence to treatment levels; Keck et al., 1996, carried out a study with bipolar disorder patients and observed that those presenting an extremely severe condition at admittance showed the lowest adherence levels. Other authors (Vocisano et al., 1996) reported that patients presenting functional deterioration showed the worse adherence to the treatment.

Compliance should be understood as a complex set of behaviors caused by different contingencies. Effective strategies employed in certain patients, may be ineffective for others (Monteiro, 2001). Thus, when a higher number of treatment modalities are involved, probabilities that the individual will follow professional recommendations are scarce (Malerbi, 2000). Based in behavioral analyses of different therapeutic modalities, intended to evaluate treatment adherence levels in patients diagnosed with anxiety disorders, Monteiro (2001), stated that 83.3% of the studied subjects failed to perform at least one of the expected behaviors during the treatment. Adherence rate showed an inverse variation related to the number of prescribed medical drugs, daily drug intake, and number of prescribed activities.

Some studies tried to identify which factors could be associated to the higher levels of adherence to treatment in social phobia patients, either during the follow up period or in the course of the treatment. In order to identify which factors might be associated with improved adherence shown by social phobia patients treatments, Edelman et Chambless (1995) compared patients´ results soon after being submitted to cognitive-behavioral group treatment focused on self-instructional training. No compliance differences were observed concerning patients´ disorder severity. However, patients presenting avoidant personality traits showed to be less responsive to the therapeutic process, while the more dependent patients tried diligently to carry out their homework tasks, paranoid patient's tendency was to leave exposition tasks unfinished.

Turner et al., 1994 related the specific or generalized subtype of social phobia with treatment compliance, withdrawing rate, and improved status following the treatment. Findings showed that the specific social phobia subtype obtained significant better results than the generalized subtype in all the analyzed items. Social skills may be related to those patients's adherence to treatment while socially phobic patients generally present ability deficits able to impair their relationship with the therapeutic team. (Beidel et al., 1999; Savoia et Vianna, 2006)

In one of the studies on social phobia it was found out a low adherence of patients submitted to group therapy. Having the patients abandoned the therapy at different stages. These differences suggested the possibility that each one of the patients had his/her own reason to leave the therapy. Renouncing patients were summoned to be interviewed in order to identify the factors able to predict the low adherence to treatment. Collected data were categorized and pointed to the following preceding common factors related to the patient's low adherence: distorted perception regarding treatment outcome, clinical status, lacking motivation for treatment acceptance, and ascribing symptoms to personality rather than face them as a disease. (Malerbi et al.,2000).

Another eventual factor associated to the patient's low adherence level to treatment may be assigned to the presence of comorbidity with depression, which seems to affect up to 70% of socially phobic patients. (Van Ameringen et al., 1991). Related literature fails to show any study on this factor. Also, no comparative studies could be found between social phobia patient's adherence to different types of treatments, and most of all, the reason for different patients to demonstrate a higher compliance degree to determined intervention modality.

Based on those findings, the present study established the following objectives:

1. Evaluate such predictive factors of adherence to the proposed treatment as personality traits, personality disorders, social abilities and depression signs and symptoms.
2. Evaluate the resulting effects caused by the following procedures: Medical (indication of a selective serotonin reuptake inhibitor- SSRI); Psychotherapy (cognitive-behavioral group therapy) and the association of both types of procedures dealing with treatment compliance of patients with primary diagnosis of social phobia without comorbidity and major depression.

METHODOLOGY

Subjects

The study included 144 patients, between 18 and 65 years of age, social phobia-diagnosed in accordance with the DSM IV criteria (1994); by spontaneously presenting themselves at the AMBAN IPQ FMUSP triage center, those subjects met the study inclusion or exclusion criteria. All the subjects signed the Informed Consent Form.

Inclusion criteria required equal or higher score than 4 in the Clinical Global Impression Scale (CGI) when considering the "severity" item (Guy, 1976); also the inclusion criteria considered scores equal or higher than 17 in the Avoidance and Social Discomfort [Distress] Scale (ASDS), and the score equal or higher than 24 in the Fear of Negative Evaluation Scale (FNE) (Watson and Friend,1969).

Exclusion criteria, included depression diagnosed patients, suicide possibility, scores equal or higher than 30 in the Beck Depression Inventory, (Beck, 1961) or equal or higher score than 21 in the Hamilton's Depression Scale (Hamilton, 1960). Patients were also excluded from the study when presenting any primary psychiatric diagnosis provided by

DSM IV as an organic disease, epilepsy, indulgence in more than 2 units of alcoholic beverages/day, or using anti-depression medications and benzodiazepines.

Instruments

The study made use of a structured diagnosis interview for DSM IV (SCID-IV, First 1997, Portuguese version Del Ben et al., 2001). Instruments used for depressive symptoms evaluation included Hamilton's Depression Scale (Hamilton 1959), and Beck Depression Inventory (Beck, 1961). In order to evaluate the social anxiety symptoms severity, instruments as the ASD scale and FNE scale were used (Watson and Friend, 1969, translation to Portuguese by Lotufo Neto, 2000). Regarding the global functioning evaluation, the CGI scale was used (Guy, 1976). Social abilities were evaluated using the Multidimensional Scale of Social Expression - motor part (Caballo, 1995). Personality disorders were evaluated and supported by the Structured Interview for Personality Disorders – (SIPD-R), DMS III-R (Pfohl et al., 1989 – adaptation to Portuguese by Torres et al., 1994). Personality traits were evaluated by the Temperament and Character Inventory (TCI) (Clonniger, 1994, translated to Portuguese by Fuentes et al., 2000). The Cloninger's Temperament and Character Inventory (TCI) (Cloninger et al., 1993) provides a theoretically based, systematic approach to personality testing, which can be experimentally tested. It describes seven independent personality dimensions. Four of them, Novelty seeking (NS), Harm Avoidance (HA), Reward Dependence (RD) and Persistence (P), are considered temperament dimensions. These involve automatic-inate responses to perceptive stimuli. In turn this inate responses influence the learning process in response to novelty, danger, reward and punishment. On the other hand, 3 of them are considered character dimensions, Self directedness (SD), Cooperativeness (C), Self-Transcendence (ST). Character is defined as an insight learning or self-concept organization, which involves individual autonomy, social and universal integration.

Procedures

Patients were submitted to an initial evaluation, which involved the application of all the instruments already described; inclusion criteria subjects were randomly distributed into four different treatment groups. Group 1 received daily doses of Sertraline, an active drug and attended the behavioral group therapy; Group 2 also received the same active drug together with support group therapy; Group 3 was administered with placebos and also attended the behavioral group therapy; and Group 4 received placebos and support group therapy. (Comparisons regarding the adopted procedures efficacy shall be soon reported). Patients could renounce participation and voluntarily leave any of the proposed therapeutic procedures.

Regarding statistical analysis, associations between adherence and putative predictive factors were evaluated using Chi-square tests. In cases where absolute frequencies were lower than 5, Fisher's exact test was applied. The identified factors in the present analysis were included within the logistic regression model (Paula, 2004) using the "backward" selection method (Neter et al., 1996) with p-value>0.10

RESULTS

From all patients, 60.3% attended the 20-week treatment period. No difference was observed between the treatment groups (Group 1= 67.6%; Group 2 = 58.3%; Group 3 = 56.1%; and Group 4 = 60%; Chi-square test = 1.128: ns).

No differences could be found concerning the studied putative predictive factors separately (table 1). However, interactions were observed between the treatment groups and the putative predictive factor. Group 4 showed lower adherence in patients with BDI scores between 11 and 29, than those patients with score 10 or lower (44.4% vs. 76.5%; p= 0.086).

Table 1. Studied putative predictive factors separately

Predictive Factor	Chi-square	p-values
Grupo	1.128	0.770
"Obs-Comp"	0.179	0.672
Histrionic	0.106	0.745
Dependent	0.080	0.777
Antisocial	0.850	0.356
Narcissistic	0.714	0.398
Avoidant	1.626	0.202
Borderline	1.642	0.200
"Passiv.Agress"	0.006	0.938
Sadistic	—	0.675[F]
Self defeating	0.107	0.743
Depression symotoms	0.613	0.893
Social abilities	0.431	0.934
Novelty seeking	3.645	0.302
Harm Avoidance	2.134	0.545
Reward Dependence	3.070	0.381
Persistence	1.404	0.705
Self directedness	5.715	0.126
Cooperativeness	1.600	0.659
Self Transcendence	2.010	0.570

[F] : Fisher's exact test.

No difference could be found in either the presence or absence of social ability related to the patient's adhesion to the proposed treatments. Social ability variable was based in 25%, 50%, and 75% percentiles according to the patient's achieved scores in the Multidimensional Scale of Social Expression: Percentile 1, 0 -130; Percentile 2, 131 -141; Percentile 3, 142- 151; Percentile 4 results were higher than 151.

Generally, personality disorders were not related to treatment compliance, although by separately analyzing each disorder, and observing the p-values in group association tests, evidences of interaction between Group 3 and the "Anti-Social" and "Borderline" personality disorders group demonstrated that these patients showed lower compliance levels (tables 2, 3, 4, and 5).

Observing the p-values shown by the group association tests, it could be suggested that personality traits, temperament, and character might disclose the existence of an interaction between group and reward–dependence (tables 6 and 7).

Using Paula's, 2004 logistic regression models, it was verified which predictive factors might conjointly influence treatment compliance and, whether this influence turned out to be different for each group.

Patients with the same self-defeating symptoms (self-defeating or not) included in the same BDI category (i.e., presence or absence of depression) and also those differing in the novelty-seeking category.(NS) showed the following results: patients with NS ≥ 16 have less than 68.6% of possibilities of adhering to the treatment when compared to the patient with 0≤ NS < 16.

Patients in the same NS and BDI categories but differing in self-defeating symptoms showed that the chance of self-defeating patients adhering to treatment is 7.028 times lower than of the no-self-defeating subjects.

The NS class patients with similar self-defeating symptoms and depression belonging to group 4 patients, had lower than 91.3% chances of adhering to the treatment than the no-depression group 1 patients (tables 8 and 9)

Table 2. Absolute and relative frequencies of adherence according to the antisocial variable by group

Group	Predictive Factor		Adherence		Total
			0	1	
1	Antisocial	0	4 (30.8%)	9 (69.2%)	13 (100.0%)
		1	1 (33.3%)	2 (66.7%)	3 (100.0%)
		Subtotal	5 (31.3%)	11 (68.8%)	16 (100.0%)
2	Antisocial	0	10 (40.0%)	15 (60.0%)	25 (100.0%)
		1	1 (50.0%)	1 (50.0%)	2 (100.0%)
		Subtotal	11 (40.7%)	16 (59.3%)	27 (100.0%)
3	Antisocial	0	9 (33.3%)	18 (66.7%)	27 (100.0%)
		1	4 (100.0%)	0 (0.0%)	4 (100.0%)
		Subtotal	13 (41.9%)	18 (58.1%)	31 (100.0%)
4	Antisocial	0	10 (41.7%)	14 (58.3%)	24 (100.0%)
		1	1 (20.0%)	4 (80.0%)	5 (100.0%)
		Subtotal	11 (37.9%)	18 (62.1%)	29 (100.0%)

Table 3. Association between adherence and antisocial variable by group

Group	p-values
1	>0.999
2	>0.999
3	0.023
4	0.622

Fisher's exact test.

**Table 4. Absolute and relative frequencies of adherence
according to the bordeline variable by group**

Group	Predictive factor		Adherence		Total
			0	1	
1	Borderline	0	4 (30.8%)	9 (69.2%)	13 (100.0%)
		1	1 (33.3%)	2 (66.7%)	3 (100.0%)
		Subtotal	5 (31.3%)	11 (68.8%)	16 (100.0%)
2	Borderline	0	9 (45.0%)	11 (55.0%)	20 (100.0%)
		1	2 (28.6%)	5 (71.4%)	7 (100.0%)
		Subtotal	11 (40.7%)	16 (59.3%)	27 (100.0%)
3	Borderline	0	6 (27.3%)	16 (72.7%)	22 (100.0%)
		1	7 (77.8%)	2 (22.2%)	9 (100.0%)
		Subtotal	13 (41.9%)	18 (58.1%)	31 (100.0%)
4	Borderline	0	9 (37.5%)	15 (62.5%)	24 (100.0%)
		1	2 (40.0%)	3 (60.0%)	5 (100.0%)
		Subtotal	11 (37.9%)	18 (62.1%)	29 (100.0%)

Table 5. Association between adherence and bordeline variable by group

Group	p-values
1	>0.999
2	0.662
3	0.017
4	>0.999

Fisher's exact test.

**Tabela 6. Absolute and relative frequencies of adherence
according to the Reward Dependence variable by group**

Group	Predictive factor		Adherence		Total
			0	1	
1	RD_cat2	1	6 (46.2%)	7 (53.8%)	13 (100.0%)
		2	3 (18.8%)	13 (81.3%)	16 (100.0%)
		Subtotal	9 (31.0%)	20 (69.0%)	29 (100.0%)
2	RD_cat2	1	2 (16.7%)	10 (83.3%)	12 (100.0%)
		2	7 (53.8%)	6 (46.2%)	13 (100.0%)
		Subtotal	9 (36.0%)	16 (64.0%)	25 (100.0%)
3	RD_cat2	1	4 (36.4%)	7 (63.6%)	11 (100.0%)
		2	8 (38.1%)	13 (61.9%)	21 (100.0%)
		Subtotal	12 (37.5%)	20 (62.5%)	32 (100.0%)
4	RD_cat2	1	4 (33.3%)	8 (66.7%)	12 (100.0%)
		2	2 (22.2%)	7 (77.8%)	9 (100.0%)
		Subtotal	6 (28.6%)	15 (71.4%)	21 (100.0%)

Table 7. Association between adherence and reward dependence variable by group

Group	p-values
1	0.226
2	0.097
3	>0.999
4	0.659

Fisher's exact test.

Table 8. Influence treatment with predictive factors conjointly

Predictive factors	estimative	Standart error	Wald's stastitic	Degree of freedom	p-value
Constante	1.810	0.538	11.299	1	0.001
Novelty seeking	-1.157	0.592	3.826	1	0.050
Self defeating	1.950	1.070	3.319	1	0.069
BDI- group	___	___	6.811	3	0.078
BDI- group(2)	-0.179	0.749	0.057	1	0.811
BDI-group(3)	-1.095	0.706	2.405	1	0.121
BDI-group(4)	-2.447	1.010	5.864	1	0.015

Table 9. Influence treatment with predictive factors conjointly confidence intervals of 90%

Variable	Odds ratio	Confidence Interval	
		lower	upper
Constante	6.109	___	___
Novelty seeking	0.314	0.119	0.832
Self defeating	7.028	1.208	40.878
BDI- group	___	___	___
BDI- group(2)	0.836	0.244	2.865
BDI-group(3)	0.335	0.105	1.069
BDI-group(4)	0.087	0.016	0.456

DISCUSSION

Since the related literature describes treatment adherence as the coincidence degree between the individual's behaviors and the healthcare professional's therapeutic recommendations, (Epstein et Cluss, 1982) we considered that no-treatment adherence patients, in this study, did not followed the protocol, either by absence to the group therapy sessions or to miss the scheduled consultations. However, even when renouncing to participate, patients would be maintained and would receive their treatment, as usual. This situation led to a significant investigative variable concerning the matter of treatment adherence. In a qualitative analysis carried out with 16 renouncing to treatment subjects, Malerbi et al., 2000, suggested that this fact could be assigned to the patients´ conviction that the treatment would not be discontinued in due to their previous commitments to the Protocol. A qualitative analysis will certainly clarify the reasons for those patients no-compliance. Factors leading to the treatment discontinuance, occurred mainly following the 10th week of treatment such as, a new job, return to academic life and different time schedules. These data might indicate that due to therapy, patients might be able to participate in activities previously avoided which corroborates the affirmation that social phobia is a psychiatric disorder affected by several factors related to low adherence levels, common to general disease occurrences and treatments as well as factors related to different psychiatric diseases and most importantly to disease peculiarities as social contact avoidance.

It is important that the adherence to the treatment be evaluated and this evaluation may be performed using either direct or indirect methods. In this study was used the indirect methods, self-reports instruments such as interviews, evaluation scales, structured questionnaires that though generally tend to overestimate the adherence level, the results shown in this study do not confirm the statement of Jordan et al., 2000. Patient reports could eventually include the patient's bias i.e., he/she may consider the adherence level adequate, just for experiencing a symptomatic relief, or fear of negative repercussions by reporting to the therapist his/her inadequate adherence levels.

Another significant variable is the treatment complexity. No treatment showed to be more advantageous than the next one when approaching the item adherence, however, when evaluating the depression item it was verified that in Group 4, the only group without active treatment, left it in large numbers. Since comorbidity events showed to be of 70% (Van Amerigen, 1991) when involving depression and social phobia patients, it was concluded that depression symptoms should be treated with pharmacological agents or CBT.

It was also possible to verify that the personality characteristics of the patients, complying or not to treatment were similar in all the items but one, the reward dependence item, thus suggesting that personality characteristics were not factors of interference in the adherence treatment. This confirms Glasgow et al., (1985) affirmation that the adherence should not be considered as a characteristic or trait inherent to the patient's personality, but accepted as a cluster of several different self-care behaviors. This latter item might be related to the group of psychotherapy modality, in which no particular patient is the main attention focus.

Regarding the personality disorder item, it was evidenced an existing interaction between the "Anti-social" and "Borderline" and patients diagnosed with those disorders had the worst adherence to treatment score in Group 3. Group 1 and 2 patients showed to have their anxiety symptoms reduced due to medication; Group 4 patients were not submitted to procedures, tasks, and any demands from the therapists; in Group 3, patients were not on medical drugs and were formally advised of how to behave socially among others. Since those patients had to report their actions, the interaction between these two personality disorders might be explained by the treatment modality.

The presence or absence of social abilities before the treatment was not related to adherence. Viewing the fact that group therapy offers better results for socially phobic patients, this variable fails to interfere in this procedure indication, different from we find in literature, because according to some authors social skills may be related to those patient's adherence to treatment while socially phobic patients generally present ability deficits able to impair their relationship with the therapeutic team. (Beidel et al., 1999; Savoia et Vianna, 2006).

Some predictive factors might conjointly influence the adherence to treatment, and may turn out to be different for each group. Significant reasons for this influence could be assigned to patients showing the presence of depression, self-defeating, and novelty seeking. Differences were found in the groups 1 (combined treatments) and 4 (no active treatment). The group 4 patients had lower than 91.3% chance of adhering to the treatment than the group 1 patients, which indicates the importance that these patients receive some sort of treatment for the adherence to occur.

Thus, we should take in consideration that compliance to treatment should be understood as a complex set of behaviors caused by different contingencies (Monteiro, 2001) and to promote effective strategies will help the health professionals with his/her patients.

CONCLUSIONS

In view of the present study, the objective is to try to estimate or to explain the probability of one individual, diagnosed with social phobia, to adhere to the pharmacological treatment with SSRI and the cognitive behavior treatment or the combined treatment correlating the above alternative with the variables such personality disorder, personality traits, social abilities, and symptoms of depression. Based on the above treatment findings, no difference in adherence was observed among the treatment groups, but a correlation between depression and active treatment was found, which indicates that the patients with signs and symptoms of depression may be treated for depression and social phobia together.

The patients with dependent personality trait adhered less to treatment, which indicates the need to promote the probability of keeping the patient in treatment. Also, the anti-social and borderline personality disorders were correlated with low adherence in just one proposed procedure – cognitive behavior therapy.

The important finding was to verify which predictive factors might conjointly influence treatment adherence and influence the different groups.

This study shows the importance of the evaluation of the adherence to the various aspects of disease characteristics. Each disease should indicate the important elements to be considered for the most effective approach.

ACKNOWLEDGMENTS

Research carried out at: Anxiety Clinic (AMBAN), Institute of Psychiatry, University of São Paulo School of Medicine, São Paulo, Brazil.

Address: Ambulatório de Ansiedade, Instituto de Psiquiatria, Hospital das Clínicas da FMUSP. R. Dr. Ovídio Pires de Campos, 785 CEP: 05403.010 – Caixa Postal 3671, São Paulo SP, Brazil.

REFERENCES

American Psychiatric Association. *Diagnostic and statistical manual of mental disorders, 4th ed.* Washington, DC, American Psychiatric Association, 1994.

Beck, A.T.; Ward, C.H.; Mendelson. M; Mock, J. ; Erbaugh, J. An inventory for measuring depression. *Arch. Gen. Pychiatry,* v. 4 pgs 53-63, 1961

Beidel, D.C.; Turner, S.M.; Taylos-Ferreira,J.C. Teaching study skills and test-taking strategies to elementary school students. The Testbusters Program. *Behav. Modif.* 1999 Oct; 23(4): 630-46.

Caballo, V.E. Manual de evaluacion y entrenamiento de las habilidades sociales Siglo Ventuno de España Ed.,1993

Cramer, J.A.; Rosenheck, R. (1998). Compliance with medication regimens for mental and physical disorders. *Psychiatric Services,* 49 (2), 196-201.

Cloniger, C.R.; Dragan, M.; Prybeck, T. A Psychobiological model of Temperament and character. *Arch. Gen. Psychiatry vol .*50, 975-990, 1993

Cloninger, C.R.; Przybeck, T.R.; Svrakic, D.M.; Wetzel, R.D.; 1994, The temperament and character inventory (TCI). A guide to its development and use. St. Louis,MO: Center of Psychobiology of Personality, Washington University.

Del-Ben, C.M.; Vilela, J.A.; Crippa, J.A.; Hallaj, J.E.; Labate, C.M.; Zuardi, A.W. Confiabilidade da "entrevista clínica estruturada para o DSM_IV – versão clínica" traduzida para o português. *Revista Brasileira de Psiquiatria,* 2001; 23(3): 156-9

Dunbar-Jacob, J.; Burke, L.E.; Puczynski, S. (1996) clinical assessment and management of adherence to medical regimens. In Nicassio,P.M.; Smith, T.W.(orgs) Manginig chronic Illness: A biopsychosocial Perspective (313-349) Washington: *American Psychological Association*

Epstein, L.A.; Cluss, P.A. A behavioral medicine perspective on adherence to long-term medical regimens. *J. Consult. Clin. Psychol.* 1982 Dec; 50(6): 950-71.

Edelman. R.: Chambless, D. Adherence during sessions and homework in cognitive-behavioral group treatment of social phobia. *Behav. Research. Therapy,* vol 33, nº 5 573-577, 1995

First, M.B.; Spitzer, M.D.; Gibbon, M.S.W.; Williams, J.Bw. *Structured clinical interview for DSM-IV axis I disorders – clinician version* (SCID_CV) Washington (DC): American Psychiatric Press, 1997

Fuentes, D.; Tavares, H.; Camargo, C.H.P.; Gorenstein, C. 2000. Inventário de Temperamento e de caráter de Cloninger – validação da versão em Português, cp 38. In Gorenstein, C.; Andrade, L.H.S.G.; Zuardi, A W. (org) escalas de avaliação clínica em Psiquiatria e psicofarmacologia, São Paulo, Editora Lemos

Glasgow, R.E..; Wilson, W.; Maccaul, K.D. (1985) Regimen adherence a problematic construct in diabetes research. *Diabetes Care,* 8 (3), 300-301

Guy, W. *Ecdeu assessment manual for psychopharmacology,* revised NIMH, Publishers, Bethesda

Hamilton, M. A. Rating scale for depression. *J. Neurol. Neurosurg. Psychiatry,* v. 23, p. 56-62, 1960.

Haynes, R.B. (1976) a critical review of the "determinants" of patient compliance with therapeutic regimens. In Sackett, D.L.; Haynes, C.B. (orgs) *Compliance with Therapeutic Regimens* (26-50). Baltimore: Johns Hopkins University Press.

Jordan, M.S.; Lopes, J.F.; Okazaki, E.; Komatsu, C.L.; Nemes, M.I.B. (2000) Aderência ao tratamento anti-retroviral em AIDS: revisão da literatura médica. In Teixeira, P.R.; Paiva.V.; Shimma.E. (orgs), Ta difícil de engolir? Experiência de adesão ao tratamento anti-retroviral em são Paulo (7-22). São Paulo: Núcleo de estudos para prevenção de AIDS.

Keck, P.; Macelroy, S.; Strakowiski, S.; West, S.; Stanton, S.P.; Kizer, D.L.; Balistreri, T.M.; Bennett, J.A.; Tugrul, K.C. (1996) Factors associated with pharmacological non-compliance inpatients with mania. *Journal of Clinical Psychiatric,* 57, 292-297.

Keck, P.; Maelroy, S. Strakowisky, S.; Wet, S.; Sak, K.W.; Hawkins, J.M.; Bourne, M.L.; Haggard, P. (1998) 12-month outcome of patients with bipolar disorder following hospitalization for a maniac or mixed epiode. *The American Journal of Psychiatry,* 155 (5), 646-652.

Lotufo Neto, F. Escalas para avaliação de fobias – cp 17 In Gorenstein, C.; Andrade, L.H.S.G.; Zuardi, A. W. (org) escalas de avaliação clínica em Psiquiatria e psicofarmacologia, São Paulo, Editora Lemos, 2000

Malerbi, F.E.K. Adesão ao tratamento. IN Kerbauy, R. *Sobre comportamento e cognição –* vol 5. Santo André: ESETEC, 2000

Malerbi, F; Savoia, M. G.; Bernik, M. Pobre aderência em tratamentos psiquiátricos: um estudo qualitativo. *Revista Brasileira de terapia comportamental cognitiva,* 2(2): 147-155. 2000

Monteiro, M.E. Adesão ao tratamento psiquiátrico: análise comportamental de pacientes com diagnóstico de transtorno de ansiedade São Paulo, 2001. dissertação de Mestrado apresentada a faculdade de psicologia da pontifícia universidade Católica de São Paulo.

Neter, J., Kutner, M. H., Nachtsheim, C. J. And Wasserman, W. (1996). *Applied linear statistical models.* 4.ed. Illinois: Mc Graw Hill. 1408p.

Paula, G. A. (2004). Modelos de regressão com apoio computacional. *Versão Preliminar.* São Paulo. 245p.

Pfohl, B.; Blum, N, Zimmerman, M. Stangl, D. *The structured interview of DSM-III-R personality disorders.* Iowa, University of Iowa hospital and clinics, 1989

Savoia,M. G.; Vianna, A.M. Especificidades do atendimento a pacientes com transtornos de ansiedade. IN Savoia, M.G. (org) a interfae entre Psicologia e Psiquiatria – novo conceito Em Saúde Mental.Pgs 78-101, São Paulo, Ed. Roca, 2006.

Skinner, B.F. (1989) The origins of cognitive tought. In skinner (org) *Recent issues in the Analysis of Behavior* (13-25). Columbus: Merrill.

Torres, A.R.; Delporto, J.A. Applicability and reliability of a Portuguese version of the Structured Interview for DSM-III-R personality disorders. *Rev. Hosp. São Paulo, Esc. Paulista de Medicina,* 1994; 5: 33-39.

Turner, S.M.; Beidel, D.C.; Jacob, R. Social phobia: a comparison of behavior therapy and Atenolol. *J. Consult. Clin. Psychol.,* V.62, P.350-358, 1994.

Van Ameringen, M.; Mancini, C.; Styan, G.; Donison, D. Relationship of social phobia with other psychiatric illness. *J. Affect. Disord.,* v.21, p.93-9, 1991.

Vocisano, C.; Klein, D.; Keefe, R.; Dienst, E.; Kincaid, Mm. (1996). Demographics, family history, premorbid functioning, development characteristics, and course of patients with deteriorated affective disorder. *The American Journal of Psychiatry*, 153, (2), 248-255.

Watson, D.; Friend, R. Measurement of social-evaluation anxiety. *J. Consult. Clin. Psychol.,* v. 33, p. 448-457, 1969.

Index

B

D

evidence, ix, xi, xii, 3, 12, 19, 26, 28, 37, 39, 44, 45, 47, 50, 51, 59, 67, 68, 78, 97, 99, 121, 124, 125, 137, 139, 143, 144, 145, 146, 148, 164, 170, 177, 180, 202, 256, 269, 285

evolution, 262

evolutionary, 258, 261

exclusion, 70, 213, 293

execution, 253, 254

exercise, vii, xiii, 20, 30, 149, 150, 152, 156, 166, 168, 169, 170, 171, 172, 178, 180, 183, 184, 185, 186, 191, 193, 197, 200, 205

exercise participation, 178

exercisers, 202

experimental design, 49, 56

expert, 10, 70

exponential, 92

exposure, 42, 52, 53, 61, 135, 143, 144, 146, 147, 148, 151, 156, 186, 189, 190, 194, 197, 201, 206, 265

expressivity, 90

externalizing behavior, viii, 17, 19, 25, 27, 54

externalizing disorders, 99

extraction, 110

extraneous variable, 49, 53

extrinsic, 92, 94, 132, 189

eye movement, 11

eye(s), 11, 212

F

factor analysis, 113, 116

failure, 42, 57, 71, 72, 84, 103, 104, 108, 109, 111, 123, 167, 277, 278

familial, x, xiii, 28, 39, 183, 197, 202

family, xii, xv, 6, 7, 20, 28, 29, 33, 48, 94, 104, 109, 121, 139, 151, 160, 161, 163, 165, 166, 190, 191, 193, 194, 195, 196, 197, 200, 203, 206, 263, 265, 268, 269, 273, 276, 277, 278, 279, 280, 281, 286, 303

family conflict, 7

family environment, 7, 190, 200, 206, 265

family history, 163, 303

family meals, 193

family members, 151, 190, 194, 196

family relationships, 160, 161

family support, 263

family therapy, 28, 33

fast food, 162

fasting, 158, 161, 169, 174, 188

fasting glucose, 158

fat, 167, 168, 169, 178, 179, 185, 191, 196, 242, 245

fatigue, 13, 15, 152

fear(s), 19, 27, 29, 58, 104, 198, 263, 275, 277, 283, 290, 299

federal government, 184

feedback, 98, 196, 206, 248, 290

feelings, xv, 6, 22, 45, 59, 92, 94, 99, 124, 125, 134, 146, 149, 164, 210, 243, 246, 251, 259, 260, 262, 264, 266

females, 20, 34, 63, 82, 95, 97, 101, 107, 108, 110, 113, 121, 128, 133, 138, 160, 162, 166, 168, 178, 184, 185, 186, 187, 188, 189, 200, 202, 203, 204, 210, 213, 215, 224, 229, 239, 240, 242, 244, 245, 247

fertility, xi, 67, 68, 77, 78, 80, 159, 171, 181

fertilization, xi, 67, 68, 69, 71, 72, 73, 74, 75, 82, 83, 84, 85, 175

fetal, 160

fidelity, 58

fight or flight response, 148

films, 91

Finland, 164, 175, 177

Finns, 177

fitness, 176, 212, 265

flexibility, 74, 93

flight, 128, 138, 148

fluctuations, 43

focusing, 89, 90, 92, 241, 260

follicle, 69, 78

follicle stimulating hormone, 78

food, 162, 163, 165, 167, 170, 172, 176, 185, 187, 190, 191, 192, 193, 194, 195, 197, 198, 200, 204, 206, 254, 263, 265, 291

food intake, 170, 172, 185

foodstuffs, 213, 263

forest fire, 48

forgetfulness, 291

fragmentation, 11

framing, 131

France, 51, 52, 60, 128, 134

freedom, 266, 298

freezing, 129

frequency distribution, 109, 120

Freud, 89, 98, 131, 132, 133

fruits, 162, 165

fulfillment, 267, 268

funding, 60

funds, 3

I

O

P

S

T

U

Z